Costs and Outcomes
of Community Services for
People with Intellectual Disabilities

Costs and Outcomes of Community Services for People with Intellectual Disabilities

edited by

Roger J. Stancliffe, Ph.D.
Research and Training Center on Community Living
University of Minnesota
and
Centre for Developmental Disability Studies
University of Sydney

and

K. Charlie Lakin, Ph.D.
Research and Training Center on Community Living
Institute on Community Integration
University of Minnesota

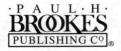
·P·A·U·L·H·
BROOKES
PUBLISHING CO.®

Baltimore • London • Sydney

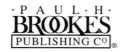

Paul H. Brookes Publishing Co.
Post Office Box 10624
Baltimore, MD 21285-0624

www.brookespublishing.com

Typeset by Auburn Associates, Baltimore, Maryland.
Manufactured in the United States of America by
Versa Press, East Peoria, Illinois.

The development of this book was supported, in part, by the National Institute
on Disability and Rehabilitation Research (NIDRR), through Grant No.
H133B031116, and by the Administration on Developmental Disabilities (ADD),
through Grant No. 90DN0064. The opinions expressed throughout the book are
those of the authors, and no endorsement by NIDRR or ADD should be presumed.

Library of Congress Cataloging-in-Publication Data

Costs and outcomes of community services for people with intellectual disabilities/
edited by Roger J. Stancliffe and K. Charlie Lakin.
    p.;   cm.
Includes bibliographical references and index.
ISBN 1-55766-718-7 (pbk.)
1. People with mental disabilities—Services for—United States—Costs.
2. People with mental disabilities—Services for—United States—Finance.
3. Community mental health services—Economic aspects—United States.
[DNLM: 1. Mental Retardation—economics.   2. Community Health
Services—economics.   3. Developmental Disabilities—economics. WM 300
C842 2005]   I. Stancliffe, Roger.   II. Lakin, K. Charlie.
RC570.5.U6C67 2005
362.2'2—dc22   2004021072

British Library Cataloguing in Publication data are available from the British Library.

Contents

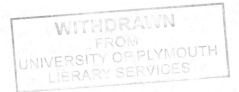

About the Editors

Roger J. Stancliffe, Ph.D., Consultant Research Associate, Research and Training Center on Community Living, University of Minnesota, and Senior Research Fellow, Centre for Developmental Disability Studies, University of Sydney, Post Office Box 6, Ryde NSW 1680, Australia

Dr. Stancliffe is Consultant Research Associate with the Research and Training Center on Community Living, Institute on Community Integration, University of Minnesota. He is also Senior Research Fellow and Clinical Senior Lecturer at the Centre for Developmental Disability Studies in Sydney, Australia. Previously, he held research posts at the University of Minnesota in Minneapolis, as well as clinical, consultative, and service management positions in intellectual disability services in Australia. He is Editor of the *Journal of Intellectual & Developmental Disability* and Consulting Editor to four other international research journals. In 2002, he was appointed Fellow of the American Association on Mental Retardation. He has written two previous books and more than 70 articles, chapters, and technical reports on issues relating to community living, deinstitutionalization, self-determination, individual planning, service outcomes and costs, and challenging behavior.

K. Charlie Lakin, Ph.D., Director, Research and Training Center on Community Living, Institute on Community Integration, University of Minnesota, 210B Pattee Hall, 150 Pillsbury Drive SE, Minneapolis, Minnesota 55455

Dr. Lakin has more than 30 years of experience in service to individuals with intellectual and developmental disabilities as a teacher, researcher, consultant, and advocate. He has directed numerous research and training projects and has authored or co-authored more than 200 publications based on that work. Dr. Lakin frequently consults with state, federal, and international agencies in matters of policy, research, and evaluation. Among recognitions for his work are appointments by President Clinton to the President's Committee on Mental Retardation, the American Association on Mental Retardation's Dybwad Humanitarian Award, and the University of Minnesota's Outstanding Community Service Award.

About the Contributors

Jerry Allen, M.A., President, Arbitre Consulting, 2017 Rollins Avenue, Cheyenne, Wyoming 82001. Mr. Allen spent 27 years in the developmental disabilities field as a clinician and manager. His company, Arbitre Consulting, is the national expert on the Inventory for Client and Agency Planning (ICAP; Bruininks, Hill, Weatherman, & Woodcock, Riverside, 1986). He divides his time between Cheyenne, Wyoming, and Barcelona, Spain.

David Braddock, Ph.D., Coleman-Turner Endowed Chair in Cognitive Disability and Professor in Psychiatry, University of Colorado School of Medicine, 4001 Discovery Drive, Suite 210, Boulder, Colorado 80304. Dr. Braddock is Associate Vice President of the University of Colorado (CU) System and Executive Director of the Coleman Institute for Cognitive Disabilities. He has contributed to cognitive disability research, public health, and social policy for more than 35 years. He received international career research awards from The Arc of the United States, the American Association on Mental Retardation, and the University Scholar Award from the President of the University of Illinois. Dr. Braddock is a former president of the American Association on Mental Retardation and a recipient of The Arc of the United States Franklin Smith Award for Distinguished National Service to the field of mental retardation, The Arc's highest honor.

Edward M. Campbell, Ph.D., President, $E = MC^2$ Consulting, 502 East Missouri, Pierre, South Dakota 57501. Dr. Campbell received degrees in psychology from the University of South Dakota. After 30 years with the South Dakota Department of Human Services, he is now retired. He currently operates an independent consulting firm.

Robert T. Clabby, II, Superintendent, Eastern Oregon Training Center, 2575 Westgate, Pendleton, Oregon 97801. Mr. Clabby is currently participating in a review of rate structures in the state of Oregon and was formerly the Developmental Disabilities Division Administrator for the state of Wyoming. He has been involved in a wide variety of state and private developmental disability services for 28 years.

James W. Conroy, Ph.D., Executive Director, Center for Outcome Analysis, 426B Darby Road, Havertown, Pennsylvania 19083. Dr. Conroy is a student of the impacts of inclusion and self-determination in services and supports for people with disabilities. His team followed more than 6,000 people as they moved out of public institutions and into community homes. The Robert Wood Johnson Foundation selected his team to measure the outcomes of self-determination on the participants, their families, and workers.

Robin E. Cooper, M.S.S.W., Director of Technical Assistance, National Association of State Directors of Developmental Disabilities Services (NASDDDS), 2222 Hollister Avenue, Madison, Wisconsin 53726. In her capacity as the Director of Technical Assistance with the NASDDDS, Ms. Cooper works with state, county, and local governments as well as with individuals with disabilities and provider organizations on issues in long-term community-based support for people with disabilities. Ms. Cooper has extensive experience in systems design that promotes effective management practices while ensuring individual choice and control. She has had the privilege of learning from and assisting individuals with disabilities for 30 years. Ms. Cooper holds bachelor's and master's degrees from the University of Wisconsin–Madison.

Kathryn Coucouvanis, Research Assistant and Data Coordinator, National Residential Information Systems Project, Research and Training Center on Community Living, University of Minnesota, 210 Pattee Hall, 150 Pillsbury Drive SE, Minneapolis, Minnesota 55455. Ms. Coucouvanis has a number of publications on the current status and long-term trends in services to people with intellectual disabilities and/or developmental disabilities in the United States. She received her bachelor's degree in sociology and has entered the doctoral program in Audiology at the University of Minnesota.

Eric Emerson, Ph.D., M.Sc., Professor of Clinical Psychology, Institute for Health Research, Lancaster University, Bowland Tower East, Lancaster LA1 4YT, United Kingdom. Before becoming Professor of Clinical Psychology at Lancaster University, Dr. Emerson was at Manchester University. He has reported extensive research relating to health and social care of people with intellectual disabilities. He is a member of the Department of Health's National Task Force on Learning Disabilities.

David Felce, Ph.D., Professor, Cardiff University, Welsh Centre for Learning Disabilities, Meridian Court, North Road, Cardiff, Wales CF4 3BL,United Kingdom. Dr. Felce's first research post, from 1973 through 1986, was at the University of Southampton, where he conducted research on the quality of residential services for people with intellectual disabilities requiring extensive or pervasive support, with a small excursion into the quality of residential accommodation for older adults with mental infirmities or who were physically frail. After 3 years as Director of the British Institute of Mental Handicap, he was appointed to his current post. He maintains research interests in the measurement of quality of life, the determinants of quality in community housing services, the analysis and amelioration of challenging behavior, and service development generally in the field of intellectual disabilities. He is a co-editor of *Journal of Applied Research in Intellectual Disabilities*, an associate editor of the *American Journal on Mental Retardation*, and on the editorial boards of seven other intellectual disability journals. In addition, he is President of the International Association for the Scientific Study of Intellectual Disability.

Jon R. Fortune, Ed.D., L.P.C., C.R.C., Deputy Administrator, Wyoming Department of Health, Developmental Disabilities Division, 186E Qwest Building, 6101 Yellowstone Road, Cheyenne, Wyoming 82002. Dr. Fortune is a 31-year veteran of intellectual disability service systems in the United States. He has published and presented regularly and is interested in individual budgets and choice implementation and the systems necessary to allow these features to develop.

Janice K. Frisch, M.S.W., Bureau Chief, Management Operations, Department of Public Health and Human Services, Disabilities Service Division, Developmental Disabilities Program, 111 Sanders, Helena, Montana 59601. Ms. Frisch has served in Montana's developmental disabilities field for more than 30 years. She assists in the design of the community services system through legislation, rules, policies, budget requests, information systems, and local service delivery development. The service system gains great support from the taxpayers and legislators due to accurately recording data, answering questions, and forecasting future needs. Developing community services to meet all of the needs of more than 4,000 adults and children with developmental disabilities and their families, independent of where they live in this very rural state, is increasingly successful.

Robert M. Gettings, M.P.A., Executive Director, National Association of State Directors of Developmental Disabilities Services, 113 Oronoco Street, Alexandria, Virginia 22314. Mr. Gettings represents the interests of 50 state developmental disabilities agencies in Washington, D.C., and facilitates communication among the states concerning the most effective means of serving citizens with lifelong disabilities. He also was on the staff of the President's Committee on Mental Retardation and the National Association for Retarded Children. He has written and lectured extensively regarding the impact of federal legislative and administrative policy on the delivery of state and local services to people with mental retardation and other developmental disabilities and is widely recognized as a leading expert in this area. He has also helped many states solve a variety of service-delivery problems. A Life Member of the American Association on Mental Retardation, Mr. Gettings recently was recognized by the National Historic Trust on Mental Retardation as one of the 36 major contributors to the field during the 20th century.

Angela Hallam, M.Sc., Principal Researcher, Mental Health Research Team, Health Department Analytical Services Division, 3rd Floor West Rear, St. Andrew's House, Regent Road, Edinburgh EH1 3DG, United Kingdom. Ms. Hallam is Principal Researcher in Social Research at the Scottish Executive in Edinburgh. She is currently responsible for the development and management of two programs of research to support mental health policy development in Scotland. Until 2002, she worked with Professor Knapp at the Centre for the Economics of Mental Health, Health Services Research Department, at the Institute of Psychiatry, specializing in the costs of care and support for people with intellectual disabilities.

Chris Hatton, Ph.D., Professor of Psychology, Health and Social Care, Institute for Health Research, Lancaster University, Bowland Tower East, Lancaster LA1 4YT, United Kingdom. Dr. Hatton has been involved in research work with people with intellectual disabilities for 15 years, largely focused on making community services work better for people with intellectual disabilities. He is the author of several books and more than 90 articles in academic and professional journals.

Michael J. Head, M.S.W., Director, Office of Consumer-Directed Home and Community-Based Services, Michigan Department of Community Health, 6th Floor, Lewis Cass Building, Lansing, Michigan 48913. Mr. Head is a consultant with more than 30 years of experience in the public mental health and long-term care fields. He is trained as a mental health clinician and has also worked as an administrator, legislative specialist, and service system developer at the state and local agency levels. Mr. Head has been extensively involved with public policy development since the 1970s, which has promoted Michigan's evolution to a full community-based system of services for people with intellectual disabilities. Mr. Head has directed Michigan's efforts to develop self-determination as a viable option and as a policy since 1996.

Laird W. Heal, Ph.D., (Deceased) Professor Emeritus, University of Illinois (Urbana/Champaign).

Kenneth B. Heinlein, Ph.D., Associate Director, Wyoming INstitute for Disabilities (WIND), University of Wyoming, College of Health Sciences, 1000 East University Avenue, Laramie, Wyoming 82071. Dr. Heinlein is the former director of Wyoming's Department of Health. He has 27 years of experience in the field of developmental disabilities. He currently is Associate Director at WIND, a University Center for Excellence in Developmental Disabilities Education, Research, and Service. WIND's services include teaching, conducting research, and providing information about disabilities.

Richard Hemp, M.A., Senior Professional Research Assistant, Department of Psychiatry, School of Medicine, University of Colorado, 4001 Discovery Drive, Suite 210, Boulder, Colorado 80303. Mr. Hemp has worked on the State of the States in Developmental Disabilities project at the University of Illinois at Chicago (1983–2001) and University of Colorado (2001 to present). He has authored or co-authored more than 60 journal articles, books, book chapters, monographs and technical reports on the structure, financing, and quality assurance of long-term care services for individuals with developmental disabilities in the United States.

Amy Hewitt, Ph.D., Research Associate and Director of Interdisciplinary Teaching, Institute on Community Integration, University of Minnesota, 150 Pillsbury Drive SE, Minneapolis, Minnesota 55455. Dr. Hewitt has worked in the field of developmental disabilities for more than 20 years. Her primary areas of interest include direct-support professionals and community inclusion for adults with disabilities. As Research Associate at the University of Minnesota, Institute on Community Integration, she directs several federal and state research, evaluation, and demonstration projects in the area of direct-support professional workforce development and community services for people with disabilities. Dr. Hewitt is a national leader in the area of workforce development and community supports to individuals with developmental disabilities.

David R. Johnson, Ph.D., Professor, Department of Educational Policy and Administration, College of Education and Human Development, University of Minnesota, 102 Pattee Hall, 150 Pillsbury Drive SE,

Minneapolis, Minnesota 55455. Dr Johnson is Director of the Institute on Community Integration, a federally designated center on disabilities research, training, and outreach. He is also Director of the National Center in Secondary Education and Transition, which provides technical assistance and consultation to all 50 states and U.S. territories. His research interests include investigations of the postschool outcomes and status of young adults with disabilities, evaluations concerning access and participation of young adults with disabilities in postsecondary education programs, studies on systems change, cost–benefit analysis, and other policy-related research. Dr. Johnson has also served as consultant to several national, regional, and state organizations including the Office of Special Education Programs, the National Institute on Disability and Rehabilitation Research, the Office of Disability Employment Policy, the Rehabilitation Services Administration, the National Alliance of Business, and several Congressional committees. He has published numerous journal articles, book chapters, research monographs, technical reports, and products on topics concerning secondary education, special education, rehabilitation, transition, and other themes.

Martin Knapp, Ph.D., M.Sc., Director, Centre for the Economics of Mental Health, Institute of Psychiatry, Health Services Research Department, The David Goldberg Centre, De Crespigny Park, Denmark Hill, London SE5 8AF, United Kingdom. Professor Knapp is Director and Professor of Health Economics in the Centre for the Economics of Mental Health at the Institute of Psychiatry. He is also Professor of Social Policy at the London School of Economics, where he is Director of the Personal Social Services Research Unit. His research focuses on the application of economic techniques and policy analysis of health care systems, social care, and support for people with intellectual disabilities.

Sheryl A. Larson, Ph.D., Research Director and Principal Investigator, Research and Training Center on Community Living, University of Minnesota, 214B Pattee Hall, 150 Pillsbury Drive SE, Minneapolis, Minnesota 55455. Dr. Larson has worked for the past 16 years at the Research and Training Center on Community Living, where she has directed projects involving survey and intervention research; secondary analysis of large data sets; and research synthesis on residential services, personnel issues, disability statistics, and community integration for people with intellectual and developmental disabilities. She has authored or co-authored more than 100 publications and has made more than 150 presentations on those topics. She is an American Association on Mental

Retardation (AAMR) Fellow, President of the AAMR Community Services Division, a consulting editor of *Mental Retardation* and *Journal of Intellectual & Developmental Disability*, and has participated in grant review panels for the National Institute on Disability and Rehabilitation Research and the Centers for Disease Control and Prevention.

Darrell R. Lewis, Ph.D., Professor of Educational Policy, University of Minnesota, 86 Pleasant Street SE, Minneapolis, Minnesota 55455. Dr. Lewis's research interests include economic assessment and evaluation of disability policies and economic productivity in higher education. He also provides technical assistance to countries that are grappling with issues of decentralization and reformation of their higher educational systems. Dr. Lewis is author of more than 14 books and monographs and 120 articles.

Robert M. Lynch, Ph.D., Professor, Kenneth W. Monfort College of Business and Public Policy, University of Northern Colorado, Greeley, Colorado 80639. Dr. Lynch received his doctorate from the University of Northern Colorado. He has published regularly in academic and professional journals and has authored several books. His interests include linear models and sampling.

Charles R. Moseley, Ed.D., Director of Special Projects, National Association of State Directors of Developmental Disabilities Services, 113 Oronoco Street, Alexandria, Virginia 22314. Prior to his current position, Dr. Moseley was Co-Director of the National Program on Self-Determination for Persons with Developmental Disabilities, funded by the Robert Wood Johnson Foundation at the University of New Hampshire Institute on Disability. Before coming to the university, Dr. Moseley was the Director of the Vermont Division of Developmental Services, where he led efforts to close the state's institution, transition services to individualized community-based alternatives, and restructure service delivery to incorporate self-directed services. He consults nationally and internationally on the design of individualized service options, institutional closure, public policy, and system change.

Susan L. Parish, Ph.D., M.S.W., Assistant Professor of Social Work, University of North Carolina at Chapel Hill, Tate-Turner-Kuralt Building, 301 Pittsboro Street, Campus Box 3550, Chapel Hill, North Carolina 27599. Dr. Parish received her master's degree in social work from Rutgers University and her doctorate in public health from the University of Illinois at Chicago. She also completed an NIH postdoctoral fellowship at the University of Wisconsin's Waisman Center. Her central research interest is the impact of disability, health, and poverty policy on low-income families affected by disability. She teaches courses in social welfare policy and research methods. Prior to beginning her doctoral work, Dr. Parish ran residential and family support programs for people with developmental disabilities and their families in New York and New Jersey.

Robert W. Prouty, M.S., Research Fellow and Co-Director, National Residential Information Systems Project, Research and Training Center on Community Living, University of Minnesota, 210 Pattee Hall, 150 Pillsbury Drive SE, Minneapolis, Minnesota 55455. Mr. Prouty has been an elementary and high school special education teacher, executive director of a preschool/clinic for young children with severe disabilities, a state manager of disability services, and consultant to many disability policies and programs. He received his bachelor's degree from the State University of New York and his master's degree from Syracruse University.

Mary C. Rizzolo, M.A., Associate Director, Institute on Disability and Human Development (IDHD), M/C 626, 1640 W. Roosevelt Road, Room 245, Chicago, Illinois 60608. Ms. Rizzolo is Associate Director of IDHD, the University Center for Excellence in Developmental Disabilities for the state of Illinois. Ms. Rizzolo has worked on the State of the States in Developmental Disabilities project at the University of Colorado. She is currently working on her doctorate in public health sciences at the University of Illinois at Chicago.

Janet Robertson, Ph.D., Lecturer, Institute for Health Research, Lancaster University, Alexandra Square, Lancaster LA1 4YT, United Kingdom. Dr. Robertson is a researcher specializing in the field of intellectual disabilities. Her work has included the evaluation of services, service recipient quality of life, the use of psychotropic medication, health issues, social networks, the needs of South Asian caregivers, and the mental health needs of children.

Donald D. Severance, M.Sc., Program Manager, Nebraska Developmental Disabilities System, West Campus No. 14, Folson and West Prospector, Lincoln, Nebraska 68509. Mr. Severance has worked in the developmental disabilities field for 25 years. He is currently responsible for developing funding methodology and a quality improvement system for the Nebraska Developmental Disabilities System.

John R. Shea, Ph.D., Partner, Allen, Shea, & Associates, 1780 Third Street, Napa, California 94559. Dr. Shea has conducted several cost–outcome studies, including a cost–benefit analysis of supported employment in California. He is also the author of *Fiscal Analysis of Assembly Bill 896: California's Developmental Services System Unification, Finance and Economic Issues,* which was published in 2001. Dr. Shea received his doctorate in economics from The Ohio State University.

Gary A. Smith, Senior Project Director, Human Services Research Institute, 8100 SW Nyberg Road, Suite 205, Tualatin, Oregon 97062. Mr. Smith has served as a state developmental disabilities administrator for almost 20 years. He has provided technical assistance to states and other organizations concerning Medicaid policy, system management, and rate-setting methods.

Patricia Noonan Walsh, Ph.D., Professor, Centre for Disability Studies, University College Dublin, John Henry Newman Building D-005, Belfield, Dublin 4, Ireland. Dr. Walsh has authored publications in the areas of aging, inclusive employment and education, and the health and quality of life of people with disabilities. She is co-author, with Barbara LeRoy, of *Women with Disabilities Aging Well: A Global View* (Paul H. Brookes Publishing Co., 2004). Dr. Walsh is a Fellow of the International Association for the Scientific Study of Intellectual Disability (IASSID).

Foreword

I am part of a generation of professionals that has focused on the costs of community services and supports for people with intellectual and developmental disabilities within the context of eliminating the horrid and inhumane conditions we saw in state institutions in the 1970s. By focusing on the greater costs of public institutions relative to those of private community services—especially after states began to make massive investments in those institutions to meet at least minimal standards of tolerability and to garner federal funds through the Medicaid Intermediate Care Facilities for Persons with Mental Retardation (ICFs/MR) program—we were able to convince state governments to commit to affording people with intellectual and developmental disabilities the opportunity to receive the support they needed while living in the community. Even when state governments did not despair over wretched conditions in their institutions, or even accept that the human rights and full citizenship promised their states' residents applied to people with disabilities, they did understand "cheaper," and, as this concept got us where we wanted (i.e., people with disabilities living in the community), we took it as success. In hindsight, the simplicity of our contentions created expectations that today haunt us.

Costs and Outcomes of Community Services for People with Intellectual Disabilities, edited by Roger J. Stancliffe and K. Charlie Lakin, fills an important void in the literature. It uses original research, reviews of existing knowledge, and policy analysis to explore how budget limitations interact with federal mandates for more individualized services. The contributors to this volume offer policy recommendations and suggestions for allocating individual funding in a rational, equitable way. This volume focuses on the issues currently facing disability services at the family, state, and federal levels.

Today, most people with intellectual and developmental disabilities live in the community. Depending on the prevalence rates that one accepts, only about 10%–15% of people with intellectual and developmental disabilities live in service settings (e.g., group homes) with formal supports that are financed by the government. Most individuals with intellectual and developmental disabilities live independently or with members of their families. Even at the height of institutionalization, only a small percentage of people were living in formal government-financed care settings.

While statistics on the populations of public and private institutions are ample and show that residents have decreased by 59% in the 20-year period from 1982 to 2002 (see Chapter 1), the number of people with intellectual and developmental disabilities living with their families or on their own is still largely deduced by subtracting the number receiving public supports from the estimated prevalence of intellectual and developmental disabilities. Many in the disabilities field suspect that the number of people supported in homes shared with family members is at an all-time high, due in part to 1) the preference of the family, 2) the long waiting lists for publicly funded supports, 3) the fact that family support services are more readily available, and 4) the better health and increased life span of people with intellectual and developmental disabilities and the family members who support them.

It would be nice, after three decades of deinstitutionalization, if people with intellectual and developmental disabilities could feel secure in a guarantee of a supported place in our communities. Unfortunately, we are still far from our goal. Nine states have closed all of their public institutions, but an unholy alliance between certain public employee unions, institution employees, and some families has kept many public institutions open long beyond the time when they should have been closed. Nearly every day, I see notices of new "farms," ranches, gated communities, and schools that segregate people with intellectual and developmental disabilities. We have barely scratched the surface of the private institutions that receive state and federal funds, primarily through ICF/MR, to provide an outmoded model of congregate care. Although the ICF/MR program has been slowly shrinking, it remains both an expensive way to meet the needs of the individuals who live in those places and an "entitlement" as much for the providers of services as for people with intellectual and developmental disabilities.

Despite the promise of placement in the most inclusive setting outlined in the Americans with Disabilities Act (ADA) of 1990 and confirmed by the U.S. Supreme Court decision that "integrated means integrated," community services and supports remain "optional" under Medicaid. Many of the same battles for inclusion into community life are fought today as were fought three decades ago. I use the word battle purposely, as this is a war for freedom; for independence; and for deciding who controls the lives of people with intellectual and developmental disabilities—the state, the provider of services, or the person and his or her family and friends.

In the United States, we are haunted by the approaches we have taken toward deinstitutionalization and the development of community services

and supports since the 1970s. We have tended to bundle deinstitutionalization and community service development as a single process when we
should have acknowledged them as notably different processes and
achievements. We have demonstrated well that it is possible to be successful with one and not the other. Getting people out of institutions has been
one effort. We know how to do it and are doing it successfully in most
places.

It is as much a political effort as it is a programmatic one. Many of
our efforts to move people out of institutions have been little more than a
change of real estate. People have been moved from 24-hour per-day
supervision by shift staff in big buildings to pretty much the same experiences in smaller buildings, from large-group homes to smaller group
homes. The extent of change in people's lives, at least the daily routine of
their lives, often is smaller than our enthusiasm for the accomplishment
suggested.

In time, as the places in which people lived changed, so too did the
possibilities for their lives. With experience, we realized that deinstitutionalization and supporting people to find valued roles and relationships in
the day-to-day life of their communities were altogether different.

Focusing much of our advocacy for deinstitutionalization on the
lower costs of services and supports in the community may have been
unfortunate because of the legacy it has left us. In large measure, those
lower costs were established on the basis of direct-support personnel who
could be recruited to contribute to the emancipation of people with intellectual and developmental disabilities at wages far below those of their
institutional counterparts and, of course, the rapid escalation of the comparative costs of per-person institutional care as a result of court orders,
higher standards, and low occupancy. In the advocacy for community supports, we focused on that comparative cost differential and in the process
created an enduring expectation that community support costs less and,
through some inherent capacity for flexibility in resource use, could get by
on less.

State governments have continued to support state institutions as a
fixed component of state budgets. In most states, state employees get a
raise every year—sometimes modest, and sometimes including a "step"
increase, an additional salary increment due to working for another year in
their jobs. Legislatures have felt a different obligation to the community
services that have been developed and operated almost entirely by private
organizations. In supporting community services, state legislators tend to
appropriate money each year to the broad whole of community supports.

The pressure to respond to the waiting lists for community services and to increase supports for families, coupled with the intolerability for most families of using the institutional alternatives despite their steady increase in per-resident expenditures, means that almost all the new resources allocated to community services are used to develop new services. As a result, the per-person average expenditure for Medicaid Home and Community-Based Services (HCBS) Waiver program increased by 19% during the 5 years between 1998 and 2003, while the average Medicaid ICF/MR expenditure increased by 34% (in fiscal year 2003 the averages were $36,558 and $104,741, respectively) (Lakin, Prouty, Coucouvanis, & Polister, 2004).

While average per-person HCBS Waiver expenditures increased by 19% between 1998 and 2003, total HCBS Waiver expenditures nearly doubled from $7.1 to $14.0 billion dollars. This total growth in public expenditures for community services has masked the severe pressures on existing service programs to deal with rising costs with very limited new revenues. While total community expenditures rapidly rose yearly, the funding for sustaining existing services and supports fell behind the escalating costs of doing business.

The primary cost of providing community supports is that of paying and insuring direct-support staff. Costs of community supports have been driven by wages required to recruit and hire direct-support staff and by significant and ongoing increases in the costs of health, liability, and workers' compensation insurance. They have been exacerbated by other, often uncontrollable, cost increases. In the face of zero annual to small annual payment increases provided by state government, the balance of controllable costs—notably wage increases, but also staff development and service recipient activities—have had to absorb the difference. The results have been disastrous.

The effects of service revenues that have not kept pace with service costs have fallen primarily on direct-support staff. The result is a crisis in the recruitment and retention of the very people most directly related to the quality of life of people with intellectual and developmental disabilities. It is also just plain unfair. We are, in essence, favoring those working in environments we want to eliminate and discriminating against those working in environments we wish to promote! These workers, who are in short supply due to labor force demographics, are bearing the brunt of the lack of legislative responsibility to fully fund community services, a problem for which we advocates also share some blame.

The wages of direct-support professionals in the community are lower than institutional staff in every state in which data have been recently gathered (see Lakin, Polister, & Prouty, 2003), despite the greater responsibility demanded of them and less direct supervision provided to them. The result is high turnover and increasing difficulty in recruitment at the salaries available for the work required. Some 25% of these workers live below or near the poverty line and qualify for food stamps and housing vouchers. This national crisis was recognized by the U.S. House and Senate in the 2003 "Direct Support Professional Recognition Resolution" (U.S. House of Representatives, 2003). But the crisis might well have been unnecessary.

Although approximately 80% of people with intellectual and developmental disabilities live with their families, there has been relatively little commitment of funding to support these individuals and families (see Chapter 2). There has also been a paucity of data on the costs incurred by families, individuals, and other nonformal supporters. Lewis and Johnson (Chapter 4) have gathered the available data to show clearly that these costs are substantial.

If my use of the word *burden* that follows disturbs some, please note that I am referring to both the financial burden and the extra effort that is assumed, not the notion that the person with a disability is a burden in the social sense of that term. Families encounter at least three types of costs in providing support for their family member with intellectual and developmental disabilities:

1. They incur direct out-of-pocket costs for purchasing goods and services above and beyond what would have been needed for a family member without intellectual and developmental disabilities.

2. They receive less income in many cases due to the burdens of care and the lack of financial supports to provide that care where they live. A family member may work fewer hours or at a lower salary, trading flexibility for income, due to the needs of the family member with intellectual and developmental disabilities.

3. They are less mobile. Anecdotal evidence I gathered while working in the field and questions we at The Arc regularly receive indicate that families who have a child or adult family member with intellectual and developmental disabilities relocate—and therefore risk losing services and supports—less often. If a family is receiving in-home or community supports, the funding for those supports does not transfer across state lines and, if they are satisfied with the special education services in one school, moving across a school district (let alone a state line) can completely change the educational experience for a child

with intellectual and developmental disabilities. We need more data on this issue to clearly identify the trends.

Obviously, these three items are, in some ways, among the immeasurable aspects of family life. Limited attention to such experiences and costs reflects the wholly unsatisfactory result of efforts to estimate such expenditures in our national health expenditure statistical programs (e.g., National Health Interview Survey). The costs to families are real and significant. The National Health Interview Survey estimates that among parents with children with intellectual and developmental disabilities, 36% have turned down a job because of their child's disability, 17% have turned down a promotion, 29% have changed work hours, 36% have reduced the hours they work, 17% have changed jobs, and 17% have quit working altogether (Anderson, Larson, Lakin, & Kwak, 2002).

These indirect public costs result in a loss of the tax revenue, productivity, and creativity that are engines of our national economy. All families, those with and without children who have disabilities, incur significant costs in raising and supporting their children. Families assume this obligation willingly. They see it as their responsibility.

For special education services, however, we have a national policy of reimbursing 40% of the incremental costs of educating children with disabilities. Our family support expenditures in no way approach 40% of the incremental cost of supporting families, nor do they approach even 10% of the cost of all publicly funded services and supports.

We do not know if the incremental costs families assume are offset by state governments not incurring direct costs for supporting people with services and benefits. But, without question, the families who have experienced these costs are in many ways the foundation of a service system that seldom recognizes them and yet, without them, could not survive.

It is estimated that in FY 2002 a total of $35 billion was spent to provide noneducational supports to individuals with intellectual and developmental disabilities. Most advocates and government officials recognize today that, while substantial, this level of funding is inadequate even to meet the needs of 20% of the people these resources touch.

We are, in some ways, still obsessed with the study of the costs of institutions and the efforts to close them. This is one piece of the nation's unfinished business, and rightfully we want closure. Perhaps, too, we find in these studies ready-made hypotheses of long standing, like outcomes in personal and social development, safety, or the false notion of economies of scale. Perhaps it is just that institutions and paid community supports are easy to study, especially from a financial perspective.

The financing of services for people captive to one provider is clearer than that for people in dispersed settings in the community. Perhaps it is natural to focus our studies of finances on the points where most of the money is being spent. This focus cum obsession may reflect on those in leadership positions at the present time. Looking around Washington, D.C., and at leading university-based research programs, several of the leaders of national organizations representing individuals or organizations working in the field of intellectual and developmental disabilities (and many academic leaders) are products of institutional exposés, scandals, and/or closures in the 1970s and 1980s. As institutions are closed and as surviving institutions achieve higher standards, what will the next generation of leaders focus on? Will there emerge another source of outrage or inspiration?

On the one hand, we state that the issue is not cost, but quality of life (Eidelman, Pietrangelo, Gardner, Jesien, & Croser, 2003) and the beneficial outcomes for people with intellectual and developmental disabilities; on the other hand, we recognize that we are accountable for the expenditure of public dollars. Public funds for human services have historically been held to a higher level of scrutiny than, for example, public expenditures for military projects. The old "guns versus butter" debate familiar to any college freshman taking Introductory Economics is played out on a number of levels. This fosters a double standard that many people advocating for people with intellectual and developmental disabilities find objectionable.

Yet, we want to be accountable for the expenditure of public funds and, with work by the researchers featured in this volume and others, we can demonstrate that community-based services and supports utilizing those funds provide better outcomes for people with intellectual and developmental disabilities. It is sound public policy and an appropriate utilization of tax dollars to move people out of highly restrictive settings and to provide supports in settings that offer people freedom, choices, and the opportunities to participate in—and contribute to—the communities in which they live.

Of necessity, the studies that demonstrate these outcomes examine life in the community after institutionalization for a group of individuals. The studies in the United States consistently show that people released from institutions fare better on virtually every quality of life indicator, when measured over time, than they did in the institution. Of course, this is not the real argument today. No credible group argues for institutionalization. The real debate will begin when we measure, over time, the costs and outcomes for all people with intellectual and developmental disabilities and show how they fare over the life span, comparing those who were institutionalized or those in a variety of program model settings to those receiving individually determined and designed services (i.e., self-determination, individual budgeting, individualized or essential lifestyle planning). The trend is away from program "models" to individualized programs of supports and services.

When discussing costs of services and support, as is done in this volume, we must always work to compare costs on a population basis, not an individual basis. It costs more to support some people than others, based on a variety of factors, many of which are out of the people's control. The right to live in a community environment of one's choosing must not be a hard dollars-and-cents calculation on an individual basis, but rather a quality of life calculation for the cohort of people with intellectual and developmental disabilities who need publicly financed supports and services. Fortunately, for people with intellectual and developmental disabilities, the outcome of community living wins out over large segregated supports settings using quality-of-life frameworks.

Although we need to understand costs, in the end, the debate cannot center on money. Dispassionate economic and cost analyses are but one factor employed in the allocation of scarce resources (i.e., tax dollars). Daily, society makes choices not necessarily between good, better, and best for a specific group of constituents, but rather about priorities among and between constituent groups.

How can we place a value on the increased benefits derived from more inclusive settings? Is it appropriate to examine quality-of-life indicators and attempt to assess their worth? Medical care research into quality-of-life outcomes takes this approach. We need to examine it further to continue the exploration of what works and why, and to provide ammunition for increased support for the tens of thousands of people who currently get little or no support. That number increases daily, and at the extreme, there are currently 700,000 people living with families who are elderly—a budgetary and human time bomb waiting to explode.

A note of caution if I may: We seem to be repeating the past, leading with cost savings and not outcomes for people. It is dangerous to hail self-determination as the savior for cost savings (see Chapter 10). We have before been led down the primrose path of conserving public resources; legislators and the media sometimes hear the saving money part and forget the ongoing costs of supporting people in the community. Can legislators ignore such savings? Can you order self-determination to be carried out on a large scale in more than a few places and replicate these results? Are these cost savings sustainable?

We are at a point of transition, in thought if not in deed. Much of our effort to date has been focused on obtaining funds to support people, through organizations, in communities. We are in the process of transitioning to a system that supports people who may or may not purchase those supports from organizations historically involved with providing paid supports for people with intellectual and developmental disabilities: a transition to a market economy. Market economies, when consumers have data about costs, quality, and outcomes, are powerful tools—not just in the disability field. The brave new world of individualized funding holds hope and promise, and this volume also provides a solid conceptual framework to understand it, so that we may move forward to implement it universally.

Until people with intellectual and developmental disabilities are perceived as having significant power, we can scrutinize cost data to the *nth* degree. The bottom line is that there remain, in the United States at least, inadequate resources, poor resource distribution and utilization, some waste and inefficiency, a bulge in the population demanding services, and growth in budgets—a burden being placed largely on the backs of families and direct-support workers.

Finally, understanding costs is but one of the important set of data needed to create options for people with intellectual and developmental disabilities in their chosen communities. The political dimension of closing institutions and of breaking up service models and the grip some programs hold over life's choices for people with intellectual and development disabilities is the subject of other volumes and an essential skill set needed to make the promises of community living for all a reality.

Steven M. Eidelman
Executive Director
The Arc of the United States
Silver Spring, Maryland

REFERENCES

Americans with Disabilities Act (ADA) of 1990, PL 101-336, 42 U.S.C. §§ 12101 *et seq.*

Anderson, L., Larson, S.A., Lakin, K.C., & Kwak, N. (2002). Children with disabilities: Social roles and family impacts in the NHIS-D. In *DD Data Brief, 4(1).* Minneapolis: University of Minnesota, Institute on Community Integration, Research and Training Center on Community Living. Also available on-line: http://rtc.umn.edu

Eidelman, S.M., Pietrangelo, R., Gardner, J.F., Jesien, G., & Croser, D.M. (2003). Let's focus on the real issues. *Mental Retardation, 41,* 126–129.

Lakin, K.C., Polister, B., & Prouty, R.W. (2003). Wages of non-state direct support professionals lag behind those of public direct support professionals and the general public. *Mental Retardation, 41*(2), 178–182.

Lakin, K.C., Prouty, R., Coucouvanis, K., & Polister, B. (2004). Fiscal year 2003 expenditures for Medicaid long-term care services and supports: Notable but limited effects of state budget crises. *Mental Retardation, 42*(5), 407–411.

U.S. House of Representatives. (2003, November 4). Sense of the Congress on the crisis in recruiting and retaining direct support professionals. *Congressional Record.* (H10301-H10304)

Acknowledgments

We thank the many people who have contributed directly and indirectly to this book. We are extremely appreciative of the efforts of the chapter authors in describing their work and its significance to the costs and outcomes of services received by people with developmental disabilities. The success of the book is fundamentally due to their efforts.

We are deeply grateful to our colleagues at the Research and Training Center on Community Living, Institute on Community Integration, University of Minnesota, who have created a positive and knowledge-rich climate that invigorated our work and helped shape many of the ideas we have presented.

We appreciate the ongoing guidance of our Research and Training Center on Community Living's Program Advisory Committee members, several of whom also contributed to the contents of this book; they are Robert M. Gettings and Charles R. Moseley of the National Association of State Directors of Developmental Disabilities Services; Valerie J. Bradley and Gary A. Smith of the Human Services Research Institute; Steven M. Eidelman of The Arc of the United States; Renee L. Pietrangelo of the American Network of Community Options and Resources; Steven J. Taylor of the Center on Human Policy, Syracuse University; David Braddock of the Coleman Institute for Cognitive Disabilities, University of Colorado; and Clifford L. Poetz, representing the National Alliance for Direct Support Professionals and People First Minnesota.

This volume would not have been possible without the thousands of individual service recipients, families, staff members, and administrators who have contributed to the research and surveys reported throughout the book. We thank them for their thoughtful and willing participation. The book's existence is due, in part, to the initial support and encouragement of Melissa Behm, Vice President of Paul H. Brookes Publishing Co. We also thank the staff at Brookes, whose highly professional work has contributed greatly to the book's successful completion.

The development of this book was supported, in part, by the National Institute on Disability and Rehabilitation Research (NIDRR), through Grant No. H133B031116, and by the Administration on Developmental Disabilities (ADD), through Grant No. 90DN0064. We are grateful to both agencies for their ongoing support for the programs of the Research and Training Center on Community Living. We appreciate the continuing support and advice of our Project Officers, Dawn Carlson (NIDRR) and Gretchen Menn (ADD). The opinions expressed throughout the book are those of the authors, and no endorsement by NIDRR or ADD should be presumed.

CHAPTER 1

Context and Issues in Research on Expenditures and Outcomes of Community Supports

Roger J. Stancliffe and K. Charlie Lakin

Many factors influence the availability and quality of services and supports for people with intellectual disabilities and developmental disabilities (ID/DD). Economic issues should not be the primary basis for service planning and policy, but as Ashbaugh has observed, "Look behind any movement that secures a place for itself in the perennially underfunded world of developmental disabilities and you will find an economic engine" (2002, p. 417). Service provision does have an important economic dimension, and it is essential to understand as much as possible the associations among service approaches, individual needs, costs, and outcomes so that effective, equitable, and economically sustainable service systems can be developed.

In the United States, federal, state, and local governments spent almost $35 billion in fiscal year (FY) 2002 on noneducational services for people with ID/DD (Rizzolo, Hemp, Braddock, & Pomeranz-Essley, 2004; see also Chapter 2). Almost 80% of this amount was used to fund community services. In FY 2002, federal and state Medicaid Intermediate Care Facilities for Persons with Mental Retardation (ICFs/MR) and Home and Community-Based Services (HCBS) Waiver programs exceeded $24 billion in total long-term care expenditures (Prouty, Smith, & Lakin, 2003). Expenditures for home, community, and institutional services are enormous in size and highly varying 1) in the nature and quality of services they purchase (e.g., from a "bed" in an institution of several hundred residents, to companion support in a person's own home); 2) in the amounts spent for similar "models" of service in different states, communities, and/or agencies; and 3) in the methods of disbursement of expenditures (e.g., from government retrospective reimbursement of provider costs, to direct cash payments to families and/or individuals for purchasing their own services). Despite these numerous variations, there is only a limited and scattered literature on the nature and outcomes of expenditures for services for people with intellectual and developmental disabilities.

This book draws together information on costs, outcomes, and approaches to financing services for people with ID/DD and the effects on efficiency and/or effectiveness of variations in such factors. The primary focus is on community services, but because institutions continue to operate, attention is also given to the costs and outcomes of deinstitutionalization. The term *costs* encompasses both expenditures for services and the mechanisms for allocating resources that affect the nature and operation of service systems, specific service types, and ultimately the lives of service recipients. *Costs* sometimes is used to include not only public expenditures but also the substantial personal costs in time and money of family members, volunteers, and others applied to the support of people with ID/DD. Acknowledging such costs leads to distinctions among costs, personal expenditures, and public expenditures. Because accounting is rarely available on the comprehensive definition of *cost*, in this book, the terms *cost* and *expenditure* are treated as synonymous unless distinguished as different.

There are many important issues that arise when considering community services and the expenditures for them. Foremost among these is effectiveness in achieving high-quality outcomes and good quality of life. Without satisfactory outcomes, expenditures on services are a poor investment for society, resulting in deprivation, increased disability, and even danger for service recipients and their families. Therefore, this book focuses on both costs *and* outcomes.

Services' cost and cost effectiveness are important concerns for service recipients and families as well as for policy makers and service administrators. The budget crises faced by the majority of states since 2002 have demonstrated this clearly. The resulting expectation that state agencies will find ways to reduce, or to some degree control, budgets has shown how important it is to have information on costs and outcomes and their associations with different approaches to service delivery and financing. It has also shown how rarely available such information is when needed.

As a result of such funding challenges, it is now better understood that there are important consequences of not reforming ineffective, inappropriate, or excessively costly services. These undesirable consequences include limited (or nonexistent) access to appropriate services by those who are unserved, underserved, or poorly served. The public's expectation that society's limited resources are used wisely involves both effective use of public funding and assuring that those resources have maximum positive benefit for support recipients. Advocates of system reform emphasize the importance of wise use of public funding (Nerney, 1998).

At its simplest, spending on services "is affected by two factors: the number of individuals who receive such services, and the per capita costs associated with furnishing services to such individuals" (Smith, O'Keeffe, Carpenter, Doty, & Kennedy, 2000, p. 152). The implication of this simple observation is that, if service costs are not managed effectively, either total system expenditures increase sharply or costs are controlled by limiting access to services through the use of restrictive eligibility criteria, waiting lists, and the like. Therefore, careful management of costs and cost effectiveness is a crucial element of equitable, sustainable service provision for people with ID/DD.

A focus on cost should not imply that lower cost is self-evidently better, or that cost outweighs other considerations. Higher-cost services that deliver better outcomes ought to be supported strongly on cost-effectiveness grounds. For example, Emerson, Robertson, Hatton, Knapp, and Walsh (Chapter 7) found that institutional services in the United Kingdom cost significantly less than community services but concluded that the additional expenditure on community services was warranted in light of the consistent benefits of these services.

In this chapter, we provide a context for the chapters in this book. We describe the U.S. service and funding situation and examine a number of key issues drawing on selected previous research—issues such as family support, needs-based funding, individual budgets, cost comparisons between institutional and community services (including wage rates for direct-support staff), economies of scale, and the relation between expenditures and outcomes. The chapter ends with a list of 11 important issues that have helped to guide the development of this book.

UNITED STATES'S SERVICE AND FUNDING CONTEXT

Since the 1980s, major changes have taken place in the legal environment, funding, operation, and control of community services for people with ID/DD in the United States. First, a widespread shift from institutional to community provision of services took place in every state, although to substantially different degrees in each state (Prouty, Lakin, & Bruininks, 2003). A 59% decrease in public and private institution residents between 1982 and 2002 was accompanied by a 696% increase in community residences housing six or fewer people. This change has been accompanied by an operational transformation from state governments being the primary *provider* of services, to state governments being largely a *purchaser* of services.

In 1982, 49% of people with ID/DD who received residential services were supported by nonstate agencies, but by 2002, this figure had increased to 86% (Prouty, Smith, et al., 2003; see also Chapter 13). This change has had an impact on system costs because nonstate agencies typically provide services at a lower cost (Campbell & Heal, 1995; Stancliffe & Lakin, 1998). This outcome has been influenced strongly by the lower wages and other compensation of nonstate employees relative to state employees (Polister, Lakin, & Prouty, 2003).

Second, a dramatic shift occurred from state financing of community services to federal–state cost sharing of community-services expenditures. Between FY 1991 and FY 2000, inflation-controlled federal expenditures for community services increased by 227%, or about $7.36 billion expressed in FY 2000 dollars. This amount compares with a notable but much smaller increase in state expenditures of 46%, or $3.65 billion expressed in FY 2000 dollars.

Third, the total number of people with ID/DD receiving services grew substantially and proportionally. Nationally, from 287,294 in 1991, to 392,740 in 2002, the number of people served by residential services grew by 105,446 (36.7% increase relative to 1991). This expansion was due not only to a national population increase but also to a rising utilization rate that grew by 19.3%, from 114 per 100,000 of total population in 1991, to 136.2 per 100,000 in 2002 (Prouty, Smith, et al., 2003). Even so, in 2002 there were almost 60,000 people waiting for residential services. Increased life expectancy among people with ID/DD (Janicki, Dalton, Henderson, & Davidson, 1999) means that the demand for services is increasing more rapidly than would be expected based on the growth of the general population alone. Individuals who live longer remain in the community-services system longer. Consequently, new entrants to the service system increasingly require the creation of new places in addition to places relinquished by deceased service recipients.

Fourth, state governments have moved away from program funding, rate setting, and funding by numbers of people served, toward individualized funding, individual budgets, and needs-based resource allocation. These initiatives are intended not only to establish appropriate levels of funding geared to individual need, but also to support greater consumer control of service decisions (see Chapters 9, 10, 11, and 12).

Fifth, in June 1999, the U.S. Supreme Court determined in *Olmstead v. L.C.* (1991) that unnecessary segregation of people with disabilities represents discrimination that is prohibited by the Americans with Disabilities Act of 1990 (PL 101-336) and that states are required to provide services, programs, and activities developed for people with disabilities in the "most integrated setting appropriate." The decision required states to place institutionalized individuals in community settings when 1) treatment professionals determine that community placement is appropriate, 2) the individual does not oppose community placement, and 3) community placement can be reasonably accommodated when taking into account the resources and needs of other people with disabilities.

Sixth, there has been substantial growth in HCBS Waiver funding (see Chapter 2) and greater flexibility in the application of this funding (see Chapter 5). Relative to HCBS Waiver–funded residential services, poorer outcomes have been reported for community ICFs/MR (Conroy, 1996, 1998; Stancliffe, Abery, & Smith, 2000; Stancliffe, Hayden, Larson, & Lakin, 2002).

Seventh, as noted by Braddock et al. (Chapter 2), total spending on public and private 16+ person institutions has fallen each year since 1992, but the rate of decline has been far less than the rate of depopulation of these facilities. As a result, average per-person daily institutional expenditures (per diems) have continued to rise. In 2002, per diems in public institutions averaged $344.51 (i.e., $125,746 annually) as compared to raw per diems of $270 in 1997, $211 in 1992, and $90 in 1982. This substantial growth in per diems was driven, in part, by diseconomies of reduced scale associated with institutional downsizing (see Chapter 13).

Eighth, wide variation continues among states in fiscal effort (see Chapter 2) and in service provision, including progress toward deinstitutionalization (see Chapter 13). Finally, supported living and family support have grown significantly. In 2002, state and federal expenditures for family support were about $1.4 billion, roughly 26% more than in 2000 (Rizzolo et al., 2004). Medicaid HCBS Waiver recipients living with family members were an estimated 149,500 in 2002, more than twice the number of just 4 years earlier (Prouty, Smith, et al., 2003).

FUNDING PROGRAMS

Funding programs influence service configurations. Historical funding decisions have strongly influenced today's funding and service patterns. Braddock et al. (Chapter 2) look at the history of public funding of disability services as well as the contemporary funding situation. The entry of federal funding of long-term care of people with ID/DD profoundly influenced services. Federal matching of funding for skilled nursing facilities (SNFs) in 1965 saw a rapid growth in patient numbers in SNFs. Many individuals with disabilities in SNFs were receiving much more medical care, at far greater cost than was really warranted, and were being placed there because of the fiscal incentive provided by federal cost sharing.

In 1971, Congress authorized federal financial participation in a less medically oriented and less expensive ICF/MR program for people with ID/DD. The ICF/MR program had far-reaching effects on large state facilities as they were brought into conformity with ICF/MR standards to secure federal financial participation. Likewise, the Medicaid HCBS Waiver program, authorized in 1981, enabled the development of a wide variety of noninstitutional services. Lakin, Hewitt, Larson, and Stancliffe (Chapter 5) describe the range, utilization, and cost of HCBS Waiver services in Minnesota.

FAMILY SUPPORT

Most people with ID/DD live in the family home and are supported by their immediate family. Fujiura (1998) estimated that in 1991 61% of Americans with ID/DD lived in this manner, with only 11% in the formal long-term ID/DD residential service system. For some time, families, children with disabilities, and policy makers have widely agreed that children and youth with ID/DD should live with family (Roseneau, 1990; Taylor, Lakin, & Hill, 1989). Achievement of this objective has progressed since the 1970s. Nationally, in 1977, 36% (55,670) of state institution residents were age birth to 21 years. In 2002, this proportion had fallen to 5% (2,165) of a much smaller total state institution population (Prouty, Smith et al., 2003). Of course, state institutions represent only one, increasingly unpopular, out-of-home option. In Minnesota in 1999, Hewitt, Larson, and Lakin (2000) found that 8.7% of all long-term care recipients (ICF/MR and HCBS Waiver) were age birth to 17 years, with most in this age group living in community residences that were HCBS Waiver funded.

The family home continues to be the place of residence for the majority of people with ID/DD, and immediate family members still are the primary caregivers for these individuals. Despite this situation, in 2002, only 4% of expenditures of state ID/DD agencies were used for family support (Rizzolo et al., 2004). Although vastly fewer resources are available to families than to recipients of residential services, this disparity is diminishing, with an 81% real increase in family support expenditures between 1997 and 2002 associated with a rapid growth in both the number of families receiving support and the amount of support provided to each family (Rizzolo et al., 2004). In fact, in 2002, there were more recipients of family support (482,000) than of residential services (393,000) (Prouty, Smith et al., 2003). Investing early in family support that has a relatively low cost is arguably less expensive for taxpayers than paying for costly out-of-home services (see Chapter 5).

Impact on People with ID/DD

Limited information is available on comparative quality of life and lifestyle outcomes for individuals with ID/DD living with families or outside of the family home. Burchard, Hasazi, Gordon, and Yoe (1991) found distinct patterns of satisfaction and lifestyle outcomes for *adults* with intellectual disabilities in Vermont living in small-group homes, in supervised apartments, or with natural families. They characterized these settings as being agency directed, client directed, and family oriented, respectively. Residents of supervised apartments experienced significantly greater independence, lifestyle normalization, community participation, and social integration. Those living in the family home mostly enjoyed similar outcomes to group home residents, except for lifestyle normalization (age-appropriate activities, personal responsibility, autonomy in decision making), with those in family homes experiencing poorer outcomes; however, residents of family homes and supervised apartments reported greater satisfaction with their residence and personal well-being than group home residents. Family home residents had significantly fewer challenging behaviors than other participants.

The Vermont study was conducted in the late 1980s, when limited support was available for families (no families were noted by Burchard et al., 1991, as receiving support services). These data, therefore, reveal little about the impact of family support services but do delineate that individuals who live with family members experience a different lifestyle and different outcomes than residents of community residential services. Contemporary evaluation of the impact of family support services indicates that such services are generally helpful, provided the services are appropriate and of adequate quality (e.g., Romer, Richardson, Nahom, Aigbe, & Porter, 2002).

Consumer-Directed Family Support

Formal family support services, such as respite, in-home support, and parent education have tended to be agency directed. Increased interest in consumer-directed programs has also influenced provision of family support, with a number of states implementing consumer-directed family support services.

Caldwell and Heller (2003) examined outcomes for both the family and the person with disabilities associated with a consumer-directed family support program in Illinois. They found that more control by families of respite and personal assistance services was linked with increased satisfaction with services, more community participation by the person with developmental disabilities, less staff turnover, and more hours per week of employment for mothers. This last finding represents an important outcome in the context of the substantial economic costs and reduced employment opportunities experienced by families with a member with disabilities (see Chapter 4).

Caldwell and Heller (2003) reported that families tended to hire people they knew (e.g., friends, neighbors, other relatives living outside the immediate home) to provide respite and personal assistance. Hiring relatives was associated with increased community participation by the person with ID/DD. In short, consumer-directed family support was shown to have benefits for both families and people with ID/DD.

Herman (1991, 1994) examined the impact of a family cash subsidy program in Michigan for families with a child (younger than 18 years of age) with developmental disabilities. Families reported satisfaction with the program and indicated that the subsidy helped to improve family life, ease financial worries, and reduce stress. Importantly, families used the subsidy for the types of services they said were needed.

NEEDS-BASED FUNDING

Allocating available funding equitably among service recipients is a basic value that should underpin all funding arrangements. Funding distribution should be fair, consistent, and based on valid methods for determining funding levels. People often assume that expenditure on services and support provision is strongly influenced by the needs of the individuals served (Schalock & Fredericks, 1990). Individuals with fewer self-care skills, more challenging behavior, or more serious health problems are thought to need, *and are assumed to receive*, more staff support and so require greater per-person expenditure to provide appropriate services. Studies have reported widely varying relationships between expenditure on services and the characteristics of service recipients.

Findings from different U.S. service systems have ranged from a very strong association (Campbell & Heal, 1995; see also Chapter 11); through a more moderate association (Jones, Conroy, Feinstein, & Lemanowicz, 1984; see also Chapter 8); to a weak, inconsistent, or nonexistent association (Ashbaugh & Nerney, 1990; Nerney, Conley, & Nisbet, 1990; Stancliffe & Lakin, 1998; see also Chapter 6). These mixed findings suggest that funding for services can be directly linked to individualized support needs, but that such practices are far from universal. In a number of jurisdictions, funding is not related (strongly) to the individual characteristics of service recipients. Such funding arrangements may be difficult to defend on the basis of either rational or equitable allocation of public money. The issue of the relationship between service-recipient characteristics and funding is taken up by Lakin et al. (Chapter 5), Campbell et al. (Chapter 8), and Fortune et al. (Chapter 11).

Traditional funding arrangements of congregate facilities have been based on rate schedules and facility operating costs, cost caps, local negotiation with service providers, and historical reimbursement rates, with little specific attention to the individual needs and characteristics of service recipients beyond basic eligibility requirements. Such a piecemeal approach may enable state funding agencies to contain expenditures within budget limits but frequently leads to unjust variations in funding. In addition, these funding arrangements tend to lock in service recipients (and providers and funders) to existing service arrangements because the amount allocated to pay for services from one agency may not be sufficient to purchase a similar service from another provider.

INDIVIDUAL BUDGETS

A desire for more flexible, individualized, self-directed services, together with the move toward needs-based funding, has been reflected in the rapid increase in availability of individual budgets for use in purchasing services and supports. This trend has confronted state officials with the need to develop methodologies for equitable allocation of funding to individuals. Moseley, Gettings, and Cooper (Chapter 12) describe the findings of a national survey of the varied approaches taken by states to individual budget determination. Fortune et al. (Chapter 11) describe one of these approaches—a statistical model known as DOORS— used throughout Wyoming, that is based on each service recipient's individual characteristics and living, working, and service-use arrangements (but *not* the rates or characteristics of specific providers). DOORS is used to compute an *individual budget amount* for each HCBS Waiver service recipient.

Among other things, individual budgets are intended to provide service recipients and their families with more control over services and supports and to shift control away from agencies and staff (Moseley, 2001). Conroy and Yuskauskas's (1996) unpublished study of the original Robert Wood Johnson Foundation–funded "self-determination" project in New Hampshire is one of the few to examine this proposition. They found significant increases in choice and control over time following self-determination interventions that may have included an individual budget. Findings regarding the outcomes for people in programs of "consumer-directed supports" (CDS), reported in Chapter 9 by Stancliffe and Lakin and Chapter 10 by Head and Conroy, offer valuable new examinations of the effects of individual budgeting and CDS. Stancliffe and Lakin used cross-sectional data from the beginning of Michigan's self-determination initiative to evaluate freedom from staff control for a sample of service recipients from Michigan by comparing those with and without an individual budget. Head and Conroy used longitudinal data to examine control, quality of life, and service costs before and after the introduction of this program that included person-centered planning and individual budgets.

In some states, such as Wyoming, the individual budgeting approach is applied to *all* (HCBS Waiver) consumers, but in other states, individual budgets are provided as an option or are only open to some service recipients (see Chapter 12). One (unintended) consequence of the latter approach is that individual budgets may be more accessible to some service recipients than others. For example, service recipients with strong, vocal family support may obtain greater access to individual budgets. Stancliffe and Lakin (Chapter 9) also investigated whether personal characteristics, family involvement, or living arrangements distinguished service recipients with an individual budget from those without one.

The valuable information about individual budgets contained in Chapters 9–12 helps to advance our understanding of the development, utilization, availability, effects, and relative cost of individual budgets. Campbell et al. (Chapter 8) provide a clear explication of data analytic techniques that can be used to underpin resource allocation methodology for individual budgeting.

COST COMPARISONS BETWEEN INSTITUTIONAL AND COMMUNITY SERVICES

Cost Effectiveness

Available U.S. studies of both costs and outcomes of deinstitutionalization reveal a consistent pattern across states and over time of better outcomes and lower costs in the community. Jones et al. (1984) found that former institution residents now living in the community in Pennsylvania showed significantly greater improvements in adaptive behavior than matched peers who remained institutionalized, whereas the overall public per-person service cost was 14.6% lower in the community. In a much smaller longitudinal study in Oregon, Knobbe, Carey, Rhodes, and Horner (1995) also reported community services to have better outcomes and to be 5.2% less expensive than institutional services. In Minnesota, Stancliffe and Lakin (1998) found significantly better lifestyle outcomes for community residents, as well as costs that were 26.6% lower for community services as compared with institutional services. These three cost-effectiveness studies reported 1) findings on outcomes that were consistent with the broader U.S. deinstitutionalization literature on outcomes (Kim, Larson, & Lakin, 2001), and 2) results regarding costs congruent with cost comparison research showing institutional services in the United States to be more costly than community services (e.g., Campbell & Heal, 1995; Schalock & Fredericks, 1990).

Methodological Problems

Walsh, Kastner, and Green (2003) reviewed studies involving cost comparisons between community and institutional residential settings. They noted that there are a number of methodological challenges in making these comparisons including cost shifting, case mix, and staffing variables (notably differences in staff wages). Eidelman, Pietrangelo, Gardner, Jesien, and Croser (2003) argued that the issue is not whether institutional or community services are cheaper, but which array of services and supports yields the best outcomes. It is of interest to note in that regard that institution–community cost comparisons in the United Kingdom yielded different findings, with community services generally more expensive (see Chapter 3). But regardless of the cost-comparison outcomes, consistent and compelling evidence supports that community services result in better outcomes than institutions (Emerson et al., 2000; Kim et al., 2001). In the light of such evidence, cost comparisons between institutional and community services are of limited importance.

Wage Rates

The largest cost component of residential and related services is staff costs, generally representing about 77% to 87% of total expenditures (Stancliffe & Lakin, 1998). Differences in staffing costs can arise in several ways, including 1) different intensities of staffing (e.g., different staff–resident ratios, live-in versus shift staff), 2) different rates of pay for the same job tasks (e.g., marked difference in pay between state employees and those who work in nonstate services), 3) different benefits, and 4) different staffing and/or service-delivery arrangements (e.g., employing paraprofessionals versus professionals; outsourcing some services, such as health services, by using local clinics instead of having medical personnel on staff).

Nationally, in 2000, the average hourly wage of direct-support staff in state-operated services was $11.57 versus $8.72 (24.6% less) in nonstate community services (Polister et al., 2003). Such wage differentials have been reported consistently in earlier research, accompanied by differences in benefits that also favor state employees (e.g., Lakin & Bruininks, 1981; Mitchell & Braddock, 1994).

Deinstitutionalization has largely been characterized by the closure of *state* institutions with residents moving to *nonstate* community services (Lakin, Prouty, Polister, & Coucouvanis, 2003). Such consistent and substantial state–nonstate wage differentials likely have been a major driver of the lower cost of nonstate community services (Campbell & Heal, 1995; Rhoades & Altman, 2001; Stancliffe & Lakin, 1998), and have also influenced the strong trend away from direct state service provision toward states being purchasers of services from nonstate providers. Interestingly, some states (e.g., Maryland, Nebraska) have embarked on initiatives intended to eliminate the wage and benefits disparity between state and nonstate direct-support staff by increasing the compensation of nonstate employees (Polister et al., 2003).

ECONOMIES OF SCALE

Nationally, in the United States, the decrease in the average size of all residential settings for people with ID/DD (including institutions) over time is shown in Figure 1.1. The continuing trend toward smaller scale has been brought about by the downsizing and closure of institutions and by the consistently decreasing size of community settings (i.e., residences for 15 or fewer people). The typical community household is now made up of few individuals.

In 2002, half (50.5%) of all residential service recipients (62.4% of community residents) were supported in settings of 1–3 people (Prouty, Lakin, et al., 2003). This trend has been accompanied over time by increases in average service cost. Unfortunately, however, there are no good

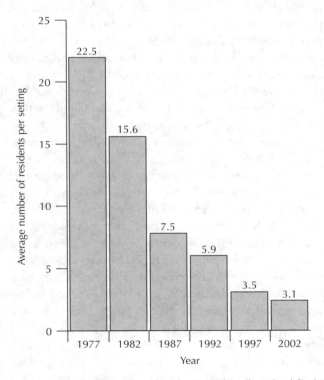

Figure 1.1.   Average number of residents per residential setting with intellectual and developmental disabilities in the United States, from 1997 to 2002 (including settings of all sizes). (From Smith, J., Coucouvanis, K., Polister, B., Prouty, R.W., & Lakin, K.C. [2003]. Services provided by state and nonstate agencies in 2002. In R.W. Prouty, G. Smith, & K.C. Lakin [Eds.], *Residential services for persons with developmental disabilities: Status trends through 2002* [p. 66]. Minneapolis: University of Minnesota, Research and Training Center on Community Living, Institute on Community Integration; reprinted by permission.)

national data sets in the United States with which to examine the effects on cost of progressing toward smaller settings while appropriately controlling for resident support needs. Lakin, Prouty, et al. (2003) noted that between 1982 and 2002 per-person ICF/MR expenditures rose by a compounded average of 6.7% per year. Between FY 1992 and FY 2002, average per-person annual ICF/MR expenditures increased from $60,370 to $95,746 while the average number of residents per ICF/MR setting decreased from 22.5 in 1992 to 16.7 in 2002 (Mangan, Blake, Prouty, & Lakin, 1993; Prouty, Smith, et al., 2003). Some observers may interpret the coincidence of these trends as evidence that services are today more costly due to the effects of *economies of scale.*

The widespread assumption that economies of scale can be expected to operate in human services, and that smaller-scale services consequently should have higher per-person costs, has strongly influenced service policy and planning. For example, the larger scale of facilities such as institutions and community ICFs/MR has been defended on the basis of fiscal responsibility because of the presumed operation of economies of scale (Erb, 1995). Similarly, very individualized living arrangements, until recently, have tended to be restricted to individuals with milder disabilities who require low levels of support, partly because people with higher support needs were believed to be too costly to serve in this way.

Actual evidence for economies of scale in ID/DD services has been equivocal and has frequently contradicted these notions. For example, the very common U.S. finding that institutional services have higher per-person costs than much smaller scale community services directly contradicts the notion of economies of scale (see Chapter 13). Rhoades and Altman (2001), in an analysis of national data on residential services for three or more residents, found that costs *increase* as residence size increases. Likewise, Campbell and Heal (1995) reported that, in South Dakota, state institutions (the largest residence type) were the most costly form of service provision. In Minnesota, Lakin and Stancliffe (1998) found medium-sized community residential settings (with 5–6 people) to be more costly than either smaller or larger community settings in the 1- to 15-person size range. Howe, Horner, and Newton (1998) found no difference in the costs of supported living and traditional community living in Oregon, even though the number of residents averaged 1.6 and 6.9 respectively.

One fundamental difficulty in evaluating economies of scale by comparing services of different size and type is that, in the U.S. context, different service types frequently also differ in terms of funding program, service ownership (state or nonstate), staff wages, and/or regulatory requirements.

Each of these factors can directly influence costs and, therefore, confound comparisons. Nerney et al. (1990) found residential service type to be the strongest determinant of service cost, with ICF/MR services being most costly, and family foster care, the least expensive. Likewise, funding sources influence cost. Cost comparisons of community ICFs/MR and HCBS Waiver–funded residences are often confounded because common national standards regulate ICFs/MR but state-designed standards regulate HCBS Waiver–funded programs. As much as standards establish staffing ratios, required hours of program participation, qualifications and training of personnel, and so forth, they have substantial effects on cost. The most meaningful evaluation of the operation of economies of scale most likely involves comparisons of services of differing *size* but the same *type*.

Nerney et al. (1990) examined costs in group homes in several states and found some weak evidence for diseconomies of very small scale in the smallest group homes; however, Nerney et al. also reported *no relationship* between number of residents and per-person cost in family foster care due to the fact that foster care providers received a specified amount per person irrespective of the number served. That is, the operation of economies of scale was *model dependent*, with some service models showing modest effects but other models experiencing no such effects.

Within-model comparisons of costs by residence size are further complicated by historical funding and service-delivery patterns. *Larger* community facilities generally were established *earlier* and have historically lower housing costs that cannot be replicated in the current market. Stancliffe and Lakin (1998) found that residence age (the number of years each residence had served people with ID/DD) was significantly negatively related to total service cost, with larger, older settings having lower raw costs. Current funding for services in the older, larger facilities homes was based on rates set at the time the home began operating. The rate of adjustment to budgets of existing facilities has grown much less rapidly than the negotiated budgets for new programs serving people with similar characteristics. Moreover, lower expenditures in older, larger facilities also derived from the lower staff ratios that established facilities were able to purchase given their low existing per-diem rate. These findings have recently been supported by research about costs in small-group homes in the United Kingdom that showed a trend toward rising cost for more recently established group homes (Felce, Jones, Lowe, & Perry, 2003).

Felce and Emerson (Chapter 3) review the U.K. evidence of economies of scale in residential services, and Stancliffe (Chapter 6) reports findings from an Australian study of group homes and semi-independent living. Both chapters report some evidence of economies of scale but only under quite specific and limited circumstances. A further facet of this topic relates to the experience that institutional per diems (average daily expenditures per person) rise as resident numbers fall. Stancliffe, Lakin, Shea, Prouty, and Coucouvanis (Chapter 13) examine the phenomenon of diseconomies of *reduced* scale when institutions are downsized but argue that it is not valid to extrapolate from the existence of such diseconomies of reduced scale and assume that economies of scale must therefore apply to facilities of differing size that are operating *at the size they were designed for.*

Clearly, the issue of economies of scale is complex. Understanding its applicability to services for people with ID/DD is important in terms of ensuring appropriate funding where economies of scale apply but avoiding unsound service-planning decisions based on the unsupported presumption that such economies will result in less costly services. The evidence shows that economies of scale do not operate in many parts of the staff-intensive world of human services.

RELATIONSHIP BETWEEN EXPENDITURES AND CONSUMER OUTCOMES

Just as household income is a powerful predictor of household expenditures, even controlling for family size and composition, so, too, the total appropriations by states to support programs for individuals with ID/DD are a major factor affecting expenditures on behalf of individuals within those states.

In the United States, there are major disparities in state allocations to services for people with ID/DD, with three states in FY 2002 spending more than $150 per year per state resident for Medicaid HCBS Waiver and ICF/MR services and three spending $40 or less per year per state resident for these same services. Of course, state appropriations are not wholly free of demands resulting from policy decisions, such as participating in the ICF/MR program, or of externally enforced requirements of court decisions or federal government reviews and required responses.

It is tempting to assume that spending more money on services to provide better staffing and improved living facilities will result in better outcomes for service recipients. In a U.S. context, the relationship between service expenditures and lifestyle outcomes for residents has mostly been examined indirectly through comparison of different types of support.

Medicaid expenditures are disproportionately higher for people in ICFs/MR than for HCBS Waiver recipients, with the 2002 U.S. average annual expenditure for ICF/MR residents being $95,746 as compared with $37,816 for each HCBS Waiver recipient (Prouty, Smith, et al., 2003).

This comparison is complicated by differences in the abilities of service recipients, in the array of services provided, and in the fact that nearly 40% of HCBS Waiver recipients live with family members who, in almost all instances, provide substantial amounts of noncompensated support and supervision. Even so, it appears that ICF/MR services consistently cost more than HCBS Waiver services for comparable levels of support (Conroy, 1998; see also Chapter 5). Of course, as with all comparisons of expenditures, whether among schools, households, or residential programs, what most determines expenditures is the amount available to be expended.

As previously noted, extensive research comparing the lifestyles and/or service costs of people living in community settings (typically HCBS Waiver funded) and institutional settings (typically ICF/MR funded) has found higher costs but poorer outcomes in institutions (Conroy & Bradley, 1985; Felce, de Kock, & Repp, 1986; Horner, Stoner, & Ferguson, 1988; Kim et al., 2001; Jones et al., 1984; O'Neil, Brown, Gordon, Schonhorn, & Green, 1981; Stancliffe & Lakin, 1998). This research is impressive both for the magnitude and the consistency of findings favoring the outcomes of community living. Likewise, despite the higher average public costs of ICFs/MR, specific comparisons between community ICFs/MR (15 or fewer residents) and HCBS Waiver–funded residences have shown better self-determination, integration, quality of life, challenging behavior, and adaptive behavior outcomes in HCBS Waiver settings (Conroy, 1996, 1998; Stancliffe et al., 2000; Stancliffe et al., 2002). Although these studies did not directly examine the relationship between expenditure and outcomes, they provided no support for the notion that increased expenditure is necessarily associated with better outcomes.

Comparisons between group homes and semi-independent living have shown more favorable outcomes in semi-independent environments (Burchard et al., 1991; Stancliffe et al., 2000; Stancliffe & Keane, 2000; see also Chapter 6). Not surprisingly, where service costs were examined, they were substantially lower for the semi-independent settings with their part-time staffing (Stancliffe & Keane, 2000; see also Chapter 6). Once again, greater expenditure was not associated with better outcomes. Rather, both expenditure and outcomes were related to service type.

These studies reveal fairly consistent differences in both outcomes and costs *between* different community-living service types, but provide limited insight into the relationships between expenditures and outcomes *within* service types. The issue of the relationship between expenditures and outcomes is taken up by Felce and Emerson (Chapter 3), who review the more extensive U.K. research on this important topic, and by Lakin et al. (Chapter 5), who examine this issue for certain HCBS Waiver services in Minnesota.

CONCLUSION

Chapters in this book bring together research findings from state and national studies in the United States and from research conducted outside North America (notably from the United Kingdom and Australia). In each of these chapters, the authors address a number of important issues, including one or more of the following.

1. What is the historical service-provision and service-funding context in which service expenditures and outcomes are to be understood?

2. What are the direct and indirect financial and social costs of family care for family members with developmental disabilities? Who meets these costs, and how have they been allocated between families and society? What implications do these findings have for public policy and family support?

3. Are there differences in outcomes and costs between community-living service models (institution versus community, community ICF/MR versus waiver, group home versus semi-independent, supported living versus traditional community services)?

4. Are larger inputs (expenditures, staffing) related to better outcomes?

5. On what basis is funding allocated to pay for community services for individuals with intellectual disabilities? Is funding allocated to individual recipients of services according to the person's support needs?

6. On what basis should funding be allocated to pay for community services for individuals with intellectual disabilities? How can an individual budgeting process be developed that is rational and equitable and that facilitates individually desired lifestyles?

7. How are states approaching the task of providing individual budgets to service recipients and their families? What are the public policy considerations involved in developing individual budgets in a statewide system of developmental disabilities services? How can an equi-

table individual funding allocation be made available while managing costs within a service system?

8. Are there differences in outcomes and costs by funding arrangements (individual budgets versus traditional funding)?

9. What is the relationship between the size of a residential setting and per-person expenditure on residential services? Is there evidence for economies of scale? Is there evidence for better outcomes in smaller settings?

10. What is the impact of institutional downsizing on the per-person expenditure on services for individuals who remain in the institution?

11. What are the policy and practice implications of the findings relating to these issues?

These 11 issues form the conceptual heart of this book. They are not the only issues that deserve consideration when discussing costs and outcomes in community services for people with intellectual and developmental disabilities; however, careful examination and better understanding of these issues can contribute significantly to guiding the evolution of service systems that provide adequately supported, individually satisfying lifestyles to a maximum number of individuals within the amount of public resources allocated to their behalf.

REFERENCES

Americans with Disabilities Act (ADA) of 1990, PL 101-336, 42 U.S.C. §§ 12101 et seq.

Ashbaugh, J.W. (2002). Down the garden path with self-determination. *Mental Retardation, 40,* 416–417.

Ashbaugh, J., & Nerney, T. (1990). Costs of providing residential and related support services to individuals with mental retardation. *Mental Retardation, 28,* 269–273.

Burchard, S.N., Hasazi, J.E., Gordon, L.R., & Yoe, J. (1991). An examination of lifestyle and adjustment in three community residential alternatives. *Research in Developmental Disabilities, 12,* 127–142.

Caldwell, J., & Heller, T. (2003). Management of respite and personal assistance services in a consumer-directed family support programme. *Journal of Intellectual Disability Research, 47,* 352–366.

Campbell, E.M., & Heal, L.W. (1995). Prediction of cost, rate, and staffing by provider and client characteristics. *American Journal on Mental Retardation, 100,* 17–35.

Conroy, J.W. (1996). The small ICF/MR program: Dimensions of quality and cost. *Mental Retardation, 34,* 13–26.

Conroy, J.W. (1998). Quality in small ICFs/MR versus waiver homes. *TASH Newsletter, 24*(3), 23–24, 28.

Conroy, J.W., & Bradley, V.J. (1985). *The Pennhurst longitudinal study: A report of five years of research and analysis.* Philadelphia: Temple University, Developmental Disabilities Center.

Conroy, J., & Yuskauskas, A. (1996, December). *Independent evaluation of the Monadnock Self-Determination Project.* Submitted to the Robert Wood Johnson Foundation. Ardmore, PA: The Center for Outcome Analysis.

Eidelman, S.M., Pietrangelo, R., Gardner, J.F., Jesien, G., & Croser, D.M. (2003). Let's focus on the real issues. *Mental Retardation, 41,* 126–129.

Emerson, E., Robertson, J., Gregory, N., Hatton, C., Kessissoglou, S., Hallam, A., Knapp, M., Järbrink, K., Walsh, P.N., & Netten, A. (2000). Quality and costs of community-based residential supports, village communities, and residential campuses in the United Kingdom. *American Journal on Mental Retardation, 105,* 81–102.

Erb, R.G. (1995). Where, oh where, has common sense gone? (Or if the shoe don't fit why wear it?). *Mental Retardation, 33,* 197–199.

Felce, D., de Kock, U., & Repp, A.C. (1986). An eco-behavioral analysis of small community based houses and traditional large hospitals for severely and profoundly mentally handicapped adults. *Applied Research in Mental Retardation, 7,* 393–408.

Felce, D., Jones, E., Lowe, K., & Perry, J. (2003). Rational resourcing and productivity: Relationships among staff input, resident characteristics, and group home quality. *American Journal on Mental Retardation, 108,* 161–172.

Fujiura, G.T. (1998). Demography of family households. *American Journal on Mental Retardation, 103,* 225–235.

Herman, S.E. (1991). Use and impact of a cash subsidy program. *Mental Retardation, 29,* 253–258.

Herman, S.E. (1994). Cash subsidy program: Family satisfaction and need. *Mental Retardation, 29,* 253–258.

Hewitt, A., Larson, S.A., & Lakin, K.C. (2000). *An independent evaluation of the quality of services and system performance of Minnesota's Medicaid home and community based services for persons with mental retardation and related conditions.* Minneapolis: University of Minnesota, Institute on Community Integration, Research and Training Center on Community Living.

Horner, R.H., Stoner, S.K., & Ferguson, D.L. (1988). *An activity-based analysis of deinstitutionalization: The effects of community re-entry on the lives of residents leaving Oregon's Fairview Training Center.* Eugene: University of Oregon, Specialized Training Program.

Howe, J., Horner, R.H., & Newton, J.S. (1998). Comparison of supported living and traditional residential services in the state of Oregon. *Mental Retardation, 36,* 1–11.

Janicki, M., Dalton, A., Henderson, C., & Davidson, P. (1999). Mortality and morbidity among older adults with intellectual disability: Health services considerations. *Disability and Rehabilitation, 21,* 284–294.

Jones, P.A., Conroy, J.W., Feinstein, C.S., & Lemanowicz, J.A. (1984). A matched comparison study of cost-effectiveness: Institutionalized and deinstitutionalized people. *Journal of The Association for the Severely Handicapped, 9,* 304–313.

Kim, S., Larson, S.A., & Lakin, K.C. (2001). Behavioural outcomes of deinstitutionalisation for people with intellectual disability: A review of U.S. studies conducted between 1980 and 1999. *Journal of Intellectual & Developmental Disability*,
   26, 35–50.
Knobbe, C.A., Carey, S.P., Rhodes, L., & Horner, R.H. (1995). Benefit–cost analysis of community residential versus institutional services for adults with severe
   mental retardation and challenging behaviors. *American Journal on Mental Retardation, 99*, 533–541.
Lakin, K.C., & Bruininks, R.H. (1981). *Occupational stability of direct care staff of residential facilities for mentally retarded people*. University of Minnesota, Research and
   Training Center on Community Living, Institute on Community Integration.
Lakin, K.C., Prouty, R., Polister, B., & Coucouvanis, K. (2003). Change in residential placements for persons with intellectual and developmental disabilities in
   the USA in the last two decades. *Journal of Intellectual & Developmental Disability*,
   28, 205–210.
Mangan, T., Blake, E.M., Prouty, R.W., & Lakin, K.C. (1993). *Residential services
   for persons with mental retardation and related conditions: Status and trends through
   1992*. Minneapolis: University of Minnesota, Research and Training Center on
   Residential Services and Community Living, Institute on Community
   Integration/UAP.
Mitchell, D., & Braddock, D. (1994). Compensation and turnover of direct care staff:
   A national survey. In M.F. Hayden & B.H. Abery (Eds.), *Challenges for a service sys-
   tem in transition: Ensuring quality community experiences for persons with developmen-
   tal disabilities* (pp. 289–312). Baltimore: Paul H. Brookes Publishing Co.
Moseley, C. (2001). Self-determination: From new initiative to business as usual.
   Common Sense, 8, 1–7.
Nerney, T. (1998). Self-determination for people with developmental disabilities.
   Doing more with less: Rethinking long-term care. *AAMR News & Notes, 11*(6),
   10–12.
Nerney, T., Conley, R., & Nisbet, J. (1990). *Cost analysis of residential systems serv-
   ing persons with severe disabilities: New directions in economic and policy research*.
   Cambridge, MA: Human Services Research Institute.
Olmstead v. L.C., 119 S. Ct. 2176 (1999).
O'Neil, J., Brown, M., Gordon, W., Schonhorn, R., & Green, E. (1981). Activity
   patterns of mentally retarded adults in institutions and communities—a longitu-
   dinal study. *Applied Research in Mental Retardation, 2*, 267–279.
Polister, B., Lakin, K.C., & Prouty, R. (2003). Wages of direct support profession-
   als serving persons with intellectual and developmental disabilities: A survey of
   state agencies and private residential provider trade associations. *Policy Research
   Brief, 14*(2). Minneapolis: University of Minnesota, Institute on Community
   Integration. Also available on-line at http://rtc.umn.edu
Prouty, R.W., Lakin, K.C., & Bruininks, R. (2003). Changing patterns in residen-
   tial service systems: 1977–2002. In R.W. Prouty, G. Smith, & K.C. Lakin (Eds.),
   *Residential services for persons with developmental disabilities: Status and trends through
   2002* (pp. 77–80). Minneapolis: University of Minnesota, Research and Training
   Center on Community Living, Institute on Community Integration. Also avail-
   able on-line at http://rtc.umn.edu

Prouty, R.W., Smith, G., & Lakin, K.C. (Eds.). (2003). *Residential services for persons with developmental disabilities: Status and trends through 2002.* Minneapolis: University of Minnesota, Research and Training Center on Community Living, Institute on Community Integration. Also available on-line at http://rtc.umn.edu

Rhoades, J.A., & Altman, B.M. (2001). Personal characteristics and contextual factors associated with residential expenditures for individuals with mental retardation. *Mental Retardation, 39,* 114–129.

Rizzolo, M.C., Hemp, R., Braddock, D., & Pomeranz-Essley, A. (2004). *The state of the states in developmental disabilities: 2004.* Washington, DC: American Association on Mental Retardation. Also available on-line at http://www.cu.edu/ColemanInstitute/stateofthestates/

Romer, L.T., Richardson, M.L., Nahom, D., Aigbe, E., & Porter, A. (2002). Providing family support through community guides. *Mental Retardation, 40,* 191–200.

Roseneau, N. (Ed.). (1990). *A child's birthright: To live in a family.* Syracuse, NY: Syracuse University, Center on Human Policy.

Schalock, M., & Fredericks, H.D.B. (1990). Comparative costs for institutional services and services for selected populations in the community. *Behavioral Residential Treatment, 5,* 271–286.

Smith, G., O'Keeffe, J., Carpenter, L., Doty, P., & Kennedy, G. (2000). *Understanding Medicaid home and community services: A primer.* Washington, DC: U.S. Department of Health and Human Services, Office of the Assistant Secretary for Planning and Evaluation.

Smith, J., Coucouvanis, K., Polister, B., Prouty, R.W., & Lakin, K.C. (2003). Services provided by state and nonstate agencies in 2002. In R.W. Prouty, G. Smith, & K.C. Lakin (Eds.), *Residential services for persons with developmental disabilities: Status and trends through 2002* (pp. 63–69). Minneapolis: University of Minnesota, Research and Training Center on Community Living, Institute on Community Integration. Also available on-line at http://rtc.umn.edu

Stancliffe, R.J., Abery, B.H., & Smith, J. (2000). Personal control and the ecology of community living settings: Beyond living-unit size and type. *American Journal on Mental Retardation, 105,* 431–454.

Stancliffe, R.J., Hayden, M.F., Larson, S., & Lakin, K.C. (2002). Longitudinal study on the adaptive and challenging behaviors of deinstitutionalized adults with intellectual disability. *American Journal on Mental Retardation, 107,* 302–320.

Stancliffe, R.J., & Keane, S. (2000). Outcomes and costs of community living: A matched comparison of group homes and semi-independent living. *Journal of Intellectual & Developmental Disability, 25,* 281–305.

Stancliffe, R.J., & Lakin, K.C. (1998). Analysis of expenditures and outcomes of residential alternatives for persons with developmental disabilities. *American Journal on Mental Retardation, 102,* 552–568.

Taylor, S.J., Lakin, K.C., & Hill, B.K. (1989). Permanency planning for children and youth: Out of home placement decisions. *Exceptional Children, 55,* 541–549.

Walsh, K.K., Kastner, T.A., & Green, R.G. (2003). Cost comparisons of community and institutional residential settings: Historical review of selected research. *Mental Retardation, 41,* 103–122.

CHAPTER 2

Public Spending for Developmental Disabilities in the United States

An Historical-Comparative Perspective

David Braddock, Mary C. Rizzolo, Richard Hemp,
and Susan L. Parish

The purpose of this chapter is to analyze trends in contemporary public spending for intellectual disabilities and developmental disabilities (ID/DD) programs in the United States within the historical context of public spending for disability programs generally. The chapter is organized into two sections. The first traces the historical foundations of governmental financing of disability programs in long-term care, general health care, income maintenance, and special education. The second section, "The State of the States in Developmental Disabilities," analyzes contemporary trends in public spending for ID/DD long-term care programs in the states.

HISTORY OF PUBLIC SPENDING FOR DISABILITIES

Public financial support for people with disabilities in the United States can be traced to early colonial America and to the adoption of derivatives of the English Poor Laws, which originally were enacted in 1601 under Queen Elizabeth I's rule. Under colonial poor laws, towns had responsibility for supporting their most impoverished citizens; however, localities often took steps to discourage vagabonds, beggars, or idle persons from settling in the town (Peterson, 1982). It was not an uncommon practice to "warn out" of town people, including those with disabilities, who were likely to become public charges. In colonial America, Puritans still held to the ancient belief that disabilities were a result of God's divine displeasure (Covey, 1998).

In 1637, the first petition was approved by King Charles I providing public payment for the guardianship of Benoni Buck, a resident of colonial Virginia with intellectual disabilities (Hecht & Hecht, 1973). The earliest evidence of public support for disabilities in the provincial colony of Pennsylvania dates to 1676. In that year, the Upland County Court in Delaware County, Pennsylvania, ordered "a small levy be laid to pay for the buildings of ye house and the maintaining of ye said madman according to the laws of ye government" (Morton, 1897, p. 4).

A century later, in 1776, the Continental Congress authorized a public pension for the first group of people with disabilities to receive compensation for their war service impairments (Obermann, 1968). Kentucky became the first U.S. state to authorize a statewide disability-related cash subsidy family support program for people with mental disabilities. The state passed legislation in 1793 that provided pension payments to families too impoverished to continue caring for their family members with mental disabilities at home. A trial system for determining the person's identity as an "idiot" or "lunatic," as well as his or her need for such support, was established. This pension system continued throughout the 19th century and was still in existence in 1928 (Estabrook, 1928).

Until the 1820s, another public-sector response to disabilities was the practice of "bidding out." This approach, commonly employed by counties and local governments, involved auctioning off the care of people with mental disabilities to the lowest bidder. Breckinridge (1939) noted that the practice was discontinued when it was perceived to be too expensive. In sum, provincial, state, and local control of spending was the characterizing feature of disability financial assistance programs in colonial America and in the early years of the United States.

Rise of State Hospitals and Special Schools

In 1752, with leadership from the physician Thomas Bond and from Benjamin Franklin, the first general hospital in the American colonies was established in Philadelphia. Care for people with mental disabilities was a major motive in the founding of this hospital. The principal argument expressed in the petition filed with the Pennsylvania Provincial Assembly, and subsequently embodied in the authorizing legislation of May 11, 1751, was to address the growing problem of mental disabilities in the colony (Morton, 1897). Initially, cells in the basement of the hospital's temporary quarters were set aside for people with mental disabilities. Four years later, a special wing in the hospital was utilized for this purpose, and in 1836, the cornerstone of a separate building was laid for the Pennsylvania Hospital for the Insane ("A sketch," 1845).

Virginia was the first colony to establish and finance an asylum exclusively for people with mental disabilities (Dain, 1971). The establishment of this facility, which opened in 1773 in Williamsburg, did not, however, influence other colonies to follow suit. Maryland opened the nation's second state-operated mental institution in 1798—a full 25 years after the Williamsburg institution—and Kentucky opened the third public facility in 1824 (Grob, 1973). The Quakers opened a private asylum in Frankford, Pennsylvania, in 1814 (Hamilton, 1944).

The first state-financed residential school for deaf people, the American Asylum for the Education of the Deaf and Dumb, opened in Hartford, Connecticut, in 1817 (Fay, 1893). The first residential schools for the blind were established in Boston and New York City in 1832 (Allen, 1914; Farrell, 1956). State government and private philanthropy had prominent roles in financing the construction and operation of the early asylums and residential schools. In a unique action, however, the federal government also assisted Connecticut and Kentucky, through land donations, to finance their first schools for the deaf (Breckinridge, 1939).

The social reformer Dorothea Dix's advocacy in the 1840s dramatically accelerated the development and public funding of state-operated asylums for people with mental disabilities (Brown, 1998; Gollaher, 1995). In her first memorial to the Massachusetts legislature, written after reviewing conditions in the Commonwealth, Dix described conditions there as follows:

> The present state of Insane Persons confined within this Commonwealth, in cages, closets, cellars, stalls, pens! Chained, naked, beaten with rods, and lashed into obedience! . . . Irritation of body, produced by utter filth and exposure, incited [one woman] to the horrid process of tearing off her skin by inches; her face, neck, and person, were thus disfigured to hideousness. (1843, p. 7)

Between 1840 and 1870, Dix's advocacy led directly to the construction or expansion of more than 30 mental asylums in the states and in Great Britain, as well (Brown, 1998). Coupled with the growth in the establishment of residential schools for deaf and blind people in the United States, disability programs emerged in the mid-19th century as one of the most important and costly state government responsibilities. When President Franklin Pierce vetoed a bill that was championed by Dorothea Dix and passed by both houses of Congress to set aside several million acres of federal lands to help finance the development of mental asylums in the states, he helped to ensure that disability programs would be almost exclusively the province of state and local governments for several subsequent generations (Grob, 1991).

Between 1824 and 1851, 19 state-operated asylums for people with mental disabilities were opened, as well as the first residential schools exclusively for people with intellectual disabilities. Between 1850 and 1890, 55 additional asylums for people with mental illness were opened in the United States, and by 1910, the residential census of these facilities doubled the 1890 level. Thus, at the close of the 19th century, nearly every U.S. state government was financing asylums and residential schools for people who were deaf, blind, mentally retarded, and mentally ill (Braddock & Parish, 2002). At the local level, during the first years of the 20th century several American cities, including New York, Providence, Boston, and Chicago, also began to publicly finance the provision of special education services for children and youth with disabilities (Weintraub, Abeson, & Braddock, 1971).

Evolution of the Federal Role

In 1864, President Abraham Lincoln signed into law legislation authorizing the creation of Gallaudet College, to specialize in the education of deaf people. The college, which has operated continuously for 140 years, continues to be supported with federal appropriations. The nation's oldest federal program authorizing rehabilitation services to nonveteran citizens with disabilities—the Civilian Vocational Rehabilitation Act of 1920 (PL 236)—was enacted shortly after World War I ended. Two years earlier, Congress had authorized rehabilitation services for discharged military personnel with physical disabilities (Soldier's Rehabilitation Act of 1918, PL 65-178). PL 236, part of the Smith-Fess Act (PL 66-236), initially established vocational rehabilitation as a federal reimbursement program requiring a dollar-for-dollar state match. PL 236 did not, however, provide eligibility for people with mental disabilities until the enactment of the Vocational Rehabilitation Act Amendments of 1943 (PL 79-113) (Braddock, 1986). In 1935, PL 236 was incorporated into Title V of the landmark Social Security Act of 1935 (PL 74-271). Title V also contained a provision authorizing $2.85 million in grants to the states for "crippled children's services."

PL 74-271 did not originally authorize public assistance on the basis of disability, except through a modest Aid to the Blind Program, authorized by Title X. Legislation amending PL 74-271 and authorizing public assistance to people with disabilities under "Aid to the Permanently and Totally Disabled" (APTD) was enacted in 1950. A few years later, the Social Security Act Amendments of 1956 (PL 84-880) authorized benefit payments to be paid from Social Security Trust funds for adults disabled in childhood. "Disabled Adult Child (DAC) benefits" were authorized under Title II to continue beyond age 18 if a surviving child of a retired, deceased, or disabled worker was classified as having a disability. *Disability* was defined in terms of an inability to engage in substantial gainful activity that originated prior to age 22. In 1972, the APTD legislation of 1950 was superceded and expanded through the Social Security Act Amendments of 1972 (PL 92-603) authorizing the Supplemental Security Income (SSI) Program.

The principal foundations of the federal role in disability-related research were authorized in 1946, 1950, and 1962 with the enactment of legislation creating the National Institute of Mental Health, the National Institute of Neurological Disorders and Blindness, and the National Institute of Child Health and Human Development, respectively. The federal role in mental health and intellectual disability services was dramatically expanded with the enactment of the Mental Retardation Facilities and Community Mental Health Centers Construction Act of 1963 (PL 88-164), which authorized grants to develop community facilities, university-affiliated programs (now University Centers for Excellence in Developmental Disabilities), and research centers to train personnel (Boggs, 1971, 1972; Braddock, 1987). Related legislation, the Maternal and Child Health and Mental Retardation Planning Amendments of 1963 (PL 88-156), doubled appropriations for the Maternal and Child Health program and authorized planning grants to the states for improving intellectual disability residential and community services. PL 88-156 was instrumental in stimulating many states to study how to reform their deteriorating public institutions and develop community-based alternatives.

In 1971, federal courts entered the intellectual disability field with landmark rulings confirming the right to education (*Pennsylvania Association for Retarded Citizens v. Commonwealth of Pennsylvania*) and the right to habilitation in the least restrictive environment (*Wyatt v. Stickney*) (Herr, 1992). Class action litigation strongly influenced subsequent growth in state and federal public spending for intellectual disability services (Braddock & Fujiura, 1987).

Several Great Society programs enacted during the 1960s, including Head Start, Medicaid, Medicare, and Titles I and III of the Elementary and Secondary Education Act of 1965 (ESEA; PL 89-10), provided programmatic vehicles for the subsequent expansion of federal, state, and local partnerships to finance a variety of health, educational, and social welfare services for people with disabilities, including people with intellectual disabilities. In 1975, the Education for All Handicapped Children Act (PL 94-142) amended PL 89-10 and dramatically expanded the federal role in financing special education in local schools. This legislation is known today as the Individuals with Disabilities Education Act Amendments of 1997 (PL 105-17). The fiscal year (FY) 2004 President's Budget requested $9.5 billion in federal funding for this program (U.S. Department of Education, 2003). If this funding request becomes law, federal funding for special education will comprise approximately 15% of the total costs of special education.

The 1970s also featured the continuing diffusion of special federal disability provisions attached to general-purpose federal legislation. Key legislative enactments included

- Medicaid Intermediate Care Facilities for the Mentally Retarded amendment to Title XIX of the Social Security Act (part of the Social Security Act Amendments of 1971, PL 92-223), which greatly expanded federal resources for residential intellectual disability institutions in the states

- Mandating 10% of all Head Start enrollment opportunities for children with disabilities (Economic Opportunity Act Amendments of 1972, PL 92-424)

- Small business loans for entrepreneurs with disabilities (Small Business Act Amendments of 1972, PL 92-595)

- Authorization of the Housing and Urban Development (HUD) loan and rental subsidy programs (Housing and Community Development Act of 1974, PL 93-383), accompanied by HUD amendments in 1977 (PL 95-128) and 1978 (PL 95-557)

- Authorization of food stamp eligibility for people with mental disabilities living in community residential programs (Food Stamp Act Amendments of 1979, PL 96-58)

The 1970s also saw the rise of independent living in the United States (DeJong, 1979a, 1979b; Stewart, Harris, & Sapey, 1999). This movement, primarily stimulated by advocacy efforts of people with physical and sensory disabilities, culminated in the promulgation of Section 504 antidiscrimination rules in the Rehabilitation Act of 1973 (PL 93-112). Initial catalysts for the independent living movement were drawn from a critical analysis of the processes of medicalization and professionalization in the rehabilitation system (Lysack & Kaufert, 1994; Zola, 1979). The independent living movement embraced the concept that the barriers that confront people with disabilities are less related to individual impairment than to prevailing negative and stereotypical social attitudes, interpretations of disability, architectural barriers, legal barriers, and lack of access to appropriate education (American Disabled for Attendant Programs Today, 1995; Bowe, 1978). The creation in the early 1970s of the nation's first Independent Living Center in Berkeley, California, served as a model for the development of such centers across the country (DeJong, 1979b; Roberts, 1989).

The culmination of the nation's civil rights protections for people with disabilities was the enactment of the Americans with Disabilities Act of 1990 (PL 101-336), which prohibited discrimination in employment, public services, public accommodations, and telecommunications (Blanck, 2000).

Disability Programs at the State and Local Level

Although there was very little federal government activity concerned with disabilities during the 19th century and the first six decades of the 20th century, hundreds of large residential institutions for people with mental disabilities were opened by state governments during this period. The census of state and county psychiatric hospitals for people with mental illness peaked in 1955 at 559,000 residents. Approximately 35,000 of these residents were individuals with intellectual disabilities (Smith, Polister, Prouty, Bruininks, & Lakin, 2002). The census of state-operated institutional facilities for people with intellectual disabilities peaked at 195,000 residents 12 years later, in 1967 (Braddock, 1981).

Many of these institutions were truly immense. Hamilton (1944) reported that, in 1941, 10 public psychiatric institutions housed over 5,000 residents (one had 9,177 residents); 22 had over 4,000 residents; 40 housed over 3,000 individuals; and 102 of the nation's 475 mental illness hospitals at that time housed more than 2,000 patients. Even though costs per resident in public psychiatric and intellectual disability facilities were artificially held down by chronic programmatic deficiencies, understaffing, and the practice of peonage, the sheer volume of residents in these facilities coupled with the need to maintain massive physical plants led states to expend a substantial proportion of their quite limited overall tax revenues on maintenance costs for people residing in these facilities.

The community services movement for people with mental illness began to gain strength in numerous states in the 1950s with the introduction of antipsychotic drugs and the development of community treatment and habilitation models. The parent movement for people with intellectual disabilities began to grow in many states in the 1950s, as well, and group homes and employment programs were implemented on a modest basis during that decade. In 1962, President John F. Kennedy's Panel on Mental Retardation issued its landmark report, offering 95 recommendations for a comprehensive program of "national action to combat mental retardation" (The President's Panel on Mental Retardation, 1962). Most of these recommendations—in research, prevention, community services, institutional reform, and special education—were implemented during the course of the next two decades. Class action litigation in federal courts in the 1970s rapidly accelerated the reform movement for intellectual disability services and presented states with a demanding budget challenge: how to pay for upgrading institutions to meet new legal and professional standards while developing and paying for an array of new and comprehensive services in the community. The states, with their limited tax base, had little choice but to turn to the federal government for financial assistance.

The legislative consequences of the move to improve institutional conditions included the 1971 enactment of the aforementioned Medicaid Intermediate Care Facility Services for Persons with Mental Retardation Program Amendment (ICF/MR; Amendments to Title XIX of the Social Secutity Act, PL 92-223), the Medicaid Home and Community-Based Services (HCBS) Waiver Program Amendment (Omnibus Budget Reconciliation Act of 1981, PL 97-35), and the Community Mental Health Services Block Grant (enacted 1981). These three programs were launched to provide financial assistance to the states and to build capacity among local community-service providers. In the 1970s, for the first time in the nation's history, the federal government emerged as a major partner with states and localities in financing the provision of residential and community services for people with mental disabilities. The long era of virtually exclusive state provision and financing of long-term care for people with mental disabilities had come to an end.

Modern Spending for Disabilities in the United States

Public spending for disability-related programs in the United States for people with intellectual disabilities, mental illness, and physical and sensory disabilities totaled $373.2 billion in FY 2001. An estimated 64% of these funds ($238.8 billion) was allocated by the federal government, 31% ($115.7 billion) was allocated by the states, and 5% of the funding ($18.7 billion) emanated from local units of government, primarily local school districts providing special education services.

The income-maintenance component of total disability spending accounted for $107.6 billion (29%) of all public funds committed in 2001. Income-maintenance programs included Social Security Disability Insurance (DI), authorized by Title II of the Social Security Act as Amended, SSI, the Adult Disabled Child (ADC) program, Veteran's Compensation, HUD payments/subsidies, and the Food Stamp program.

General health care represented $74.6 billion (20%; see Figure 2.1) of total spending and consisted of 1) Medicare, which supports hospital insurance and supplemental medical insurance, including home health care, hospital care, and time-limited skilled nursing facility care; 2) Medicaid, which provides general health-care services to people with disabilities; and 3) veteran's medical care.

Special education spending totaled $49.8 billion in 2001. An estimated 32% of the special education funding was derived from local school district sources, 55% from state governments, and 13% from the federal government. Most of the federal funds are authorized by the Individuals with Disabilities Education Act of 1990 (PL 101-476).

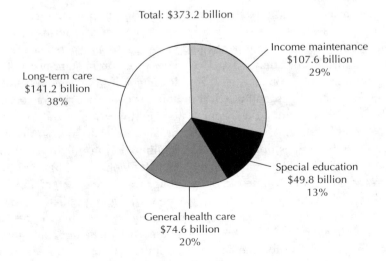

Total: $373.2 billion

Income maintenance
$107.6 billion
29%

Long-term care
$141.2 billion
38%

Special education
$49.8 billion
13%

General health care
$74.6 billion
20%

Figure 2.1. Public-sector spending for disability programs in the United States, 2001. (*Source:* Braddock, 2002a.)

Long-term care accounted for $141.2 billion (38%) of total spending and included three institutional program elements: nursing homes, institutions for people with ID/DD, and institutions for people with mental illness. An institution was defined in this analysis of spending to refer to a 24-hour facility providing residential services and related program support for 16 or more people in a public or private setting.

In terms of disabilities generally, the United States remains quite oriented toward institutional long-term care. In 2001, approximately one half of the $141.2 billion in total long-term care spending was associated with institutional-scale settings, even though the vast majority of people with disabilities reside in home and community-based settings (Braddock, 2002b).

This institutional bias is particularly evident for people with physical disabilities—approximately 70% of total expenditures for this group was allocated for institutional care in nursing facilities, whereas less than one third was allocated for home and community-based long-term care services. Surprisingly, based on 1997 data, no state allocated a majority of its long-term care funding base for community services and supports for people with physical disabilities. In contrast, approximately three fourths of total public funding for long-term care services for people with mental disabilities (intellectual disabilities and mental illness) is allocated for community services and supports, and every state with one exception (i.e., Mississippi) is allocating a majority of its public funding for community services (Braddock, 2002b).

Financial commitments for community long-term care services for people with disabilities varied greatly across the states in terms of funds budgeted for such programs per $1,000 of aggregate state personal income ("fiscal effort"). In a study using 1997 data, variation in state fiscal effort commitments for people with disabilities generally (i.e., mental illness, intellectual disabilities, and physical disabilities combined) was associated with two key predictors: the extent of state participation in the Medicaid Waiver and Personal Assistance programs, and early adoption in the state of civil rights statutes promoting nondiscrimination in public accommodation, public housing, and employment (Braddock, 2002b). However, when the data for the three disability groups was disaggregated and analyzed separately by disability category, the civil rights predictor variable was statistically significant only with long-term care spending for intellectual disability services. This finding suggests that financing community-based long-term care for people with disabilities in the United States has become more of an entitlement for people with intellectual disabilities than it has for people with physical disabilities or mental illness.

THE STATE OF THE STATES IN DEVELOPMENTAL DISABILITIES

In this section, we summarize recent trends in the financing of intellectual and developmental disabilities services in the United States (Rizzolo, Hemp, Braddock, & Pomeranz-Essley, 2004). The State of the States in Developmental Disabilities Project, now located at the University of Colorado, has been studying the financial and programmatic structure of long-term care services for people with intellectual disabilities in the states since 1982. The project has published over 170 journal articles, books, monographs, and reports. These resources are cited on the project's web site at http://www.cu.edu/ColemanInstitute/stateofthestates/.

Total public spending for ID/DD long-term care services in the United States was $34.6 billion in 2002, representing approximately 9% of total estimated disability spending of $393.0 billion. Inflation-adjusted spending for community services grew by an average increment of 10% per year during 1977–2002 (see Figure 2.2). Community services were defined in this study as residential settings for 15 or fewer people and day programs. Individual and family supports, a subcomponent of community services, includes family support, supported living, personal assistance, and supported employment.

Spending for community services first surpassed institutional spending in 1989 (see Figure 2.2); however, if community services are defined as residential settings for six or fewer people, community spending did not surpass institutional spending until 1994 (Rizzolo et al., 2004). In contrast with the vigorous growth of community spending, inflation-adjusted spending for public and private 16+ person institutions posted average annual growth rates of less than 1% during the 25-year period.

Spending for public and private institutions constituted 22% of total ID/DD system-wide spending in 2002, although these settings served only 17% of service recipients. Of the $7.7 billion total in institutional spending, 78%, or $6.0 billion, was allocated for the 44,252 residents of publicly operated state institutions. The remaining $1.7 billion (22%) was spent for the 32,333 people residing in private 16+ institutional facilities.

Spending for community services in 2002 totaled $27.0 billion—78% of total ID/DD spending for residential and community services nationally. In 2002, all states except Mississippi were spending more for community services than for institutional services. Nationwide, 298,170 people were served in settings for 1–6 people in 2002, and 55,187 individuals lived in settings for 7–15 people. Sixteen percent of total spending for commu-

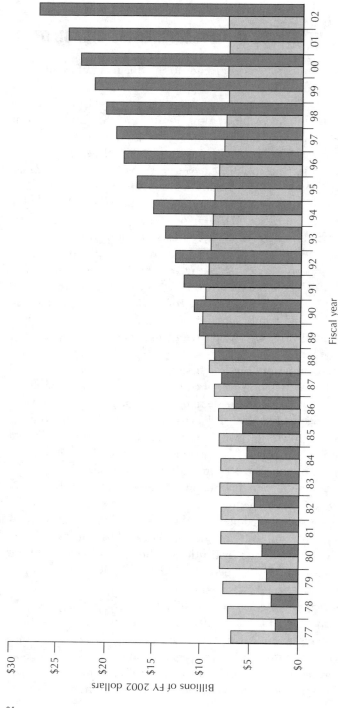

Figure 2.2. United States: Trends in intellectual disabilities/developmental disabilities spending, FY 1977 through FY 2002.
(*Key* = ■ Public/private institutions [16+]; ■ Community services[1].)

[1]*Community services* includes residential settings for 15 or fewer people, day programs, and individual and family support services (family support, supported living, and supported employment).

(*Source:* Rizzolo, Hemp, Braddock, and Pomeranz-Essley, 2004.)

nity services ($4.4 billion) was allocated for Individual and Family Support (IFS), including $2.3 billion for supported living/personal assistance, $1.4 billion for family support, and $663 million for supported employment (Rizzolo et al., 2004). IFS spending ranged from less than 1% of total ID/DD spending in the District of Columbia, to 40% or more in Alaska, New Mexico, Oklahoma, and Washington state.

Sources of Revenue

Medicaid is the primary source of revenue for financing ID/DD services in the United States. Combined federal and state Medicaid spending in 2002 constituted 77% of all ID/DD spending of $34.6 billion (99% of spending for institutions). States rely on the Medicaid program's size and stability, especially when implementing service-system reform efforts such as institutional downsizing and closure. The ICF/MR program has historically exhibited an "institutional bias" in favor of financing large, institutional settings (Braddock, 1987); however, in 2001, for the first time in the program's 20-year history, federal and state funding for the Medicaid HCBS Waiver for people with developmental disabilities surpassed funding for Medicaid ICFs/MR (Lakin, Prouty, Smith, Polister, & Smith, 2002).

Federal funds have played an increasing role in the financing of community ID/DD services across the nation, as shown in Figure 2.3. In 1977, federal funds represented 23% of total allocations for community services. By 2002, that proportion had increased to 50% of total community services spending. State government general revenues, including optional state augmentation of federal SSI payments, comprised 46% of total community services revenues in 2002, while local funds comprised the remaining 4% (see Figure 2.4).

The HCBS Waiver

Figure 2.4 illustrates the instrumental role the HCBS Waiver program plays in the provision of community ID/DD services in the United States. First authorized by Congress in 1981, HCBS Waiver spending grew from $1.2 million in federal reimbursements in 1982 to $7.2 billion in 2002. Waiver services, including case management; assistive technology; homemaker assistance; home health aides; personal care; residential habilitation; day habilitation; respite care; transportation; supported employment; adapted equipment; home modification; and occupational, speech, physical, and behavioral therapy, were provided to 367,456 participants in FY 2002.

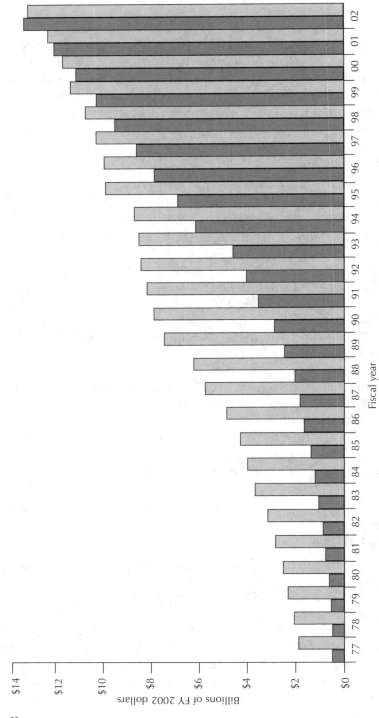

Figure 2.3. United States: Trends in spending for community intellectual disabilities/developmental disabilities services by level of government, FY 1977 through FY 2002. (*Key* = ■ Federal government; ☐ State/local government.)

(*Source*: Rizzolo, Hemp, Braddock, and Pomeranz-Essley, 2004.)

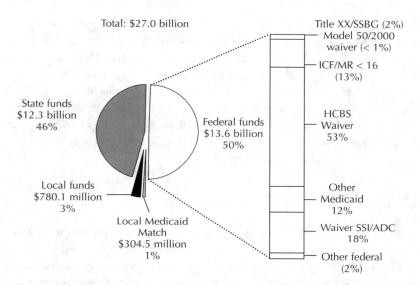

Figure 2.4. United States intellectual disabilities/developmental disabilities community services revenue sources, FY 2002. (*Source:* Rizzolo, Hemp, Braddock, and Pomeranz-Essley, 2004.)

The HCBS Waiver was established in every state by 2000, although Washington, D.C., did not utilize federal HCBS Waiver dollars until 2001. The role played by the HCBS Waiver seems likely to grow even larger in the years ahead due to the increasing flexibility of the federal government's Centers for Medicare & Medicaid Services (CMS) in permitting innovation in the states and due to states' efforts to utilize currently unmatched state and local funds to draw down additional federal HCBS Waiver revenue (Hemp, Braddock, Parish, & Smith, 2001).

In addition, the Supreme Court's landmark ruling in the *Olmstead* case (*Olmstead v. L.C.*, 1999) is likely to stimulate increased utilization of the HCBS Waiver to finance community long-term care supports. Judge Ruth Bader Ginsburg, writing for the 6 to 3 Court majority, described the essence of the Supreme Court's ruling: "We confront the question of whether the proscription of discrimination may require placement of people with mental disabilities in community settings rather than in institutions. The answer, we hold, is a qualified yes" (*Olmstead v. L.C.*, 1999).

State Spending Patterns

There were wide variations in fiscal effort for ID/DD services among the states in 2002. Fiscal effort, as previously noted, is a ratio that can be uti-

lized to rank states according to the proportion of their total statewide
personal income devoted to the financing of developmental disabilities
services (Braddock & Fujiura, 1987). Under the federal Medicaid statute,
states are required to allocate funding for matching purposes in order to
receive federal HCBS Waiver reimbursement. Much of the variation
across the states in community services fiscal effort for intellectual disability programs is associated with state utilization of the HCBS Waiver.
Figure 2.5 presents state-by-state fiscal effort data for community, institutional, and total ID/DD spending in 2002.

CONCLUSION

In this chapter, we review the evolution of disability programs in the United
States since the early 17th century and note the particularly rapid growth of
public spending for long-term care services in developmental disabilities
since the 1970s. On a national basis, in the near-term future, we expect a
significant slowing in the rate of growth of ID/DD spending due to the
severe budget reductions being implemented in most states during FY 2002
through FY 2004 (Ku, Nathanson, Park, Cox, & Broaddus, 2003).

In the first quarter of 2001, many states began to confront significant
economic challenges. By fiscal year 2004, state budget deficits were projected to reach $70 billion to $85 billion.

> These new deficits are on top of the $50 billion in deficits that states closed
> when they enacted their fiscal year 2003 budgets. The new deficits for fiscal
> year 2004 are also on top of at least $17.5 billion in additional deficits that
> have opened up in 2003 budgets since those budgets were enacted. (Lav &
> Johnson, 2003, p. 1)

States are required to balance their budgets each year. In order to
meet these mandates, states are currently under intense pressure to reduce
their budgets (Ku et al., 2003). Many states addressed their FY 2003 deficits by tapping into their rainy-day funds or tobacco-litigation settle-
ments. These options were one-time opportunities, however, and many
states will need to initiate programmatic cutbacks or raise taxes to close
future funding gaps.

Though the immediate outlook on state budgets is grim, powerful
forces are at work in the United States to increase pressure on the national
and state governments to continue to increase public financial commitments for ID/DD services and for disability programs generally. For
example, the rapid aging of U.S. society will increase the demand for

Figure 2.5. Fiscal effort for intellectual disabilities/developmental disabilities spending, 2002. (*Source:* Rizzolo, Hemp, Braddock, and Pomeranz-Essley, 2004.)
Note: Fiscal effort is defined as community, institutional, and total mental retardation/developmental disabilities spending, respectively, per $1,000 of total statewide aggregate personal income.

State	Community spending	Institutional spending	Total spending	State	Community spending	Institutional spending	Total spending
Alabama	$1.57	$0.61	$2.18	Montana	$3.39	$0.77	$4.17
Alaska	$4.22	$0.00	$4.22	Nebraska	$2.83	$1.07	$3.90
Arizona	$3.01	$0.18	$3.19	Nevada	$0.94	$0.32	$1.26
Arkansas	$3.05	$1.78	$4.83	New Hampshire	$3.47	$0.05	$3.52
California	$2.68	$0.62	$3.30	New Jersey	$2.18	$1.32	$3.49
Colorado	$2.30	$0.11	$2.41	New Mexico	$4.80	$0.04	$4.84
Connecticut	$4.67	$1.57	$6.24	New York	$6.05	$0.97	$7.02
Delaware	$3.01	$1.15	$4.16	North Carolina	$3.13	$1.23	$4.35
D.C.	$4.43	$0.08	$4.51	North Dakota	$5.58	$1.35	$6.93
Florida	$1.57	$0.55	$2.12	Ohio	$3.91	$1.32	$5.23
Georgia	$1.69	$0.55	$2.24	Oklahoma	$3.75	$1.23	$4.98
Hawaii	$1.84	$0.03	$1.87	Oregon	$4.14	$0.40	$4.54
Idaho	$3.99	$0.70	$4.69	Pennsylvania	$4.04	$1.09	$5.13
Illinois	$1.93	$1.34	$3.27	Rhode Island	$6.99	$0.11	$7.10
Indiana	$2.70	$0.86	$3.56	South Carolina	$3.15	$1.16	$4.31
Iowa	$3.83	$2.49	$6.32	South Dakota	$3.90	$0.91	$4.81
Kansas	$3.65	$0.70	$4.35	Tennesee	$2.55	$1.15	$3.71
Kentucky	$1.42	$1.01	$2.43	Texas	$1.75	$0.86	$2.61
Louisiana	$3.29	$2.08	$5.37	Utah	$2.43	$0.97	$3.40
Maine	$7.26	$0.12	$7.39	Vermont	$5.31	$0.00	$5.31
Maryland	$2.04	$0.35	$2.39	Virginia	$1.58	$0.80	$2.38
Massachusetts	$3.92	$0.92	$4.84	Washington	$2.60	$0.83	$3.43
Michigan	$3.21	$0.10	$3.31	West Virginia	$4.82	$0.13	$4.95
Minnesota	$6.84	$0.36	$7.19	Wisconsin	$3.42	$1.43	$4.84
Mississippi	$1.62	$2.47	$4.09	Wyoming	$4.52	$1.01	$5.53
Missouri	$2.24	$1.21	$3.45	**United States**	**$3.07**	**$0.87**	**$3.94**

developmental disabilities services because the majority of people with these conditions reside with family caregivers and the number of people older than 65 will double by 2035 (U.S. Census Bureau, 2002). As these caregivers age beyond their caregiving capacities, supervised living arrangements will need to be established to support their relatives with disabilities (Braddock, 1999).

There are also growing pressures internationally promoting the rapidly increasing development of services for people with disabilities in general. In the United States, 36% of people 65 years of age and older have one or more functional limitations, as opposed to 8% of the population younger than age 65 (Fujiura, 2002). By 2050, the number of people 60 years or older in the world is projected to exceed the number of people 59 years or younger for the first time in history.

The oldest old, or those 80 years or older, are expected to be the fastest growing age group (United Nations, 2002). Many countries will be affected by this demographic trend, particularly Japan, Germany, and Italy. For example, the United Nations estimates that, by 2050, the percentage of Japan's citizens older than 60 will increase from 23% to 42%. At least 10% of their population will be older than 80 (United Nations, 1999). By 2050, the global "support ratio" (the number of people age 15–64 in proportion to people age 65 or older) is projected to decline by an estimated 56%. This trend will have significant international implications for the solvency of traditional social security, retirement, and health care programs, and consequently for financial support for people with disabilities (United Nations, 2002).

Another key factor promoting a growing demand for developmental disabilities long-term care services is an increasing life span. The mean age at death for people with intellectual disabilities in the United States was 66 years in 1993—an increase from 59 years in the 1970s. The mean age at death for the general population in 1993 was 70 years. Janicki (1996) noted that with continued improvement in their health status, individuals with intellectual disabilities—particularly those without the most severe impairments—are expected to have a life span equal to that of the general population. The increased life expectancy of people with developmental disabilities accounts for an estimated 10%–20% of the growth in demand for residential services since 1970.

Class-action litigation has also emerged once again in the United States as a force shaping the funding and development of service-delivery systems for people with developmental disabilities. In the 1990s, three types of class-action litigation emerged: lawsuits filed to force states to expand services to people on waiting lists; lawsuits filed to force states to meet the requirements of the community integration mandate in the

Olmstead Supreme Court decision; and lawsuits filed on behalf of individuals eligible for Medicaid services, but who did not receive them. As of April 2004, 26 waiting list lawsuits, 10 *Olmstead* lawsuits, and 19 Medicaid-access lawsuits had been filed (Smith, 2004).

Thus, as a consequence of demographic dynamics and civil rights initiatives, states will be pressed to expand long-term care services for people with developmental disabilities and, simultaneously, in a cutback budgetary environment, to develop cost-effective means of providing such support. In addition, as suggested by the cross-disability analysis presented earlier in this chapter, budgetary demands on the states to expand home and community-based long-term care services for people with physical disabilities and with severe, persistent mental illness are also likely to intensify in the future. Confronting this increasingly competitive context of budgetary stringency, coupled with a rapidly growing demand for long-term care across the entire spectrum of disability, will be a formidable challenge for advocates and policy makers in the first decade of the 21st century and beyond.

REFERENCES

Allen, E.E. (1914). *Progress of the education of the blind in the United States in the year 1912–1913: Chapter XXII. Vol. I. 1913.* Washington, DC: Government Printing Office.

American Disabled for Attendant Programs Today. (ADAPT). (1995). *Long term care policy. It's good to have the facts when you choose (statistics, sources, a call to action).* Rochester, NY: Free Hand Press.

Americans with Disabilities Act (ADA) of 1990, PL 101-336, 42 U.S.C. §§ 12101 *et seq.*

Blanck, P.D. (2000). Studying disability, employment policy, and the ADA. In L.P. Francis & A. Silvers (Eds.), *Americans with disabilities* (pp. 209–220). New York: Routledge Press.

Boggs, E.M. (1971). Federal legislation. In J. Wortis (Ed.), *Mental retardation: An annual review* (Vol. 3, pp. 103–127). New York: Grune & Stratton.

Boggs, E.M. (1972). Federal legislation (Conclusion). In J. Wortis (Ed.), *Mental retardation: An annual review* (Vol. 4, pp. 165–206). New York: Grune & Stratton.

Bowe, F.G. (1978). *Handicapping America: Barriers to disabled people.* New York: Harper & Row.

Braddock, D. (1981). Deinstitutionalization of the retarded: Trends in public policy. *Hospital and Community Psychiatry, 32,* 607–615.

Braddock, D. (1986). Federal assistance for mental retardation and developmental disabilities: II. The modern era. *Mental Retardation, 24*(4), 175–182.

Braddock, D. (1987). *Federal policy toward mental retardation and developmental disabilities.* Baltimore: Paul H. Brookes Publishing Co.

Braddock, D. (1999). Aging and developmental disabilities: Demographic and policy issues affecting American families. *Mental Retardation, 37*(2), 155–161.

Braddock, D. (Ed.). (2002a). *Disability at the dawn of the 21st Century and the state of the states*. Washington, DC: American Association on Mental Retardation.

Braddock, D. (2002b). Public financial support for disability at the dawn of the 21st century. *American Journal on Mental Retardation, 107*(6), 478–489.

Braddock, D., & Fujiura, G. (1987). State government financial effort in mental retardation. *American Journal of Mental Deficiency, 91*(5), 450–459.

Braddock, D., & Parish, S. (2002). An institutional history of disability. In D. Braddock (Ed.), *Disability at the dawn of the 21st century and the state of the states* (pp. 3–61). Washington, DC: American Association on Mental Retardation.

Breckinridge, S.P. (1939). *The Illinois Poor Law and its administration*. Chicago: University of Chicago Press.

Brown, T.J. (1998). *Dorothea Dix: New England reformer.* Cambridge, MA: Harvard University Press.

Civilian Vocational Rehabilitation Act of 1920, PL 236.

Covey, H.C. (1998). *Social perceptions of people with disabilities in history.* Springfield, IL: Charles C Thomas.

Dain, N. (1971). *Disordered minds: The first century of Eastern State Hospital in Williamsburg, Virginia, 1766–1866.* Williamsburg, VA: The Colonial Press.

DeJong, G. (1979a). Independent living: From social movement to analytic paradigm. *Archives of Physical Medicine and Rehabilitation, 60,* 435–446.

DeJong, G. (1979b). *The movement for independent living: Origins, ideology, and implications for disability research.* East Lansing: Michigan State University, University Center for International Rehabilitation.

Dix, D. (1843). *Memorial: To the legislature of Massachusetts.* Boston: Munroe & Francis.

Economic Opportunity Act Amendments of 1972, PL 92-424, 42 U.S.C. §§ 2701 *et seq.*

Education for All Handicapped Children Act of 1975, PL 94-142, 20 U.S.C. §§ 1400 *et seq.*

Elementary and Secondary Education Act of 1965, PL 89-10, 20 U.S.C. §§ 241 *et seq.*

Estabrook, A.H. (1928). The pauper idiot pension in Kentucky. *Journal of Psycho-Asthenics, 33,* 59–61.

Farrell, G. (1956). *The story of blindness.* Cambridge, MA: Harvard University Press.

Fay, E.A. (1893). *Histories of American schools for the deaf, 1817–1893.* Washington, DC: Volta Bureau.

Food Stamp Act Amendments of 1979, PL 96-58, 7, U.S.C. 2012. C.F.D.A.: 10.551.

Fujiura, G.T. (2002, September). *Emerging policy issues for public health and disability.* Plenary presentation at the CDC Center on Birth Defects and Developmental Disabilities National Conference, Atlanta.

Gollaher, D. (1995). *Voice for the mad: The life of Dorothea Dix.* New York: Free Press.

Grob, G.N. (1973). *Mental institutions in America: Social policy to 1875.* New York: Free Press.

Grob, G.N. (1991). *From asylum to community: Mental health policy in modern America.* Princeton, NJ: Princeton University Press.

Hamilton, S.W. (1944). *One hundred years of American psychiatry.* New York: Columbia University Press.

Hecht, I.W.D., & Hecht, F. (1973). Mara and Benomi Buck: Familial mental retardation in colonial Jamestown. *Journal of the History of Medicine & Allied Sciences, 28,* 171–176.

Hemp, R., Braddock, D., Parish, S.L, & Smith, G. (2001). Trends and milestones: Leveraging federal funding in the states to address Olmstead and growing waiting lists. *Mental Retardation, 39*(3), 241–243.

Herr, S.S. (1992). Beyond benevolence: Legal protection for persons with special needs. In L. Rowitz (Ed.), *Mental retardation in the year 2000* (pp. 279–298). New York: Springer-Verlag.

Housing and Community Development Act of 1974, PL 93-383, 42, U.S.C.5301. C.F.D.A.: 14.218.

Housing and Community Development Act Amendments of 1977, PL 95-128, 42, U.S.C.5301. C.F.D.A.: 14.218.

Housing and Community Development Act Amendments of 1978, PL 95-557, 42, U.S.C.5301. C.F.D.A.: 14.218.

Individuals with Disabilities Education Act Amendments of 1997, PL 105-17, 20 U.S.C. §§ 1400 *et seq.*

Individuals with Disabilities Education Act (IDEA) of 1990, PL 101-476, 20 U.S.C. §§ 1400 *et seq.*

Janicki, M.P. (1996, Fall). Longevity increasing among older adults with an intellectual disability. *Aging, Health, and Society, 2,* 2.

Ku, L., Nathanson, M., Park, E., Cox, L., & Broaddus, M. (2003, January 6). *Proposed state Medicaid cuts would jeopardize health insurance coverage for one million people.* Center on Budget and Policy Priorities. Available on-line at http://www.cbpp.org/12-23-02health.htm

Lakin, K.C., Prouty, R., Smith, J., Polister, B., & Smith, G. (2002). Fiscal year 2001 Medicaid Home and Community-Based Services expenditures exceed those of ICFs/MR. *Mental Retardation, 40*(4), 336–339.

Lav, I.J., & Johnson, N. (2003, January 23). *State budget deficits for fiscal year 2004 are huge and growing.* Center on Budget and Policy Priorities. Available on-line at http://www.cbpp.org/12-23-02sfp.htm

Lysack, C., & Kaufert, J. (1994). Comparing the origins and ideologies of the independent living movement and community-based rehabilitation. *International Journal of Rehabilitation Research, 17,* 231–240.

Maternal and Child Health and Mental Retardation Planning Amendments of 1963, PL 88-156, 77 Stat. L. 273.

Mental Retardation Facilities and Community Mental Health Centers Construction Act of 1963, PL 88-164, 44 U.S.C. §§ 2670 *et seq.*

Morton, T.G. (1897). *The history of Pennsylvania Hospital 1751–1895.* Philadelphia: Times Printing House.

Obermann, C.E. (1968). *A history of vocational rehabilitation in America* (5th ed.). Minneapolis, MN: T.S. Dennison.

Olmstead v. L.C., 119 S. Ct. 2176 (1999).

Omnibus Budget Reconciliation Act of 1981, PL 97-35, 95 Stat. 357.

Pennsylvania Association for Retarded Children v. Commonwealth of Pennsylvania, 334 F. Supp. 1257 (E.D. Pa. 1971).

Peterson, D. (1982). *A mad people's history of madness.* Pittsburgh: University of Pittsburgh Press.

President's Panel on Mental Retardation, The (1962). *Report to the President. A proposed program for national action to combat mental retardation.* Washington, DC: Author.

Rehabilitation Act of 1973, PL 93-112, 29 U.S.C. §§ 701 *et seq.*

Rizzolo, M.C., Hemp, R., Braddock, D., & Pomeranz-Essley, A. (2004). *The state of the states in developmental disabilities: 2004.* Boulder: University of Colorado.

Roberts, E.V. (1989). A history of the Independent Living Movement: A founder's perspective. In B.W. Heller, L.M. Flohr, & L.S. Zegans (Eds.), *Psychosocial interventions with physically disabled persons* (pp. 231–244). New Brunswick, NJ: Rutgers University Press.

"Sketch of the history, buildings, and organization of the Pennsylvania Hospital for the Insane, A" extracted principally from the reports of Thomas S. Kirkbride, M.D., Physician to the institution. (1845). *American Journal of Insanity, 2,* 97–114.

Small Business Act Amendments of 1972, PL 92-595, 15 U.S.C. 636. C.F.D.A.: 59.021.

Smith, G. (2004, April). *Status report: Litigation concerning home and community services for people with disabilities.* Tualatin, OR: Human Services Research Institute.

Smith, J., Polister, B., Prouty, R.W., Bruininks, R.H., & Lakin, K.C. (2002). Current populations and longitudinal trends of state residential settings (1950–2001). In R.W. Prouty, G. Smith, & K.C. Lakin (Eds.), *Residential services for persons with developmental disabilities: Status and trends through 2001* (pp. 3–28). Minneapolis: University of Minnesota, Research and Training Center on Community Living, Institute on Community Integration.

Smith-Fess Act of 1920, PL 66-236, 29 U.S.C. §§ 31 *et seq.*

Social Security Act of 1935, PL 74-271, 42 U.S.C. §§ 301 *et seq.*

Social Security Act Amendments of 1956, PL 84-880, 42 U.S.C. §§ 101 *et seq.*

Social Security Act Amendments of 1972, PL 92-603, 42 U.S.C. §§ 301 *et seq.*

Soldier's Rehabilitation Act of 1918, PL 65-178.

Stewart, J., Harris, J., & Sapey, B. (1999). Disability and dependency: Origins and futures of "special needs" housing for disabled people. *Disability & Society, 14,* 5–20.

United Nations. (1999). *Population ageing, 1999.* Sales No. E.99.XIII.11.

United Nations. (2002). *World population ageing: 1950–2050.* United Nations Population Division, Department of Economic and Social Affairs. Available on-line at http://www.un.org/esa/population/publications/worldageing19502050/index.htm.

U. S. Census Bureau. (2002). *International database. Table 094. Midyear population, by age and sex.* Available on-line at http://www.census.gov/population/www/projections/natdet-D1A.html

U. S. Department of Education. (2003). *Fiscal Year 2004 budget summary.* Available on-line at http://www.ed.gov/offices/OUS/Budget04/04summary/section1.html

Vocational Rehabilitation Act Amendments of 1943, PL 79-113, 29 U.S.C. §§ 3141 *et seq.*

Weintraub, F., Abeson, A., & Braddock, D. (1971). *State law and the education of handicapped children: Issues and recommendations.* Arlington, VA: Council for Exceptional Children.

Wyatt v. Stickney, 325 F. Supp. 781 (M.D. Ala.1971), 334 F. Supp. 1341 (M.D. Ala. 1971), 344 F. Supp. 373 (M.D. Ala. 1972), sub nom Wyatt v. Aderholt, 503 F. 2d 1305 (5th Cir. 1974).

Zola, I.K. (1979). Helping one another: Speculative history of the self-help movement. *Archives of Physical Medicine, 60*(10), 452–456.

CHAPTER 3

Community Living

Costs, Outcomes, and Economies of Scale: Findings from U.K. Research

David Felce and Eric Emerson

Large-scale institutional care for people with intellectual disabilities in England and Wales reached its greatest extent at the end of the 1960s with about 65,000 people with intellectual disabilities living in specialized intellectual disability or psychiatric institutions. Community services had co-existed on a small scale with these institutions for a number of years but it was not until this time that the first systematic attempts were made to provide community-based alternatives for those receiving institutional care. Service development, often accompanied by research, continued throughout the following decade, until the 1980s when the governments of both England and Wales adopted deinstitutionalization policies. As a result of these policies, the combined institutional population of the two countries fell to about 1,500 by 2003, with a complementary development of supported accommodations in the community as well as other forms of care, such as new campus-based facilities.

The replacement of institutional services with community-based services in the United Kingdom has been defined as much by a reduction in the size of living unit and an increase in resource inputs[1] as by the physical move to the community itself. Dehumanizing scale and insufficient resources were two strands of the common explanation of why quality of care and quality of life were so poor in the traditional institution (Martin, 1984). As a result, the achievement of small living unit size has been seen

---

[1]In resource inputs, we include all material (e.g., buildings, possessions, food) and human resources (e.g., staffing levels, staff skills) involved in providing a service.

as integral to the achievement of high-quality care and a decent quality of life. Moreover, perceptions have changed over time, and what was at first regarded as small soon appeared too large. Hence, more recent provision either tends to be smaller or is advocated to be so. When looking for reasons why the reality of deinstitutionalization may not have fully lived up to initial expectations, the idea that residential groupings need to be smaller continues to be pressed. Small size of residence is widely held to be a prerequisite for high-quality outcome (e.g., Office of the Deputy Prime Minister and Department of Health, 2003).

The fact that genuinely small community residential services were not immediately adopted as the preferred model for institutional replacement was in part attributable to another widespread belief that economies of scale were bound to be present in the operation of residential services. Service planners showed a reluctance to commit themselves to what they predicted would be the additional resource consequences of adopting small-scale community living. As deinstitutionalization was in any case characterized by a major change in the scale of provision, it was predicted, at least in the United Kingdom, that a system of community care would prove more expensive. There was, however, some tolerance of escalating costs, as institutional care was generally regarded as under-resourced, and such under-resourcing was widely viewed as another contributing factor to poor outcome (Martin, 1984).

In particular, low budget allocations and difficulties in recruiting staff meant that staff-to-resident ratios were generally seen as inadequate. The idea that better outcomes would be associated with greater resource input was commonly assumed. Thus, there was an acceptance that reform of institutional care in the United Kingdom should be accompanied by increasing costs per resident as this additional investment was necessary to avoid replicating in the community the often scandalous conditions found in U.K. institutions.

Three common assumptions are intertwined in this introductory account:

1. Smaller scale provision will produce better outcomes.

2. Smaller scale provision will be more expensive than larger scale provision due to the operation of economies of scale.

3. Greater resource input (i.e., more expensive provision per person usually involving more favorable staff-to-resident ratios) will produce better outcomes.

Residential services are complex organizations, and isolating the impact of single provision characteristics on the quality of the service is often difficult. For example, deinstitutionalization has generally been evaluated as leading to better outcomes (e.g., Emerson & Hatton, 1994, 1996; Felce, 2000; Kim, Larson, & Lakin, 2001; Young, Sigafoos, Suttie, Ashman, & Grevell, 1998). Although the community services being compared with institutional services in this literature would certainly have been smaller and likely to have had higher staff-to-resident ratios, such associations do not necessarily provide evidence relevant to these three propositions. Reduction in size or greater resource input are not necessarily drivers of the improved outcome associated with community services. Whether or at what point economies of scale begin to operate is also not clear.

This chapter is an attempt to distil evidence from the U.K. research literature on the relationships between size, resource input (i.e., cost[2]), staff-to-resident ratios, and outcome. Our starting point is the deinstitutionalization literature; however, we do not intend to review the impact of deinstitutionalization on reduced size of living unit or on outcome. The former will be readily accepted, and the latter has been done adequately by the reviews cited previously. Rather, the first section of this chapter simply addresses whether deinstitutionalization was associated with increased cost per resident. The second section of the chapter summarizes research that has compared community housing costs to those of other service models. The third section explores research on costs both within community services and between community services and other service models for any evidence of economies of scale. In the fourth section, we explore research on outcomes within community services for any evidence of the impact of size of resident grouping or resource input per person. The concluding section summarizes the evidence in relation to the following three questions:

- Does size of living unit affect outcome?

- Does size of living unit affect cost per person?

- Does cost per person and/or staff-to-resident ratio affect outcome?

---

[2]We have decided not to quote actual costs in this chapter because 1) studies vary in the aspects of care (e.g., accommodation, day services, professional treatment) costed, 2) price inflation over time means that costs are specific to a date, and 3) changing exchange rates means that costs are specific to a given country at a particular time. Rather, we have concentrated on general findings concerned with the relationships between service model, relative costs, and quality of outcome.

COSTS OF DEINSTITUTIONALIZATION

A number of studies have compared the costs of community-based and institutional services in the United Kingdom. Early studies showed that the costs of 25-person residential facilities and 6- to 8-person group homes tended to be more expensive than equivalent large institutions, albeit only slightly, when resident characteristics and occupancy levels were taken into account (Davies, 1987, 1988; Felce, 1986; Felce, Mansell, & Kushlick, 1980). Later and more extensive studies also reported an increase in cost associated with relocation to the community. On the basis of studying the costs of one large institution and those of a number of smaller community settings, Wright and Haycox (1985) estimated that the consequences of transferring residents to community care would result in a 22% increase in expenditure. Glennerster and Korman (1990) reported that the costs to public funds of small homes developed in the wake of the closure of a large institution were about twice as much as a poorly staffed institution when it was working at full capacity. Knapp, Cambridge, Thomason, Beecham, Allen, and Darton (1992) showed that costs in a number of community care demonstration projects were on average 17% greater than equivalent institution costs, and Felce et al. (1998) found community housing services for people with the most severe challenging behavior in Wales to be about twice as expensive as institutional provision.

Markedly different results have been found in the United States, where service costs in the community have been found to be about 66% to 95% of those in institutions (Campbell & Heal, 1995; Knobbe, Carey, Rhodes, & Horner, 1995; Schalock & Fredericks, 1990; Stancliffe & Lakin, 1998). In particular, Stancliffe and Lakin (1998) reported that community services for people with severe or profound intellectual disabilities in one U.S. state were less costly than institutional services, even though they had more favorable staffing. One can only speculate on why studies from the United States and the United Kingdom differ. Reasons could include the possibility that institutional services in the United States became more costly than they did in the United Kingdom prior to or during the process of deinstitutionalization. Alternatively, differences may relate to differences in service funding mechanisms and entitlements.

The United Kingdom traditionally has had a national service system, and the development of community services has generally been funded by reinvesting the resources withdrawn from institutions as people moved. In addition, new funding in Wales has been available for the development of community services but not for institutional services. In contrast, institutional funding levels in the United States have increased, even as most residents have moved to the community. Data reported by Prouty, Smith, and Lakin (2003) indicate that between 1970 and 2002, state institution "real dollar" (inflation-adjusted) expenditures increased from $4.0 billion to $5.6 billion, even as the average daily populations of state institutions decreased from 186,700 to 44,300 people. The finding from the United States that community services may be cheaper while being more favorably staffed derives from a wage differential between institution and community staff not found in the United Kingdom. Polister, Lakin, and Prouty (2003) reported that the average direct-support staff wage for employees of nonstate community service agencies was 74.4% of the average for state institution direct-support staff.

Finally, Braddock, Emerson, Felce, and Stancliffe (2001) showed that the prevalence of residential services in the United States expanded (by at least 44%) during the period when deinstitutionalization occurred, whereas it remained static or even declined in the United Kingdom. They also showed that a significantly higher proportion of the population are identified as having intellectual disabilities in the United States than in the United Kingdom, and the rate of residential provision is about 27% higher. Differences in the characteristics of people receiving support may underlie the different findings from the two countries. Whatever the reasons, the overriding point is that issues concerning service costs are particularly likely to be bound up in prevailing national circumstances and differ from country to country.

COMPARISON BETWEEN COMMUNITY AND OTHER SERVICE MODELS

Not all newly provided services in the United Kingdom that have replaced the traditional institutions have involved community housing. A number of new campus-based facilities have been opened, typically smaller in scale than the old institutions. They tend to provide for people with multiple impairments or high support needs. Hatton, Emerson, Robertson, Henderson, and Cooper (1995) compared the costs of 1) institution-based "specialized" units, 2) a campus-based "specialized" service, 3) "specialized" community houses, and 4) "ordinary" community houses for people with intellectual disabilities and sensory impairments. (*Specialized* refers to environments in which all of the people in the residential group had additional sensory impairments; *ordinary* refers to environments in which one or two people with additional sensory impairments shared with others without such additional impairments). In contrast to the general United Kingdom deinstitutionalization literature, they found that the specialized institution-based units and campus-based service had higher average annual costs per person than ordinary group homes,[3] although the study did not appear to control for the severity of the disability of co-residents, whose costs were averaged. The two service types also had slightly higher costs than the specialized community houses, although the differences were not statistically significant.

Emerson et al. (2000) studied the costs, quality of care, and outcomes associated with community living, village communities, and new campus-based facilities (see also Hallam et al., 2002, and Chapter 7). Multivariate analyses indicated that accommodation and total costs were significantly greater in community-living schemes than residential campuses, which were in turn significantly greater than in village communities, once costs were adjusted to control for between-model differences in adaptive behavior, challenging behavior, and age. The results derived from an analysis of matched samples of participants were broadly consistent with the multivariate analyses in that significantly higher total costs per week were found in community-living schemes than residential campuses, although differences in total costs between community-living schemes and village communities were not statistically significant.

The two studies reported in this section that have compared the costs of "newly" established institutional provision with community-living services provide contradictory results: Hatton et al. (1995) reported that community-living services were less costly, and Emerson et al. (2000) reported that community-living services were more costly. This discrepancy may reflect the highly specialized nature of provision investigated by Hatton et al. (1995).

EVIDENCE OF ECONOMIES OF SCALE WITHIN AND BETWEEN MODELS

Considerable evidence from the literature cited previously shows that costs vary widely both within and across different forms of residential service. Notwithstanding the general agreement in the U.K. deinstitutionalization literature that community services tend to be more expensive than

---

[3]Both the specialized institution and the campus-based services were recently provided and resourced at a higher level than was typical of longer-established institutional settings.

institutional care, size has not been found to be a strong influence on cost across much of the possible size spectrum. For example, Felce (1986) described 6- to 8-resident houses that had annual costs per resident similar to the average of two institutions with several hundred residents each. Differences in size did not contribute greatly to the explanation of costs in the studies by Wright and Haycox (1985) or Davies (1987). Although Wright and Haycox (1985) suggested that a system of community care would prove to be more expensive than institutional care, they considered that the increase in costs would arise primarily from ensuring that inadequate staffing levels existing within the institutions were not replicated in new community services. Cost inflation was a matter of meeting minimum standards that could not be met at that time within many institutions because of staff recruitment difficulties. It was not seen as arising from diseconomies of small scale. Felce, Lowe, Beecham, and Hallam (2000) demonstrated that setting size was a less good predictor of residential accommodation costs of adults with the most severe challenging behavior than a dummy service-model variable (institution or community setting). This finding suggests that the relationship between costs and setting size across the institution–community divide may be due to a number of variables that define the service dichotomy rather than size per se.

Knapp et al. (1992) found a significant effect for size of setting in analyzing the costs of care of 109 people living in a range of community settings (including residential homes and hostels, staffed group homes, independent living, foster placement, and living with minimal support). They concluded that size of setting did influence costs, with smaller settings being more expensive; however, number of residents was one of five variables that in total accounted for only 23% of cost variation. Moreover, in the light of the Felce et al. (2000) analysis mentioned previously, it is not possible to tell whether size was simply acting as a proxy for the different residential models within the range of community settings included. Analysis within a single community service model is required to address this limitation.

Raynes, Wright, Shiell, and Pettipher (1994) studied the costs of 150 community settings with between 2 and 31 places. They concluded that there were no economies of scale apparent within facilities larger than six and that, in general, there were no cost disadvantages in providing smaller settings. They added a caution, however, that a discontinuity in relationship may occur with very small size, leading to cost increases at a certain point. Too few settings with five or fewer places existed in their sample for them to be confident about the relationship between cost and size within this range.

As part of their wider study of community living, village communities, and new campus-based facilities referred to earlier, Emerson et al. (2001; see also Chapter 7) analyzed the costs for 63 participants in supported living schemes (1–3 residents), 55 participants in small-group homes (1–3 residents), and 152 participants in larger group homes (4–6 residents). There were no statistically significant differences in either raw or adjusted costs between models; however, once the data were pooled, there was a significant inverse association between size and both total and accommodation costs after controlling for differences in adaptive behavior, challenging behavior, and age. After the data were analyzed differently, Emerson et al. found a significant association between size and cost within the community schemes for participants with more severe disabilities (AAMR Adaptive Behavior Scale Part 1 score < 140) but not for participants with less severe disabilities (AAMR Adaptive Behavior Scale Part 1 score ≥ 140).

Robertson et al. (2002) conducted a longitudinal study of 50 people with severe challenging behaviors living in either community-based congregate provision ($n = 25$; at least 50% of residents in the setting had challenging behavior) or noncongregate provision ($n = 25$; less than 50% of residents in the setting had challenging behavior). Settings ranged in size between 2 and 6 residents. Additional analyses of these data for the present chapter failed to find any association between costs and size across both models combined or within congregate care. Within noncongregate care, 2-person services were found to be significantly more costly than services for 3 to 6 people after controlling for adaptive and challenging behavior.

Finally, Felce, Jones, Lowe, and Perry (2003) investigated the variation in staff-to-resident ratios and staff costs in a sample of 51 staffed houses accommodating 6 or fewer people with intellectual disabilities in Wales.[4] They found that there was a significant inverse relationship between size of residence and both measures, after first controlling for resident characteristics. Size explained an additional 11% of the variation in allocated staff hours per resident, per week and an additional 16% of the variation of actual staff costs per resident, per week.

Thus, these within-model analyses appear to show that diseconomies of scale do set in within very small settings, dependent on the level of support needs of residents (see Chapter 7) or the specific model of provision

---

[4]Although total costs were not analysed, this study is considered relevant as staff costs comprise about 60%–80% of community residential service costs in the United Kingdom (Felce et al., 1998; Hallam et al., 2002; Netten, Dennett, & Knight, 1999; Raynes et al., 1994).

(Robertson et al., 2002). Interestingly, Stancliffe (Chapter 6) also reported that diseconomies of scale in very small settings may be model dependent, with such diseconomies being apparent in group homes with relatively fixed staffing requirements but not in semi-independent living, where staff allocations can be individualized. These results are consistent with a view that diseconomies of scale will occur within models/settings at a point at which costs associated with specific support practices (e.g., on-site staff presence across the night, continuous daytime staff presence during times when residents are present) can no longer be reduced in a manner proportionate to the numbers of residents. Thus, for example, in a situation requiring modest but continuous staff presence, one member of staff on duty at a time might be both necessary and sufficient for a group home in which four people live together; however, one member of staff on duty would be similarly necessary if only two or three of the individuals lived together, at consequently greater per-capita costs. In contrast, allocating a set amount of staff input per person is more feasible when continuous staff presence is not required. For example, one might allocate 40 hours of staff support to a group home in which four people lived together, but only 20 or 30 respectively for a group home in which only two or three people lived together, thereby keeping per-capita costs constant.

IMPACT OF SIZE AND RESOURCE INPUT ON OUTCOMES WITHIN COMMUNITY SERVICES

Apparent associations exist between improved outcomes and both the higher costs and smaller scale of community settings within the U.K. comparative institution–community research literature; however, there is no basis within this literature to link the improvement in quality specifically to either factor. Research that has analyzed variation in outcome within community services provides an uncertain picture for the impact of residence size. A similar body of research suggests that the relationship between resource input and quality of outcome is weak or nonexistent.

Outcome and Size of Residence

Emerson et al. (2001; see also Chapter 7) found that residents in small-group homes (1–3 residents) had larger and more diverse social networks than those in large-group homes (4–6 residents). Settings defined as *supported living* (1–3 residents) were associated with increased choice and more frequent community activities, but because both small- and large-group homes were used as the basis of comparison, increased choice and more frequent community activities may be a consequence of service model rather than size. In Emerson et al.'s regression analysis of predictors of outcome in the combined community sample, living in a smaller setting size was unrelated to choice, social integration, being "healthily active," and overall risk, although it was associated with being underweight, having a lower risk of abuse, and enjoying greater participation in community activities (see Chapter 7).

Perry, Felce, and Lowe (2000) analyzed predictors of choice and participation in household, social, and community activities in 47 staffed group homes for 154 residents living in groups of 6 residents or fewer. After controlling for resident characteristics, size of residence was not a factor in accounting for variation in choice reported by staff for the sample as a whole; however, fewer residents living together was a significant predictor of higher choice as reported by a restricted sample of 56 people who could respond to the self-report version of the measure. Size was not a significant factor in relation to the extent of participation in household activity or observed engagement in activity (i.e., the combination of social, personal, household, leisure, and other constructive activity). Greater size predicted a greater range of social and community activities (i.e., a higher proportion of a given list of social and community activities being undertaken in the previous month) but it was not a factor in the explanation of variation in the frequency of social and community activities.

Felce, Lowe, and Jones (2002) analyzed predictors of participation in household, social, and community activities in 29 group homes for 97 residents living in groups of 2–6 residents. After controlling for resident characteristics, larger size of residence was positively associated with observed engagement in activity but was otherwise unrelated to extent of participation in household activity or the frequency of social or community activities. Felce et al. (2003) found engagement in activity unrelated to residence size in their study of 51 group homes accommodating 6 or fewer people. Hatton, Emerson, Robertson, Henderson, and Cooper (1996) found that residence size was not a factor in the prediction of observed engagement in activity or the frequency of activities outside the home in their study of settings for people with additional sensory impairments.

In summary, although a few analyses within community housing services suggest that certain positive outcomes are associated with small size, an approximately equal number suggest the opposite. The greatest number of findings show an absence of impact of residence size on outcome.

This mixed picture is mirrored in the international research literature. For example, smaller size was found to be associated with more choice or greater individualization by Stancliffe (1997) and Tøssebro (1995) but not by Stancliffe and Lakin (1998). Stancliffe and Lakin also found that access to leisure and community activities was unrelated to residence size. It should be emphasized, however, that these reports of a weak or nonexistent association between size and outcomes have largely been derived from studies of relatively small settings. The literature comparing outcomes associated with moving from large-scale community provision (e.g., hostels) to small-scale community living services is relatively consistent in reporting that such moves are associated with a range of benefits for people with intellectual disabilities (Emerson & Hatton, 1994, 1996).

Resource Input and Outcome

Research in the United Kingdom has found that about a quarter to two fifths of the variation in costs between settings can be related to resident characteristics such as adaptive or challenging behavior or age (Cambridge, Hayes, & Knapp, 1994; Felce et al., 2003; Knapp et al., 1992). Therefore, the investigation of the relationship between costs and outcome should control for such differences in resident characteristics. In a model that also took account of resident adaptive behavior and age, provider agency, and staff qualifications, Raynes et al. (1994) found that a composite measure of quality predicted variation in the costs of their sample of 150 community settings, albeit at only $p < .10$ significance. One might infer that resource input would be a significant predictor of quality of outcome, but no such analysis was undertaken. Cambridge et al. (1994, p. 77), however, concluded that there were "no links between costs and outcomes" in their 5-year follow-up of people in the community placements originally evaluated by Knapp et al. (1992). Moreover, Hatton et al. (1996) found no association between service costs and any indicator of quality in their analysis of settings for people with additional sensory impairments.

Emerson et al. (Chapter 7) demonstrated that links between costs and outcome in their study of community living, village communities, and new campus-based facilities were found in only a minority of analyses. First, using partial correlation controlling for the effects of adaptive and challenging behavior, increased costs were only associated with increased performance on 1 of 13 quality indicators within village communities (physical activity), 3 of 13 quality indicators within residential campuses (physical activity, number and variety of community activities), and 6 of 13 quality indicators within community housing schemes (choice; variety of community activities; size of social network; number of people other than staff, relatives, or people with intellectual disabilities in social network; number of days and hours of scheduled activity; reduced perceived risk of exploitation).

Moreover, among a subsample of relatively able participants, there were no significant bivariate associations between costs and any domain of service recipient satisfaction. Furthermore, in an analysis of supports provided to people with the most severe and complex disabilities, the association between cost and outcome was again explored using partial correlation coefficients, controlling for the effects of levels of adaptive behavior. Increased total costs were associated with just four process or outcome variables: poorer procedures for assessment and teaching, less block treatment, greater variety of community-based activities, and greater receipt of praise. Second, in a series of more complex multivariate analyses, resource inputs (either costs or staffing ratios) were associated with outcomes in four domains for the full sample but just two domains for the community-based sample.

Robertson et al. (2002) also explored the relationship between costs and outcome in their study of congregate and noncongregate group homes for people with severe challenging behavior. Across both types of settings combined, higher total costs were significantly correlated with fewer community-based activities; more use of sedation and physical restraint for the immediate control of challenging behavior; increased receipt of antipsychotic medication; and receipt of a greater number of injuries from co-tenants. There was no association between either accommodation or total costs and any observed measure of staff attention to residents or resident activity. Within each type of setting, increased cost in congregate provision (after controlling for adaptive and challenging behavior) was associated only with less choice, and increased cost in noncongregate provision was only associated with increased use of sedation.

On the whole, the previously mentioned results are consistent with research that has failed to demonstrate any clear link between staff-to-resident ratios, a major component of costs, and outcome.[5] Felce et al. (2000) found that higher staff-to-resident ratios in Wales predicted lower autonomy among people with the most severe challenging behavior, but

---

[5]The four studies cited in this paragraph all first take account of a range of resident characteristics, including adaptive and challenging behavior.

more staff per resident did not affect observed engagement in activity, household participation, or community involvement. Perry et al. (2000) found that variation in choice, household participation, observed engagement in activity, and the range and frequency of social and community activities was independent of variation in staff-to-resident ratios. Felce et al. (2002) found that staff-to-resident ratios predicted lower participation in household activities but more frequent community activities. Variation in observed engagement in activity and the frequency of social activities were independent of variation in staff-to-resident ratios. The former absence of relationship was also found by Felce et al. (2003).[6]

These results are consistent with research from other countries. Thus, for example, Stancliffe (Chapter 6) and Stancliffe and Keane (2000) reported that, once resident characteristics had been controlled for, semi-independent living was associated with significantly lower costs and better outcomes in some areas (choice, community and domestic participation) than staffed group homes (see also Stancliffe, Abery, & Smith, 2000). Indeed, research has a long-standing record of showing that there are diminishing marginal returns from adding staff to a given situation and that staff deployment may be more important than staff numbers per se (e.g., Felce, Repp, Thomas, Ager, & Blunden, 1991; Harris, Viet, Allen, & Chinsky, 1974; Landesman-Dwyer, Sackett, & Kleinman, 1980; Mansell, Felce, Jenkins, & de Kock, 1982), so much so that Landesman (1988, p. 109) was prompted to refer to the "myth of understaffing."

CONCLUSION

This chapter explores the U.K. research literature in order to throw light on the three propositions listed at the beginning of the chapter. The empirical support for these propositions is, at best, equivocal. Large living environments, such as institutions and hostels, provide poorer outcomes than domestic-scale settings; however, among domestic-scale community residences (for 1–6 residents), the relationship between size and outcomes is ambiguous or nonexistent.

The existing evidence suggests that diseconomies of scale are only likely to occur in settings supporting 3 or fewer people, and their opera-

---

[6]In some of the studies cited in this paragraph, higher staff-to-resident ratios have predicted greater staff attention or assistance being given to residents, which in turn has predicted higher resident engagement in activity; however, a direct relationship between staff-to-resident ratios and resident activity was not found.

tion at all may be dependent on the level of support needs of residents or the specific model of provision. These results are consistent with a view that diseconomies of scale will occur within models/settings at a point at which costs associated with specific support practices (e.g., on-site staff presence across the night or continuous daytime staff presence during times when residents are present) can no longer be reduced in a manner proportionate to the number of residents due to either the level of support needs of residents or the inflexibility of the service model.

Results from the United Kingdom (and elsewhere) suggest that there are no robust associations between outcomes and measures of resource input or the structural characteristics of community-living services such as size (see also Emerson & Hatton, 1994; Felce, 2000). This assumption does not suggest, of course, that either resources or size are irrelevant. Clearly, a sufficient level of resources is necessary to deliver any service. The lack of association between resources and outcomes may reflect two types of failing within U.K. services. First, resources may not be entirely allocated on the basis of need (Emerson, 1999; Felce, 2000; Felce et al., 2003). As a result, some services may be over-resourced, with the addition of excess resources failing to result in further benefits (or indeed reducing benefits by reducing the opportunities and demands for independent action; see Chapter 6). Second, major inefficiencies may be present in the use of the available resources (Emerson, 1999; Felce, 2000). This latter view is supported by evidence that changes in staff training, organization, and management practices can, without additional resources, result in significant improvements in outcome (e.g., Jones et al., 2001). Whatever the reasons, basing policy decisions on either the level of resources or the structural characteristics of residential services provides no guarantee of delivering better outcomes for people with intellectual disabilities.

Our consideration of the United States and the United Kingdom demonstrates that countries differ in whether the costs of new community services are less than, no different from, or more than those of the institutional services that they have replaced. Service systems and funding mechanisms, the baseline commitment to investment within institutional services prior to reform, and the models of community services adopted to replace them are likely to be specific to each country; however, research findings about the relationship between resource inputs and service characteristics, on the one hand, and outcomes, on the other hand, might be more generalizable. The fact that we have been able to discuss consistencies between U.K. research findings and those from overseas supports this conjecture.

REFERENCES

Braddock, D., Emerson, E., Felce, D., & Stancliffe, R. (2001). The living circumstances of children and adults with mental retardation or developmental disabilities in the United States, Canada, England and Wales, and Australia. *Mental Retardation & Developmental Disabilities Research Reviews, 7,* 115–121.

Cambridge, P., Hayes, L., & Knapp, M. (1994). *Care in the community: Five years on.* Aldershot, United Kingdom: Ashgate Publishing.

Campbell, E.M., & Heal, L.W. (1995). Government cost of providing services for individuals with developmental disabilities. *American Journal on Mental Retardation, 100,* 17–35.

Davies, L. (1987). *Quality, costs and "an ordinary life."* London: King's Fund Centre.

Davies, L. (1988). Community care: The costs and quality. *Health Services Management Research, 1,* 145–155.

Emerson, E. (1999). Residential supports for people with intellectual disabilities: Questions and challenges from the UK. *Journal of Intellectual & Developmental Disability, 24,* 309–319.

Emerson, E., & Hatton, C. (1994). *Moving out: The impact of relocation from hospital to community on the quality of life of people with learning disabilities.* London: Her Majesty's Stationary Office (HMSO).

Emerson, E., & Hatton, C. (1996). Deinstitutionalization in the UK: Outcomes for service users. *Journal of Intellectual & Developmental Disability, 21,* 17–37.

Emerson, E., Robertson, J., Gregory, N., Kessissoglou, S., Hatton, C., Hallam, A., Knapp, M., Järbrink, K., Walsh, P., & Netten, A. (2000). The quality and costs of village communities, residential campuses and community-based residential supports in the United Kingdom. *American Journal on Mental Retardation, 105,* 81–102.

Emerson, E., Robertson, J., Gregory, N., Hatton, C., Kessissoglou, S., Hallam, A., Järbrink, K., Knapp, M., Netten, A., & Walsh, P. (2001). The quality and costs of supported living residences and group homes in the United Kingdom. *American Journal on Mental Retardation, 106,* 401–415.

Felce, D. (1986). Accommodating adults with severe and profound mental handicaps: Comparative revenue costs. *Mental Handicap, 14,* 104–107.

Felce, D. (2000). *Quality of life in supported housing in the community: A review of research.* Exeter, United Kingdom: University of Exeter, Centre for Evidence-based Social Services.

Felce, D., Jones, E., Lowe, K., & Perry, J. (2003). Rational resourcing and productivity: Relationships among staff input, resident characteristics and group home quality. *American Journal on Mental Retardation, 108,* 161–172.

Felce, D., Lowe, K., Beecham, J., & Hallam, A. (2000). Exploring the relationships between costs and quality of services for adults with severe intellectual disabilities and the most severe challenging behaviours in Wales: A multivariate regression analysis. *Journal of Intellectual & Developmental Disability, 25,* 307–326.

Felce, D., Lowe, K., & Jones, E. (2002). Association between the provision characteristics and operation of supported housing services and resident outcomes. *Journal of Applied Research in Intellectual Disabilities, 15,* 404–418.

Felce, D., Lowe, K., Perry, J., Baxter, H., Jones, E., Hallam, A., & Beecham, J. (1998). Service support to people with severe intellectual disabilities and the most severe challenging behaviours in Wales: Processes, outcomes and costs. *Journal of Intellectual Disability Research, 42,* 390–408.

Felce, D., Mansell, J., & Kushlick, A. (1980). Evaluation of alternative residential facilities for the severely mentally handicapped in Wessex: Revenue costs. *Advances in Behaviour Research and Therapy, 3,* 43–47.

Felce, D., Repp, A.C., Thomas, M., Ager, A., & Blunden, R. (1991). The relationship of staff:client ratios, interactions and residential placement. *Research in Developmental Disabilities, 12,* 315–331.

Glennerster, H., & Korman, N. (1990, April 26). Success costs money. *Community Care, 30–31.*

Hallam, A., Knapp, M., Järbrink, K., Netten, A., Emerson, E., Robertson, J., Gregory, N., Hatton, C., Kessissoglou, S., & Durkan, J. (2002). The costs of residential supports for people with intellectual disabilities. *Journal of Intellectual Disability Research, 46,* 394–404.

Harris, J.M., Viet, S.W., Allen, G.J., & Chinsky, J.M. (1974). Aide-resident ratio and ward population density as mediators of social interaction. *American Journal of Mental Deficiency, 79,* 320–326.

Hatton, C., Emerson, E., Robertson, J., Henderson, D., & Cooper, J. (1995). The quality and costs of services for adults with multiple disabilities: A comparative evaluation. *Research in Developmental Disabilities, 16,* 439–460.

Hatton, C., Emerson, E., Robertson, J., Henderson, D., & Cooper, J. (1996). Factors associated with staff support and user lifestyle in services for people with multiple disabilities: A path analytic approach. *Journal of Intellectual Disability Research, 40,* 466–477.

Jones, E., Felce, D., Lowe, K., Bowley, C., Pagler, J., Gallagher, B., & Roper, A. (2001). Evaluation of the dissemination of Active Support training in staffed community residences. *American Journal on Mental Retardation, 106,* 344–358.

Kim, S., Larson, S.A., & Lakin, K.C. (2001). Behavioral outcomes of deinstitutionalization for people with intellectual disabilities: A review of studies conducted between 1980 and 1999. *Journal of Intellectual & Developmental Disability, 26,* 35–50.

Knapp, M., Cambridge, P., Thomason, C., Beecham, J., Allen, C., & Darton, R. (1992). *Care in the community: Challenge and demonstration.* Aldershot, United Kingdom: Ashgate Publishing.

Knobbe, C.A., Carey, S.P., Rhodes, L., & Horner, R.H. (1995). Benefit–cost analysis of community residential versus institutional services for adults with severe mental retardation and challenging behaviors. *American Journal on Mental Retardation, 99,* 533–541.

Landesman, S. (1988). The changing structure and function of institutions: A search for optimal group care environments. In S. Landesman & P. Vietze (Eds.), *Living environments and mental retardation* (pp. 79–126). Washington, DC: American Association on Mental Retardation.

Landesman-Dwyer, S., Sackett, G.P., & Kleinman, J.A. (1980). Small community residences: The relationship of size to resident and staff behavior. *American Journal of Mental Deficiency, 85,* 6–18.

Mansell, J., Felce, D., Jenkins, J., & de Kock, U. (1982). Increasing staff ratios in an activity with severely mentally handicapped people. *British Journal of Mental Subnormality*, *18*, 97–99.

Martin, J.P (1984). *Hospitals in trouble*. Oxford, United Kingdom: Blackwell Publishers.

Netten, A., Dennett, J., & Knight, J. (1999). *The unit costs of health and social care*. Canterbury, United Kingdom: University of Kent, Personal Social Services Research Unit.

Office of the Deputy Prime Minister and Department of Health. (2003). *Housing and support services for people with learning disabilities*. London: Office of the Deputy Prime Minister and Department of Health.

Perry, J., Felce, D., & Lowe, K. (2000). *Subjective and objective quality of life assessment: Their interrelationship and determinants*. Cardiff, United Kingdom: University of Wales College of Medicine, Welsh Centre for Learning Disabilities.

Polister, B., Lakin, K.C., & Prouty, R. (2003). Wages of direct support professionals serving persons with intellectual and developmental disabilities: A survey of state agencies and private residential provider trade associations. *Policy Research Brief*, *14*(2). Minneapolis: University of Minnesota, Institute on Community Integration. Also available on-line at http://rtc.umn.edu

Prouty, R.W., Smith, G., & Lakin, K.C. (Eds.). (2003). *Residential services for persons with developmental disabilities: Status and trends through 2002*. Minneapolis: University of Minnesota, Research and Training Center on Community Living, Institute on Community Integration. Also available on-line at http://rtc.umn.edu

Raynes, N.V., Wright, K., Shiell, A., & Pettipher, C. (1994). *The cost and quality of community residential care: An evaluation of the services for adults with learning disabilities*. London: David Fulton Publishers.

Roberston, J., Emerson, E., Pinkney, L., Cesar, E., Felce, D., Lowe, K., Meek, A., Knapp, M., & Hallam, A. (2002). *Quality and costs of community-based residential supports for people with learning disabilities and severe challenging behaviour*. Lancaster, United Kingdom: University of Lancaster, Institute for Health Research.

Schalock, M., & Fredericks, H.D.B. (1990). Comparative costs for institutional services and services for selected populations in the community. *Behavioral Residential Treatment*, *5*, 271–286.

Stancliffe, R.J. (1997). Community living-unit size, staff presence and resident's choice-making. *Mental Retardation*, *35*, 1–9.

Stancliffe, R.J., Abery, B.H., & Smith, J. (2000). Personal control and the ecology of community living settings: Beyond living-unit size and type. *American Journal on Mental Retardation*, *105*, 431–454.

Stancliffe, R.J., & Keane, S. (2000). Outcomes and costs of community living: A matched comparison of group homes and semi-independent living. *Journal of Intellectual & Developmental Disability*, *25*, 281–305.

Stancliffe, R.J., & Lakin, K.C. (1998). Analysis of expenditures and outcomes of residential alternatives for persons with developmental disabilities. *American Journal on Mental Retardation*, *102*, 552–568.

Tøssebro, J. (1995). Impact of size revisited: Relation of number of residents to self-determination and deprivization. *American Journal on Mental Retardation*, *100*, 59–67.

Wright, K., & Haycox, A. (1985). *Costs of alternative forms of NHS care for mentally handicapped persons.* York, United Kingdom: University of York, Centre for Health Economics.

Young, I., Sigafoos, J., Suttie, J., Ashman, A., & Grevell, P. (1998). Deinstitutionalisation of person with intellectual disabilities: A review of Australian studies. *Journal of Intellectual & Developmental Disability, 23,* 155–170.

CHAPTER 4

Costs of Family Care for Individuals with Developmental Disabilities

Darrell R. Lewis and David R. Johnson

The family has historically played a central role in the care of individuals with developmental disabilities. The vast majority of people with disabilities live with their families, many for their entire lives. Fewer than 20% of the U.S. population with intellectual disabilities and developmental disabilities (ID/DD) live in any form of out-of-home placement (Fujiura & Braddock, 1999). Although the risk of out-of-home placement increases throughout the age cycle, the rate of placement even in adulthood is not high. The American family is simply the largest "provider" of care in the nation; yet, it receives the lowest form of public assistance.

Surprisingly, little research, public policy initiatives, or public resources have been directed to family care throughout the life cycle of individuals with developmental disabilities. Rather, most efforts have been directed at providing support for and understanding about those individuals who live outside their natural family homes. To the extent that family care has been examined, it has largely focused on early childhood or the developmental years of high school (Seltzer, 2000). The lack of information about home care costs and services is more surprising when one realizes that the overwhelming majority of individuals with developmental disabilities live at home with their families (Jaskulski, Lakin, & Zierman, 1995). This lack of information was also highly evident and important in the 1996 "welfare reform" legislation—the Personal Responsibility and Work Opportunity Reconciliation Act of 1996, PL 104-193—that brought discontinuation of Supplemental Security Income to about 100,000 children with ID/DD and their families. As noted by Fujiura and Braddock (1999), the needs of families caring for relatives with disabilities can be characterized as numerous, diverse, and generally ill served by the formal systems of care, and much of the current research on public policy for family home care is inadequate for policy development, management, and decision making (Lewis & Bruininks, 1994).

In spite of this neglect of the role of family care for individuals with developmental disabilities, public policy since the 1980s has had differing cost and benefit consequences for both the family and society. For a long time, families had to choose between institutionalizing their children with disabilities or bearing almost the entire burden of care within the home. An all-or-nothing trade-off in costs and burden was imposed on the family, the individual, and the state. Although the introduction of a variety of public assistance programs since the 1970s has had significant influence on families' ability to support family members with disabilities at home, eligibility requirements, family members' general availability, and other limitations still make families' decisions about home care difficult.

Public policy, funding patterns, and service-delivery models have historically focused on out-of-home placements. Most forms of public funding for people with intellectual disabilities have continued to be directed toward services received outside the family home. Less than 8% of all community-based services for people with intellectual disabilities in the late 1990s were directed to family care (Braddock, Hemp, Parish, & Westrich, 1998). Although references to this dilemma are fairly common and well documented in the literature (Bradley & Agosta, 1985; Fujiura & Braddock, 1999; Gallagher & Vietze, 1986), surprisingly little has been written or developed relative to the identification, measurement, and distribution of the cost of care within the family home.

The decision to maintain a child with intellectual disabilities in the immediate family home or to seek out-of-home placement has been confirmed in the literature as a function of family adaptation to financial and other perceived burdens of home care and to the availability of family support services (Black, Molaison, & Smull, 1990; Bruns, 2000; Castellani, Downey, Thusig, & Bird, 1986; Llewellyn, Dunn, Fante, Turnbull, & Grace, 1999; Seltzer & Krauss, 1989). The decision is affected by numerous child-related stressors, family resources, and the availability of other sources of support from outside the home. Cole and Meyer (1989) used these variables to survey parents of children with intellectual disabilities still living at home and also explored the parents' plans for future child placement. Multiple regression analyses revealed that both child-related stress and financial pressures (i.e., limited family resources) contributed to family decisions about placing children outside of the home. Most important, Cole and Meyer found that the availability of external services and resources was related to plans for maintaining the child at home more than both child-related stressors and family resources. The amount and type of external support services and financial help largely determines whether children and young adults with disabilities will remain within home-based caring units.

DEFINING FAMILY AND FAMILY CARE

Before delving into the goals and purposes of this chapter, it is important to first have a clear notion about how one defines *family* in the provision of services to families and members with disabilities. Many states have begun to develop diversified forms of residential living arrangements within communities, and many of these residences are described as forms of "family" living. The expansion and effect of the national Medicaid Home and Community-Based Services (HCBS) Waiver programs have encouraged this transformation. Until the late 1960s, whenever families decided to place individuals with ID/DD outside the immediate family residential setting, they could choose to place the individuals in either a large state institutional setting or a community-based foster family setting.

Medicaid HCBS Waiver programs offer greater choices for funding services. An individual with ID/DD (i.e., service recipient) can continue to live at home with his or her "immediate *family*" or an "extended *family*" member (e.g., grandparent, sibling), or the service recipient can move into his or her "own *family* home," a residential setting that is owned or rented by the service recipient or by the service recipient's family. The service recipient can also move into a small "private foster care *family*," which is the family home of people who are not immediate or extended family members and who are providing services and support to service recipients.

Service recipients also have the choice of moving into "corporate foster care," which is a home of four or fewer people in which services are provided by paid staff in a setting that is under the control of a service provider agency. Corporate foster care has been characterized by some as having a family care setting, but we will not include corporate foster care in our taxonomy of "family care."

A service recipient could also move into other types of community-based nonfamily residences, such as variously sized licensed group homes. In 1997, in the United States, there were more than 300,000 people with developmental disabilities living in their family homes and receiving services from publicly funded sources (Prouty & Lakin, 1998). Other individuals with developmental disabilities were also living in family homes and receiving services funded through private insurance or through family out-of-pocket expenses (Fujiura, Roccoforte, & Braddock, 1994).

ISSUES EXAMINED

This chapter reviews the literature since 1980 and focuses on several questions:

- What are the social and family costs of care for family members with developmental disabilities?
- Are there costs of care beyond just financial resources?
- Who bears the financial burden of these costs?
- How have these costs been allocated between families and society?

A related set of questions deals with comparisons of the costs of family care in alternative care settings within the community. For example, how do family costs of care differ from those within alternative settings, such as in foster homes and in other community-based small- and large-group homes? Using the answers to these questions, we examine appropriate implications for public policy.

This analysis of cost information and links with outcomes is important for several reasons. First, it is useful in the development of public policy concerning the care of people with developmental disabilities. Information on the costs of home-based care, including those borne by the family, is essential for any realistic cost comparisons between home-based and alternative care systems. Without these data comparisons, making informed judgments about the balance of care and funding between residential options is impossible. A second major reason for developing cost information on the outcomes and effects of family care is for public agency and family welfare purposes. State agencies must have such information about the costs involved in caring for children with disabilities 1) if they are to provide benefit payments that adequately recompense families, and 2) if they are to provide the types and amounts of services most needed by these families. The current levels and types of state services and financial supports appear to be based on an ad hoc system seriously constrained by outdated legislation and the availability of agency funds.

ACCOUNTING FOR FAMILY COSTS IN THE LITERATURE

Many authors have pointed out the crucial role played by families in the care of dependent family members; however, few studies have systematically examined and measured the financial burden involved. With some notable exceptions, most studies have ignored individual families' expenses to focus on the public expenses of the state, county, or other governmental jurisdiction. They have also focused on various themes relating to services, such as the costs of a specific medical disability (e.g., Hogan, Rogers, & Msall, 2000), the comparative costs of differing residential facilities (e.g., Haycox, 1995; Hewitt et al., 2000; Hill, Lakin, Bruininks, Amado, Anderson, & Copher, 1989; Lewis & Bruininks, 1994; Stancliffe & Lakin, 1998), or the correlates of the costs of developmental disabilities services (e.g., Campbell & Heal, 1995), but they have seldom focused on the direct resource use and costs of in-home family care.

The U.S. Department of Agriculture (Lino, 1998) estimated in the late 1990s that raising a child without disabilities from birth to age 17 would average at least $180,000 in 1997 dollars depending on regions of the country, household incomes, and number of siblings. Edwards and Beckham (1984) have estimated that these direct-cost figures triple when indirect costs are taken into account. Indirect costs refer to the value of the time spent by parents in child care and additional household tasks (e.g., added laundry) as well as *opportunity costs* (e.g., loss of earnings by the caregiving parent who could have been otherwise employed). Moreover, it has been estimated that family members invest three to four times as much time each day in caring for an infant than a 10-year-old. Part of this difference, of course, is accounted for by the caring functions of formal schooling.

Fujiura et al. (1994) estimated that the extra nonreimbursed (i.e., out-of-pocket) spending by families supporting an adult family member with intellectual disabilities or related developmental disabilities would total at least $6,300 in additional expenditures each year. This estimation computes to at least a 60% increase in family costs for raising a child with disabilities. Moreover, the indirect and opportunity costs of caring for a child with disabilities would add dramatically to the family's financial burden.

Without a doubt, care of a family member with disabilities costs more in both cash expenditures and extraordinary indirect costs than care for a family member without disabilities. If child care of an infant, for example, takes 5–6 hours per day and child care of a typically developing 10-year-old requires only 1 hour, a physically dependent 10-year-old or a 10-year old with intellectual disabilities (whose high mobility combined with disregard for personal danger requires continuous supervision) may require 5–6 hours a day. Surprisingly, little has been done to measure these differential or extraordinary costs, many of which are not out-of-pocket but in-kind or psychological in nature.

The adverse effects, or costs, on the families of individuals with disabilities are many and varied. Baldwin (1985), for example, drew a distinction between direct financial costs (e.g., extra spending in the household and on health care), opportunity financial costs (e.g., loss of earnings), and psychological costs (e.g., restricted social life, raised stress levels). From such distinctions, a useful taxonomy of the literature on family costs can be constructed and is represented in the following review.

Direct Financial Costs Met by Families

Boggs (1979) recommended a conceptually useful and detailed taxonomy for measuring the costs and family expenditures for the care of family members with developmental disabilities. She first outlined the typical distribution of family expenditures for typical child care needs (e.g., food, clothing, shelter), then identified extraordinary expenditures relevant to the disability circumstances (e.g., home therapy, home modification), all in a matrix by sources of support (e.g., family income, family in-kind, country and state). Unfortunately, this matrix has never been reported with real data.

Several small-scale costs of care studies in the literature have involved families and focused on selected types of care with limited populations, but only a few studies employed national survey data. Moreover, most of the small-scale studies have emerged from the health care literature (Jacobs & McDermott, 1989) and have focused on the impact of having disabilities rather than specific financial or family consequences.

Only seven studies that have specifically focused on families who had members with developmental disabilities can be characterized as true cost or expenditure studies (Baldwin, 1985; Birenbaum, Guyot, & Cohen, 1990; Chetwynd, 1985; Fujiura et al., 1994; Gunn & Berry, 1987; Hyman, 1977; Rees & Emerson, 1983). Rees and Emerson (1983) investigated the costs of caring for 51 Australian children with disabilities living at home whose families had indicated the need for residential care. The children came from a wide range of social groups; the majority were selected at random from waiting lists for residential care, and their disabilities included intellectual as well as physical and sensory limitations. The authors reported on monthly expenditures per child on 11 items, which included medication, special equipment and aids, medical insurance, transport, child care or school fees, domestic help, temporary care, special food, extra items, and extra clothing. Another Australian study (Gunn & Berry, 1987) also investigated the extent to which families with a child with Down syndrome incurred additional financial expenses. Over a 4-week period, 37 families with a child with Down syndrome and 20 comparison families recorded the expenses involved in rearing their children. Expenditure data were collected on medication and health expenses, special foods, transport, activities, specialists, school fees and child care, special programs, special toys, and special equipment. In both studies, large and important costs were incurred by families supporting children with disabilities.

A similar type of study by Chetwynd (1985) also showed that raising a child with intellectual disabilities at home in the United States incurs extra financial burdens on families. This study involved 91 families with a child with intellectual disabilities and showed that these families had additional weekly expenditures on household items (e.g., food, electricity, household supplies), special equipment, health care, and substantial expenses for house alterations. Hyman's (1977) case study of the extra costs of living with disabilities for 56 adults who use wheelchairs also attempted to obtain a comprehensive picture of the costs imposed by disabilities. Her study in England not only included detailed estimates of earning losses and all extra expenses, but also estimated the opportunity costs of close relatives and friends and the costs borne by the community at large in the form of services.

Baldwin (1985) reported on one of the most carefully designed studies in the literature on determining whether and to what extent having a child with severe disabilities affects family income and expenditures. This large-scale comparative study was commissioned by the Department of Health and Social Security in the United Kingdom. The study compared information on income and expenditure patterns of a sample of 438 families who had children with disabilities and a control group of 638 families who had children without disabilities. The control sample was drawn from the national Family Expenditure Survey data set and matched on several important variables with families drawn from the national Family Fund data set. Forty-eight case studies were also conducted to further document incomes, expenditures, and family stress histories.

In this study by Baldwin, parents of children with disabilities reported that the child's condition clearly created extra financial costs. This claim was tested in relationship to everyday living costs, larger items bought less frequently, and the episodic costs associated with health care and hospital treatment. In all three areas, the child's disabilities had led to extra expense and had substantially altered families' expenditure patterns. The data indicated that children with severe disabilities caused most families in the sample to spend more than their counterparts with typically developing children on both a number of individual items and on total expenditures. The overall daily living expenses for families with a child with disabilities were estimated to be, on average, more than 8%–20% greater than matched controls. If accounts were taken of the less regular costs arising from the need for housing adaptations, the purchase and replacement of consumer durables, and hospital costs, the cost estimates and differences would be even greater.

Although the Baldwin study is one of the best family cost studies on the implications of caring for a child with disabilities at home, it—along with most other family expenditure studies—has two weaknesses with respect to design and cost estimates. First, the expenditure data in all of these studies do not typically allow spending on particular individuals to be identified; the extent to which the needs of a child with disabilities are met at the expense of other family members is clearly hidden. Changes in the purposes for which items are bought are also hidden. As a consequence, the true financial impact and family burden of the child's disabilities are clearly underestimated in the results of these studies. Second, the designs of almost all of these studies preclude estimating the full financial needs of family care for a child with disabilities. The studies typically report only on expenditures made from available family resources. Expenditures by their very nature are constrained by the budgets available to families. If earnings are less for families with a child or adult family member with disabilities, then the expenditures reported in the studies are essentially constrained by cash allowances from charitable and governmental agencies, and these allowances may be significantly inadequate. Baldwin herself noted, "as more money becomes available it continues to be directed disproportionately to the disabled child. There appears to be no income point at which the child's special needs are met within the family's normal budget" (1985, p. 132).

Most of these studies do not attempt to estimate the costs of disabilities to society but rather examine only the financial burden of disabilities borne by families. For example, all forms of direct services (e.g., therapy, hospitalization, and other medical services) provided by outside education, health, and social service agencies, and all forms of indirect social costs (e.g., case management), were ignored in the cost estimates by Baldwin and others. All of the studies were intended to focus on only family financial burden.

Although the lifelong financial problems for families with members with serious and chronic disabilities are a persistent concern among health care policy experts, only a few large-scale cost studies in the health care literature have focused on this population, and none have addressed the life-cycle needs of families. Rossiter and Wilensky (1982) reported that the 1977 National Health Care Expenditures Study in the United States suggested that families will be particularly burdened financially when they include people characterized as being in poor health. Out-of-pocket expenses for young adults in poor health, for example, were two and a half times higher than for those in excellent health; however, because this national survey of 14,000 randomly selected households did not deliberately oversample people with developmental disabilities, no expenditure data were reported for any of these sample subpopulations.

Using U.S. data from the 1981 Child Health Supplement to the National Health Interview Survey, Newacheck and Halfon found that "children with substantial health problems from low-income families continue to lag behind their higher income counterparts in similar health" as far as access to ambulatory services is concerned (1986, p. 813). Moreover, less than half of these low-income families with children reported to be in fair or poor health were Medicaid eligible in the early 1980s.

A national survey of state expenditures through ID/DD agencies also reported very limited funding for family care (Braddock et al., 1998). Braddock and his colleagues collected data for all forms of state support for families with members with disabilities and concluded that less than 8% of all intellectual disability community-based services in 1998 were to families with a member with developmental disabilities. Their study consisted of any community-based service administered by a state intellectual disability services agency that included vouchers, direct cash payments to families, reimbursement, or direct payments to service providers that the state agency itself identified as family support. It also included services other than cash subsidy, such as respite care, family counseling, equipment purchase, architectural adaptation of the home, in-home training, education, and behavior management services. Although the addition of Medicaid HCBS Waiver programs has undoubtedly increased these family support services, the totals are still very low relative to needs.

A study by Birenbaum et al. (1990) is the only attempt to focus directly on U.S. families at the national level in order to study the costs of family care for children with disabilities. The study surveyed both families of children with disabilities and providers of services, and the results present a depressing picture of America's response to family needs. Birenbaum et al. attempted to estimate all expenses related to using medical services and caring for children with autism and severe intellectual disabilities. In 1989 dollars, average annual out-of-pocket expenditures ranged from a high of $3,076 to a low of $838 for children with severe intellectual disabilities. These home-based costs were compared with Medicaid payments to care for a child in residential placement, which ranged between $16,000 and $27,000.

Birenbaum et al. (1990) reported that such comparisons do indeed support their proposition that America's expenditures on child care are not supportive of families. Results from the study indicate that families with a child with disabilities have substantial unreimbursed financial expenses beyond the direct costs of medical care and additional nonfinancial family hardships. The study records that children and youth with serious developmental disabilities require care far in excess of their healthy peers and that families bear the financial burden of this extra child care with virtually no external financial assistance. The study found that the ultimate step for an overburdened family was to place their child with severe disabilities in residential care.

Fujiura et al. (1994) reported on nonreimbursed spending among a sample of Chicago-area families supporting an adult family member with intellectual and related developmental disabilities. Through surveys and telephone interviews across 10 categories of routine, daily living expenses, and disability-related services, Fujiura et al. estimated that the average annualized out-of-pocket cost to the family was $6,348 in 1990 dollars. Although higher-income families reported higher levels of spending, the percent of household income represented by nonreimbursed expenditures increased significantly as family income decreased. The study's results were highly consistent with those reported by Birenbaum et al. (1990), and Fujiura et al.'s policy recommendations were also similar—namely, that the focus for the nation's system of care, service planning, and public policy needs to be on the importance and needs of the family. Although the family is the nation's largest provider of care for individuals with intellectual and related developmental disabilities, other than these studies, little else is known about the direct costs or expenditures of home care for children and adults with disabilities living with their families.

Indirect and Opportunity Costs

Information on the financial impact and income effects on families of children with disabilities has come from large-scale statistical studies of poverty and income distribution and from several studies looking specifically at populations of individuals with disabilities. The picture that emerges from both is remarkable in its consistency over time. Abel-Smith and Townsend (1965) in the United Kingdom used their analysis of Family Expenditure Survey data to reveal that having a family member with disabilities was strongly associated with the family's having a low income. This finding of the effects of disabilities on income has been confirmed consistently across time (Baldwin, 1985; Chiu, Tang, Shyu, Huang, & Wang, 2000; Ellis et al., 2002) and countries (Birenbaum et al., 1990).

The literature clearly shows that having a disability has a marked effect on income. Lower earnings are not offset to any great extent by government transfer payments in either the United Kingdom (Hirst, 1985) or the United States (Birenbaum & Cohen, 1993). As noted by Baldwin,

> In spite of new benefits, disabled people remain disproportionately represented among the poor, while a high proportion of the disabled have very low incomes. Even when they are not technically in poverty, disabled people are likely to find their incomes lower as a result of disablement. (1985, p. 54)

Mothers of children with disabilities are much less likely to have paid employment. When they do work, they are less likely to be employed full time. Most likely, mothers of children with disabilities are left without outside employment and income opportunities because of the additional demands for caregiving. Birenbaum et al. (1990) have reported that data from the U.S. Bureau of Labor Statistics on paid employment showed that at least 12% more mothers with young children work full time than mothers of children with severe disabilities. Other studies have similarly reported that mothers of children with disabilities, especially those in low-income families, clearly participate less in the labor force. Most notably, for low-income families, "the costs of acceptable substitute child care often outweigh the potential contribution to family income from the mother's paid work" (Breslau, Salkever, & Staruch, 1982, p. 169). Birenbaum and Cohen (1993) also reported that the proportion of full-time working mothers with a child with disabilities who were living in residential care outside of the family setting rose to just below the national average in the United States.

Baldwin (1985) also clearly indicated that U.K. mothers of children with disabilities are less free to increase their hours of work outside the home, with a consequent adverse effect on current earnings as well as lifetime earnings and employment conditions. They remain in lower paid jobs, work in part-time jobs longer, and generally work under poorer conditions than mothers of typically developing children. Baldwin found that mothers of typically developing children earned twice as much as mothers of children with disabilities. Hirst (1985) also found that U.K. mothers of young adults with disabilities had lower workforce participation, fewer hours of work, and lower earnings than U.K. women in general.

Baldwin also provided no support for the suggestion that family care of a child with disabilities leads men to increase their earnings. On the contrary, both the men's subjective accounts and the study's comparative data on the men's earnings suggested that the working lives and amount earned by most men with children with disabilities were adversely affected. When differences in the two groups' occupational classifications were taken into account, the earnings of men with children with disabilities remained on average almost 9% less per week than those of men in the control group. On the whole, families of children with disabilities had more than 18% less income when matched with families in the control group. Because mothers, and sometimes fathers, could not work, the children's chronic disabilities had substantial indirect costs on family income.

In a previous survey by Baldwin of applicants to the U.K.'s Family Fund, 303 families were asked whether the child's condition had affected the mothers' or fathers' earnings or had caused extra expenditure. When parents indicated that the condition had such effects, parents were asked to estimate their weekly earnings loss and their extra spending on a range of items. Of the families in this sample, 48% said that their earnings were less because of the child's special needs, and more than 90% claimed to be spending more on their child with disabilities than their children without disabilities.

The enhanced economic demands of having a child with disabilities place single mothers (i.e., widows, divorcees, separated or never-married mothers) in a particularly stressful situation. Regardless of the single mother's age, race, or income, the presence of a child with disabilities does not significantly affect the mother's labor-force participation (Breslau et al., 1982). The most stressed single mothers are undoubtedly those who must work to survive under PL 104-193. This Act requires welfare recipients, typically single mothers, to return to work within specified time periods or lose their benefits. These requirements, particularly for mothers of children with disabilities, produce additional emotional stress on the family situation.

Indirect Psychological Costs

Many individuals have persistently noted that the most important dimensions of family costs and stress have not necessarily been financial, but psychological (e.g., Cole, 1986; Farber & DeOllos, 2000; Minnes, 1998). A substantial body of literature written by parents describes in detail the ways in which family and personal lives are affected (e.g., Darling, 1987). In addition, considerable empirically based research shows the effects of having a child with developmental disabilities on families (e.g., Baxter, Cummins, & Yiolitis, 2000; Cole & Meyer, 1989; Cummins, 2001; Farber & DeOllos, 2000; Hirst, 1985; Taanila, Syrjala, Kokkonen, & Jarvelin, 2002; Tausig, 1985; Traute & Hiebert-Murphy, 2002; Wikler, 1986). This literature generally enumerates the negative psychosocial outcomes for such families (e.g., social isolation, loss of leisure time, increased familial stress, depression, physical burdens). In fact, there are literally hundreds of such family stress studies, and most can be grouped according to the characteristics of the child being investigated (Minnes, 1998).

Hirst (1985), for example, examined the health effects on mothers with a young adult with severe disabilities in their homes. In comparing the effects on these mothers with those of women in the general population, he found that mothers in his sample were much more likely to suffer from a severe chronic illness and to experience symptoms of psychiatric disturbance. Specific aspects of their sons' or daughters' disabilities could not explain variations in mothers' health status and employment patterns. Mothers of all young adults with disabilities, not just mothers of children with more severe disabilities, experienced the adverse effects of providing care in the family. Also, reasonably firm evidence proves that both mothers and fathers of a child with disabilities are more likely than mothers and fathers of typically developing children to suffer stress, anxiety, and depression (e.g., Minnes, 1998; Tausig, 1985; Traute & Hiebert-Murphy, 2002). Evidence even shows that such stress affects grandparents as well (Katz & Kessel, 2002). Birenbaum et al. (1990) noted that although parents and siblings of children with disabilities are good candidates for psychological counseling, such counseling was received by only one fourth to one third of family members from all family cases in their study.

One of the most profound findings from the Birenbaum et al. study (1990) was that the huge variation in the proportion of individuals in out-of-home placement depended largely on the availability of alternative services to the family. Fujiura et al. (1994) and others have found similar results. The ultimate step for an overburdened family (i.e., with both financial and psychosocial burdens) is to place their child with severe disabilities in residential care outside their family home. Although home care respite services are believed to materially minimize some of the social and psychological burdens of caring for an individual with disabilities, few families use such services. In 1998, Minnesota had a progressive system of care and reimbursement for families with members with disabilities, but only 470 respondents from a total random sample of over 6,809 families that were eligible for services took advantage of any reimbursement for such respite services—less than 7% of all families within the state's Medicaid HCBS Waiver program (Hewitt et al., 2000).

COST-ACCOUNTING FRAMEWORK
FOR ESTIMATING FAMILY COSTS

This review of the literature related to estimating and measuring the costs of family care for members with disabilities has clearly shown that there is a need for a conceptual framework that adequately addresses both the *added* costs and the *incidence* of the burden from such care. In almost all of the empirical studies to date, much confusion existed about the importance of differences between average and marginal costs and between who bears the financial and other burdens for delivering care and supporting services. Almost all studies have largely focused on the use of average costs in settings outside the family home and then only in the context of cash expenditures. In the development of an accounting framework for estimating the costs that families incur as a result of undertaking the care-giving function for their children and young adults with disabilities, the focus of concern should be on both marginal (i.e., added) and average costs and on perspective of burden. *Marginal costs* refer to the economic burden related to the care-giving functions that are in addition to those that they would have incurred in the absence of the condition. *Perspective* refers to the distribution of burden among the individual, family, and various outside agencies.

As we have already noted, costs to the family can be direct (out-of-pocket) expenditures, as well as indirect costs, which are costs resulting from lost opportunity. Direct expenditures can be for medical services (e.g., physician care, therapeutic services, hospitalization, drugs, medical supplies); training services (e.g., day activities, transportation to supported employment); other social services (e.g., legal services); direct recurring home costs (e.g., adaptive aids for toileting and feeding, special clothing); and direct nonrecurring home costs (e.g., special equipment, home renovations). When costs are incurred for a child with disabilities, the measured costs for families should be those that are in excess of the typical level of costs for a child without disabilities. In contrast, when estimating costs for adults with disabilities, the costs would be those that would be comparable to the adult living in an alternative residential setting outside the family home.

Indirect family costs, as noted earlier, can result from both forgone income and intangible, but real, additional stress. Family members give up time from work and other activities in order to provide care for the child or young adult. Only a few studies (e.g., Baldwin, 1985) have focused on the time lost from work and placed a value on it equal to how much family members would have earned had they worked. Forgone leisure time, however, is seldom included, even though family members give up many preferred activities. Several measurements can determine the value of both lost working and leisure time, but perhaps the most reasonable is to determine the hours devoted to a caregiving activity and apply a market price (i.e., the cost to purchase the activity).

Our concern is also with estimating the costs that society and others might incur as a result of providing special services outside of the family's budget. The cost of such services can be estimated from an enumeration of all services that the service recipient or family might receive in support of the individual with disabilities living within the home. Such services would include training services (e.g., day activity programs, supported employment), medical services (e.g., visiting nurse care, mental health services), and other social services (e.g., legal services, case managers). All of these out-of-pocket family expenditures, along with all direct and community-provided social services, need to be accounted for in any costing framework.

Most important, the perspective of who bears the burden of these costs needs to be clearly identified and understood. Without a proper perspective of who bears the cost burden in delivering services to individuals with disabilities, public policy is adrift. The establishment of priorities in delivering both resources and services to families in need is simply unattainable without such information. Who bears the financial burden of the service being delivered? Is it the federal or state government (and ultimately the taxpayers)? Is it the local government? Private individuals and agencies outside of government? The family itself? Such a perspective on the burden of costs is illustrated in the accounting framework of Table 4.1.

Note that in Table 4.1 all costs are distributed across all stakeholders in the delivery of services. All data in this table are illustrative for a young adult with developmental disabilities residing in a natural family setting. Several of the cost estimates (e.g., adult day/habilitation training) were drawn from averages for comparable individuals in similar studies (e.g., Hewitt et al., 2000). The cost estimates in this case would include all food, clothing, and housing that would have been provided in an alternative res-

Table 4.1. Costs of services to a family-based adult with severe intellectual disabilities

Expenditure component	Total social costs	Federal/ state govern- ment	Local govern- ment	Private contribu- tions	Client's family	Individual service recipient
			Distribution and burden of costs			
Habilitative services						
In-home food/clothing	$6,269	$0	$0	$0	$6,269	$0
Personal support	$551	$0	$0	$105	$446	$0
Adaptive aids	$46	$0	$0	$0	$46	$0
Other supplies	$390	$0	$0	$0	$390	$0
Home care assessment	$136	$136	$0	$0	$0	$0
Special equipment	$626	$626	$0	$0	$0	$0
Housing/renovations	$560	$0	$0	$0	$560	$0
Personal and attendant care (estimated market wages)	$15,382	$0	$0	$0	$15,382	$0
Training services						
Supported employment	$0	$0	$0	$0	$0	$0
Sheltered workshop	$0	$0	$0	$0	$0	$0
Adult day/habilitation training	$13,420	$9,394	$0	$4,026	$0	$0
Other special training	$780	$780	$0	$0	$0	$0
Transportation	$3,590	$2,350	$0	$0	$1,240	$0
Medical services						
Physician/dental care	$1,207	$1,207	$0	$0	$0	$0
Visiting nurse care	$678	$678	$0	$0	$0	$0
Therapeutic services	$0	$0	$0	$0	$0	$0
Other acute care	$0	$0	$0	$0	$0	$0
Hospitalization	$0	$0	$0	$0	$0	$0
Drugs and medical supplies	$1,584	$1,584	$0	$0	$0	$0
Transportation	$560	$0	$0	$0	$560	$0
Other social services						
Legal services	$93	$93	$0	$0	$0	$0
State/local administration	$2,477	$2,034	$443	$0	$0	$0
Social and case managers	$1,338	$1,338	$0	$0	$0	$0
Volunteers assistance	$834	$0	$0	$834	$0	$0
Transportation	$1,330	$0	$0	$1,180	$150	$0
Respite care	$3,345	$3,278	$67	$0	$0	
Family counseling	$64	$0	$64	$0	$0	$0
Total costs	$55,260	$23,498	$574	$6,145	$25,043	$0
Transfer payments	$0	$5,052	$0	$0	($5,052)	$0
Net costs	$55,260	$28,550	$574	$6,145	$19,991	$0

Notes: All data in this table are illustrative for a young adult with severe intellectual disabilities residing within a natural family setting. Costs for several community services are prorated from 1998 averages for comparable individuals in Minnesota (Hewitt et al., 2000).

idential facility. In the case of a child, such cost estimates may include only special food and clothing beyond regular child care, depending on the focus of the cost study. Reimbursements and budget support to the family are identified as transfer payments from various governmental agencies in determining net costs at the bottom of Table 4.1.

It is important to note that the cost estimates in Table 4.1 are only approximations and are not drawn directly from any single study, although in all cases attempts were made to approximate real average costs drawn from actual studies and are reported in nominal dollars for 1998. For example, the modest total family cost differences between Table 4.1 ($25,043) and Figure 4.1 ($26,995) are merely reflective of the differences between a young adult and a child with disabilities. Table 4.1 is only intended to illustrate the relative distribution of costs across various sources of support.

From this illustrative case, however, one can draw several inferences that are identified in the literature but seldom brought together in overall

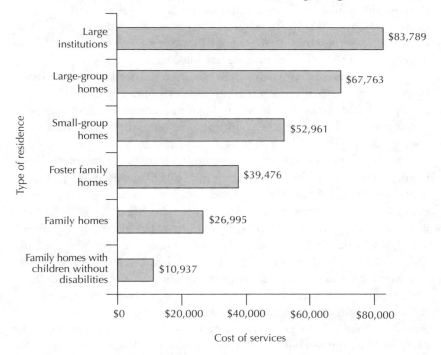

Figure 4.1. Direct annual costs of services for children with severe intellectual disabilities. *Note:* All costs are adjusted and estimated in FY 1998 prices. Bars do not represent indirect costs, such as foregone earnings, additional family stress, and lack of leisure, or special education services. These cost estimates are drawn from a variety of sources over time that include Anderson et al., 1987; Birenbaum et al., 1990; Hewitt et al., 2000; Hill et al., 1989; Lino, 1998; Nerney et al., 1991; and Stancliffe and Lakin, 1998.

view. First, almost half of the cost burden falls on the family, and this amount does *not* include foregone income and other indirect costs (e.g., stress, foregone leisure). If the service recipient lives in an alternative community setting, such as a group home, almost all of the family's financial burden is passed on to the federal and state governments. Thus, the social cost estimates in most family care studies are underestimated in rather gross terms, contributing to confusion in both public policy and the health of families and their children and adults with disabilities.

Second, the costs profiled in Table 4.1 are probably underestimated. Although evidence in Minnesota indicates that more than 20% of all Medicaid waiver community-based recipients received between $3,500 and $14,000 in emergency, therapeutic, or other extraordinary health care services (Hewitt et al., 2000), we have assumed that our illustrative recipient does not need those services. As a consequence, our estimated costs are conservative. Finally, many nongovernmental organizations independent of the family make material contributions to these services. Frequently, volunteers contribute money, services, and time in support of individuals with disabilities; these contributions are ignored when studies are conducted on behalf of governmental agencies.

Another way to view costs across community-based residential facilities is to examine their costs relative to the costs of family care. These relative profiles are frequently given in different studies by way of expressed nominal expenditures and costs, but they are seldom reported relative to each other in comparable dollars, as represented in Figure 4.1.

Notice in Figure 4.1 that costs appear to increase as one moves from natural family care without disabilities, to family care with individuals with disabilities, to foster family care, then to small-group homes, to increasing sizes of corporate group homes, and then to the largest of all residential facilities, state institutions, and hospitals. The data reported in Figure 4.1 are adjusted from their original studies and estimated in 1998 prices for the United States. The data estimates in Figure 4.1 only report on the average cost estimates and relative differences between care residences that have been reported by researchers since the 1980s. Although their methods, research designs, and accounting systems have varied a great deal over this time span, their relative cost estimates (i.e., estimates on taxpayer expenditures) are surprisingly consistent. Over time, family home care has been universally found to be the least expensive for governmental agency expenditures, with foster care a bit more and small- to large-group homes ranging between two to three times the public costs of family home care. These cost estimates have been drawn from a variety of sources, including Anderson,

Lakin, Bruininks, and Hill (1987); Birenbaum et al. (1990); Hewitt et al. (2000); Hill et al. (1989); Lakin, Hill, and Bruininks (1985); Lino (1998); Nerney, Conley, and Nisbet (1991); and Stancliffe and Lakin (1998).

The estimates reported in Figure 4.1 are intended to be averages and only illustrative of the differing residential perspectives. The baseline family costs for raising a single child without disabilities would average about $10,937 per year until the age of 17 for an average-income family (Lino, 1998). The average out-of-pocket family costs and other social costs for special services and health care for an individual with disabilities would add an additional $16,058 to these costs in a natural family-care setting (Hewitt et al., 2000). These latter costs for support services within the home residence do *not* count the additional annual average costs of approximately $5,363 for special education services within the schools (Lewis, Bruininks, & Thurlow, 1989), nor do they count foregone earnings.

The foster family care estimate of $39,476 and the small-group home estimate of $52,961 are adjusted (i.e., into 1998 prices) and are composite estimates from several study findings (Birenbaum et al., 1990; Hewitt et al., 2000; Hill et al., 1989). The larger corporate group home estimate of $67,763 (Hewitt et al., 2000) and the large institution residential facilities estimate of $83,789 also represent composites from several studies (Hewitt et al., 2000; Stancliffe & Lakin, 1998). All of these estimates are based on average expenditures for services rendered. If, for example, some services were not available or utilized, then such "costs" would also be reduced. These data do *not* provide insight into anything to do with the important dimensions of service outcomes. They report only on average cost estimates and relative differences between care residences that have been reported for the United States since the 1980s.

The data in Figure 4.1 represent only the relative magnitude of perceived social costs in average terms without regard to those variations in conditions that will undoubtedly cause variations in expenditures and costs (i.e., type and level of individual's disabilities, family income, number of siblings, stage in life cycle, location or region of country, state and local policies relative to service availability and funding). Nevertheless, one can view the relative expenditure and cost differences of differing residential facilities for 1998.

PROBLEMS IN PUBLIC POLICIES

The studies reviewed in this chapter reveal several important public policy problems that have clear implications for legislative proposals on behalf of families with both children and adults with disabilities. Although several of these were originally noted in Birenbaum and Cohen's (1993) review, the findings in this chapter and their importance merit additional mention. First, and perhaps most important for taxpayers, it is simply more cost-effective to provide greater assistance to caring families with children and adult family members with disabilities. Many writers and researchers (e.g., Birenbaum & Cohen, 1993; Fujiura et al., 1994; Meyers & Marcenko, 1989; Turnbull, Garlow, & Barber, 1991) have persuasively argued that more widespread implementation of family support programs can reduce demand for more costly out-of-home residential placement; but even if the costs of family care are not lower, the benefits are likely to be greater. Not only will the demand for lower-cost home care increase, but the quality of family life will materially increase as well (Meyers & Marcenko, 1989). As Fujiura and his colleagues note, "the marginal costs of supplementing and encouraging family-based care may represent a far more efficient use of limited service resources than the outright purchase of additional out-of-home capacity" (1994, p. 258). Why should current policies and practices continue to be counterproductive and inefficient?

The United States has successfully moved its public policies from support for large state institutions to small, community-based programs. The country now needs to move further to provide greater service support and financial incentives to families who elect to keep their children and young adults with disabilities in their natural family homes. Because of their disabilities, for example, the health care requirements of these children and adults should be viewed more broadly to include personal care and family support. Birenbaum and Cohen (1993) noted that all of the extraordinary care for children, adolescents, and adults results directly from their disabilities and that it is appropriate to regard all of these services as health-care related because, in the absence of their health condition, none of the extra care would be necessary. If these individuals were placed within an alternative residential facility within the community, such care would indeed be covered by Medicaid under much higher cost conditions. Why should a more favorable and caring environment in a natural home be discriminated against by public policy?

Public policies and funding should promote family-centered care. Birenbaum and Cohen again state the case in bold terms that "the family should be regarded as the unit for receiving services" (1993, p. 72). The proportion of individuals in residential placement outside the family home depends largely on the availability of financial support and outside services to the family (see Birenbaum et al., 1990, and Fujiura et al., 1994). The natural desire of parents to nurture their children during their growing years and on into adulthood should be especially encouraged for children and young adults who are highly vulnerable and at risk in our society. Again, why should such family nurture be discriminated against by public policy?

Perhaps the most vivid reminder of the counterproductive behavior of public policy has been the recent denial of financial support for families with a child with disabilities that arose when the U.S. Congress tightened the eligibility criteria for Supplemental Security Income (SSI) as it passed PL 104-193. Congress added within PL 104-193 the requirement for periodic continuing disability reviews (CDRs) and redeterminations for SSI children's eligibility. For example, children younger than age 18 are reviewed every 3 years to reestablish eligibility. This policy has resulted in the cessation of many cases based on the documentation of improved health status. Although ensuring the successful retention of individuals with disabilities within their own families was beginning to emerge as an important national policy, it suffered a major setback through this legislation. Thousands of families with children with disabilities lost their SSI benefits. More than two thirds of all families with members with disabilities who claim assistance under SSI are being denied such support.

PL 104-193 also required all children receiving SSI benefits to undergo a "redetermination" at age 18, even if they were still in school. At age 18, the individual must exhibit an inability to engage in any substantial paid employment because of a medically determined physical and/or mental impairment. Available reports from Social Security Administration Office (1998) reveal that very high criteria were employed in the administration of social security in 1998 and that over 56% of the initial age 18 redeterminations resulted in cessation.

Almost all of the national advocacy organizations in the field of disabilities (e.g., The Arc of the United States, Consortium for Citizens with Disabilities, Community Legal Services) and the national training and research centers have petitioned and argued strongly against the highly restrictive requirements employed in the implementation of this legislation. Nevertheless, implementation of the legislation has largely prevailed. In short, if individuals with disabilities are successful in gaining employment (i.e., their families successfully nurtured them, raised them, and facilitated their transition to work), they are not rewarded. If they do any substantial amount of work for pay, the family caregivers lose SSI as financial support. The legislation requires many low-income families to absorb the additional costs of care or place their family member in an alternative high-cost out-of-home residence. Surprisingly, during the congressional hearings on this legislation, many proponents of placing stricter limitations on SSI for children with disabilities questioned whether SSI cash benefits should have been provided in the first place.

The financing and organizing of long-term family supports and subsidies should be administratively simple and readily available (Lakin, Burwell, Hayden, & Jackson, 1992). Long-term care needs should be included in public policy thinking about children, particularly those with severe disabilities. This attention has already been given to long-term care for older adults, including new ways to expand home care, and it clearly needs to be expanded to include child home care and family services for children with chronic disabilities. The majority of children with severe disabilities cannot be left at home alone even for a few minutes; however, the only alternative that is fully supported in our public policies is to place the child or young adult in a community-based residence *outside the home.*

From the parents' perspective, residential placement is cost-effective because parents pay nothing after the first month, but the paradox is that home care may be the most cost-effective from a societal view, even though it is very costly to the family, which must either find free caregivers among their relatives or friends or pay the whole costs themselves.

> If a single source were to pay for both long-term residential care and for its substitutes, then the payer would have monetary incentive to provide a range of child care, home care, day programs, and respite services as alternatives to residential care. (Birenbaum & Cohen, 1993, p. 72)

If the current public policy focus on achieving independence for people with disabilities neglects the other members of their household, then such policies will always be minimized. Why should family care be discriminated against by federal health policy when national and state policies clearly favor more family care and reduced residential care?

Rather than continue to provide care in their family homes, parents are encouraged not only to place their children and young adults with disabilities in residential homes, but also to induce local units to prefer placements in higher cost ICF/MR types of units as well. In many states that have *not* taken full advantage of Medicaid HCBS Waiver programs, the higher costs to local political units for family placements provide incentives to these units to avoid higher-cost family placements and their fiscal impact on local budgets by emphasizing ICF/MR residences because they are federally subsidized. Again, we find that the financial burden of who pays for services has important policy implications.

Finally, both SSI and Medicaid can and should be expanded to increase the use of both home and community-based services. Although Medicaid HCBS Waivers have been available for states to adopt in order to use federal funds for services outside of institutions, more can and should be done to expand this program across all states. Surprisingly, by the mid-1990s, more than 20% of states still did not have adequate provisions for Medicaid HCBS Waivers (Lakin, Prouty, Smith, & Braddock, 1995). Similar problems exist with SSI as well; 72% of families with children with severe disabilities reportedly are being unserved or underserved through SSI benefits (Birenbaum & Cohen, 1993; Pear, 1997). Why should public policy favor tax deductions for dependent child care for all taxpayers, including middle- and upper-income groups, while denying medical and income assistance for lower-income families with children with severe disabilities? In short, families of children with intellectual disabilities deal with significant hardships, and choosing to care for their children at home is punished rather than rewarded (Hodapp & Zigler, 1993). This public policy is unacceptable in today's industrialized and democratized world.

CONCLUSION

Public policies in both taxation and expenditures in the United States should be based on the important principles of fairness and equity, efficiency, simplicity in understanding and access, and moral and human rights in delivery. Unfortunately, policies in support of family care for individuals with disabilities *fail* on all of these grounds. These policies are counterproductive relative to all of these principles. They discriminate against low-income families and effectively promote underemployment for family members and regressive forms of benefits by providing extraordinary tax benefits for child care for families with typically developing members. They also transfer much of the financial burden from taxpayers to the families themselves. They are clearly not cost-effective or efficient when promoting residential life outside of family homes. They are also often complicated and difficult for providing community services and for reimbursement support for families of individuals with disabilities. Public policies are simply wrong to deny the nurturing of family life to individuals with disabilities. In short, public policies in support of family care need to change and be more supportive, not only at the federal level, but also at state, county, and local levels.

REFERENCES

Abel-Smith, B., & Townsend, P. (1965). *The poor and the poorest*. London: Bell.

Anderson, D.J., Lakin, K.C., Bruininks, R.H., & Hill, B.K. (1987). *A national study of residential and support services for elderly persons with mental retardation*. Minneapolis: University of Minnesota, Center for Residential and Community Services.

Baldwin, S. (1985). *The costs of caring: Families with disabled children*. Boston: Routledge and Kegan Paul.

Baxter, C., Cummins, R., & Yiolitis, L. (2000). Parental stress attributed to family members with and without disability. *Journal of Intellectual & Developmental Disability, 25*(2), 105–118.

Birenbaum, A., & Cohen, H.J. (1993). On the importance of helping families: Policy implications from a national study. *Mental Retardation, 31*(2), 67–74.

Birenbaum, A., Guyot, D., & Cohen, H.J. (1990). *Health care financing for severe developmental disabilities*. Washington, DC: American Association on Mental Retardation.

Black, M.M., Molaison, V.A., & Smull, M.W. (1990). Families caring for a young adult with mental retardation: Service needs and urgency of community living requests. *American Journal on Mental Retardation, 95*, 32–39.

Boggs, E.M. (1979). Economic factors in family care. In R.H. Bruininks & G.C. Krantz (Eds.), *Family care of developmentally disabled members: Conference proceedings*. Minneapolis: University of Minnesota.

Braddock, D., Hemp, R., Parish, S., & Westrich, J. (1998). *State of the states in developmental disabilities*. Washington, DC: American Association on Mental Retardation.

Bradley, V.J., & Agosto, J.M. (1985). *Family care for persons with developmental disabilities*. Cambridge, MA: Human Services Research Institute.

Breslau, N., Salkever, D., & Staruch, K. (1982). Women's labor force activity and responsibilities for disabled dependents: A study of families with disabled children. *Journal of Health and Social Behavior, 23*, 169–183.

Bruns, D.A. (2000). Leaving home at an early age: Parents' decisions about out-of-home placement for young children with complex medical needs. *Mental Retardation, 38*(1), 50–60.

Campbell, E.M., & Heal, L.W. (1995). Prediction of cost, rates, and staffing by provider and client characteristics. *American Journal on Mental Retardation, 100*, 17–35.

Castellani, R.J., Downey, N.A., Thusig, M.B., & Bird, W.A. (1986). Availability and accessibility of family support services. *Mental Retardation, 21*(l), 71–79.

Chetwynd, J. (1985). Some costs of caring at home for an intellectually handicapped child. *Australia and New Zealand Journal of Developmental Disabilities, 11*(1), 35–40.

Chiu, L., Tang, K., Shyu, W., Huang, C., & Wang, S. (2000). Cost analyses of home care and nursing home services in the southern Taiwan area. *Public Health Nursing, 17*(5), 525–535.

Cole, D.A. (1986). Out-of-home child placement and family adaptation: A theoretical framework. *American Journal of Mental Deficiency, 91*, 226–236.

Cole, D.A., & Meyer, L.H. (1989). Impact of needs and resources on family plans to seek out-of-home placement. *American Journal on Mental Retardation, 93*(4), 380–387.

Cummins, R. (2001). The subjective well-being of people caring for a family member with a severe disability at home. *Journal of Intellectual & Developmental Disability, 26*(1), 83–100.

Darling, R.B. (1987). The economic and psychosocial consequences of disability: Family social relationships. *Marriage and Family Review, 11*(1–2), 45–61.

Edwards, C.S., & Beckham, L.J. (1984). Child cost user data updated to 1983. *Family Economics Review, 3,* 13–19.

Ellis, J., Luiselli, J., Amirault, D., Byrne, S., O'Malley-Cannon, B., Taras, M., Wolongevicz, J., & Sisson, R. (2002). Families of children with developmental disabilities: Assessment and comparison of self-reported needs in relation to situational variables. *Journal of Developmental and Physical Disabilities, 14*(2), 191–202.

Farber, B., & DeOllos, I. (2000). Increasing knowledge on family issues: A research agenda for 2000. In L. Rowitz (Ed.), *Mental retardation in the year 2000.* New York: Springer-Verlag.

Fujiura, G.T., & Braddock, D. (1999). Fiscal and demographic trends in mental retardation services: The emergence of the family. In L. Rowitz (Ed.), *Mental retardation in the year 2000.* New York: Springer-Verlag.

Fujiura, G.T., Roccoforte, J.A., & Braddock, D. (1994). Costs of family care for adults with mental retardation and related developmental disabilities. *American Journal on Mental Retardation, 99*(3), 250–261.

Gallagher, J.J., & Vietze, P.M. (1986). *Families of handicapped persons: Research, programs, and policy issues.* Baltimore: Paul H. Brookes Publishing Co.

Gunn, P., & Berry, R. (1987). Some financial costs of caring for children with Down syndrome at home. *Australia and New Zealand Journal of Developmental Disabilities, 13*(4), 187–193.

Haycox, A. (1995). *The costs and benefits of community care: A case study of people with learning difficulties.* Aldershot, United Kingdom: Avebury.

Hewitt, A., Larson, S., Lakin, C., Kwak, N., Sauer, J., Jendro, J., & Lightfoot, E. (2000). *An independent evaluation of the quality of services and system performance of Minnesota's Medicaid Home and Community-Based Services for persons with mental retardation and related conditions.* Minneapolis: University of Minnesota, Institute on Community Integration.

Hill, B.K., Lakin, K.C., Bruininks, R.H., Amado, A.N., Anderson, D.J., & Copher, J.I. (1989). *Living in the community: A comparative study of foster homes and small group homes for people with mental retardation* (Report No. 28). Minneapolis: University of Minnesota, Center for Residential and Community Services.

Hirst, M. (1985). Young adults with disabilities: Health, employment and financial costs for family caregivers. *Child: Care, Health & Development, 11,* 291–307.

Hodapp, R.M., & Zigler, E. (1993). Comparison of families of children with mental retardation and families of children without mental retardation. *Mental Retardation, 31*(2), 75–77.

Hogan, D.P., Rogers, M.L., & Msall, M.E. (2000). Functional limitations and key indicators of well-being in children with disability. *Archives of Pediatrics and Adolescent Medicine, 154*(10), 1042–1048.

Hyman, M. (1977). *The extra costs of disabled living*. London: National Fund for Research into Crippling Diseases and Disablement Income Group.

Jacobs, P., & McDermott, S. (1989). Family caregiver costs of chronically ill and handicapped children: Method and literature review. *Public Health Reports, 104*(2), 158–163.

Jaskulski, T.M., Lakin, K.C., & Zierman, S.A. (1995). *The journey to inclusion: A resource guide for state policymakers*. Washington, DC: U.S. Department of Health and Human Services, Presidential Committee on Mental Retardation.

Katz, S., & Kessel, L. (2002). Grandparents of children with developmental disabilities: Perceptions, beliefs and involvement in their care. *Issues in Comprehensive Pediatric Nursing, 25*(2), 113–128.

Lakin, K.C., Burwell, B.O., Hayden, M.F., & Jackson, M.E. (1992). *An independent assessment of Minnesota's Medicaid Home and Community-Based Services Waiver programs*. Minneapolis: University of Minnesota, Research and Training Center on Community Living, Institute on Community Integration.

Lakin, K.C., Hill, B., & Bruininks, R. (Eds.). (1985). *An analysis of Medicaid's intermediate care facility for the mentally retarded (ICF-MR) program*. Minneapolis: University of Minnesota, Research and Training Center on Community Living, Institute on Community Integration.

Lakin, K.C., Prouty, R., Smith, G., & Braddock, D. (1995). Places of residence of Medicaid HCBS recipients. *Mental Retardation, 33*(6), 406.

Lewis, D., & Bruininks, R. (1994). Costs of community-based residential services to individuals with mental retardation and other developmental disabilities. In M.F. Hayden & B.H. Abery (Eds.), *Challenges for a service system in transition: Ensuring quality community experiences for persons with developmental disabilities* (pp. 231–263). Baltimore: Paul H. Brookes Publishing Co.

Lewis, D., Bruininks, R., & Thurlow, M. (1989). Cost analysis for district level special education planning, budgeting and administrating. *Journal of Education Finance, 14*(4), 466–483.

Lino, M. (1998). *Expenditures on children by families: 1997 annual report* (Publication Number 1528–1997). Washington, DC: U.S. Department of Agriculture, Center for Nutrition Policy and Promotion.

Llewellyn, G., Dunn, P., Fante, M., Turnbull, L., & Grace, R. (1999). Family factors influencing out-of-home placement decisions. *Journal of Intellectual Disability Research, 43*(3), 219–233.

Meyers, J.C., & Marcenko, M.O. (1989). Impact of a cash subsidy program for families of children with severe developmental disabilities. *Mental Retardation, 27*(6), 383–387.

Minnes, P.N. (1998). Mental retardation: The impact upon the family. In J.A. Burack, R.M. Hodapp, & E. Zigler (Eds.), *Handbook of mental retardation and development* (pp. 693–712). Cambridge, United Kingdom: Cambridge University Press.

Nerney, T., Conley, R., & Nisbet, J. (1991). *A cost analysis of residential systems serving persons with severe disabilities: New directions in economic and policy research*. Cambridge, MA: Human Services Research Institute.

Newacheck, P.W., & Halfon, N. (1986). Access to ambulatory care services for economically disadvantaged children. *Pediatrics, 78*, 813–819.

Pear, R. (1997, November 16). Disabled youths are wrongly cut from aid program. *The New York Times National Sunday*, pp. 1, 30.

Personal Responsibility and Work Opportunity Reconciliation Act of 1996, PL 104-193, 42 U.S.C. §§ 1305 *et seq.*

Prouty, R., & Lakin, K.C. (1998). *Residential services for persons with developmental disabilities: Status and trends through 1997.* Minneapolis: University of Minnesota, Institute on Community Integration.

Rees, S., & Emerson, A. (1983). The costs of caring for disabled children at home. *Australian Rehabilitation Review, 7,* 26–31.

Rossiter, L.F., & Wilensky, G.R. (1982). *Out-of-pocket expenditures for personal health services* (Data Preview 13). Washington, DC: National Center for Health Services Research.

Seltzer, M.M. (2000). Family caregiving across the full life span. In L. Rowitz (Ed.), *Mental retardation in the year 2000.* New York: Springer-Verlag.

Seltzer, M.M., & Krauss, M.W. (1989). Aging parents with adult mentally retarded children: Family risk factors and sources of support. *American Journal on Mental Retardation, 94,* 303–312.

Social Security Administration Office, Office of Disability. (1998). *Review of SSA's implementation of new SSI child disability legislation* (SSA Pub. No. 64-070). Baltimore: Author.

Stancliffe, R.J., & Lakin, K.C. (1998). Analysis of expenditures and outcomes of residential alternatives for persons with developmental disabilities. *American Journal on Mental Retardation, 102*(6), 552–568.

Taanila, A., Syrjala, L., Kokkonen, J., & Jarvelin, M. (2002). Coping of parents with physically and/or intellectually disabled children. *Child: Care, Health & Development, 28*(1), 73–86.

Tausig, M. (1985). Factors in family decision-making about placement for developmentally disabled individuals. *American Journal of Mental Deficiency, 89,* 352–361.

Traute, B., & Hiebert-Murphy, D. (2002). Family adjustment to childhood developmental disability. *Journal of Pediatric Psychology, 27*(3), 271–280.

Turnbull, H.R., Garlow, J.E., & Barber, P.A. (1991). A policy analysis of family support for families with members with disabilities. *Kansas Law Review, 39,* 739–782.

Wikler, L. (1986). Family stress theory and research on families of children with mental retardation. In J.J. Gallagher & P.M. Vietze (Eds.), *Families of handicapped persons: Research, programs, and policy issues.* Baltimore: Paul H. Brookes Publishing Co.

CHAPTER 5

Home and Community-Based Services

Costs, Utilization, and Outcomes

*K. Charlie Lakin, Amy Hewitt, Sheryl A. Larson,
and Roger J. Stancliffe*

Medicaid Home and Community-Based Services (HCBS) Waiver programs have become the most widely used and by far the most rapidly growing programs for financing long-term services and supports for individuals with intellectual and developmental disabilities in the United States. HCBS Waiver programs are intended to support people in their homes and communities as an alternative to more costly institutional care. This chapter, based on comprehensive evaluation by the University of Minnesota, describes Minnesota's HCBS Waiver program and participants and those living in Intermediate Care Facilities for Persons with Mental Retardation (ICFs/MR), factors associated with variations in HCBS utilization and expenditures, and the association between service costs and quality-of-life outcomes. It discusses the implication of the findings for HCBS policy in Minnesota, in particular, and for long-term care systems, in general.

MINNESOTA'S HCBS WAIVER PROGRAM

Medicaid HCBS Waiver for people with intellectual and developmental disabilities began in Minnesota in 1984. In June 2002, there were 14,735

The full report of the study described here (Hewitt, Larson, & Lakin, 2000) can be found at http://rtc.umn.edu

The research and analysis reported in this chapter were supported by the Minnesota Department of Human Services (Agreement #5402455T53) and the National Institute on Disability and Rehabilitation Research, U.S. Department of Education (Grant #H133B031116). The contents of this chapter do not necessarily reflect the official position of these agencies.

HCBS Waiver recipients in Minnesota, or 293.5 HCBS Waiver recipients per 100,000 state residents, which was the fifth largest per-capita utilization rate in the nation. In fiscal year (FY) 2002, Minnesota spent $699.7 million for HCBS, or $139.39 per state resident (Prouty, Smith, & Lakin, 2003), which was the second-highest amount in the United States. In FY 2003, total HCBS expenditures in Minnesota increased to $796.8 million (Prouty et al., 2003). Figure 5.1 shows the relative growth in out-of-family home residential services in Minnesota funded through the ICF/MR and HCBS Waiver programs.

In its original and subsequent applications for federal approval to provide HCBS, Minnesota has been authorized to provide a wide array of

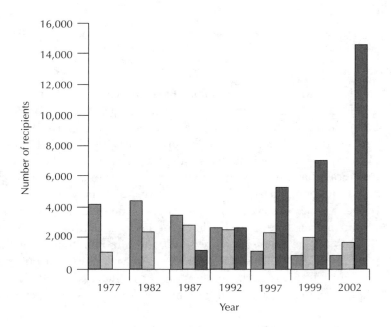

	1977	1982	1987	1992	1997	1999	2002
■ ICF/MR large (16+)	4,251	4,187	3,702	2,618	1,331	1,056	1,023
☐ ICF/MR small (4–15)	1,052	2,412	2,847	2,584	2,273	2,045	1,733
■ HCBS Waiver	0	0	1,423	2,890	5,422	7,102	14,735

Number of recipients

Figure 5.1.   Medicaid-funded long-term care service recipients by program, 1977–2002.

HCBS, including case management, residential habilitation (supported living services and in-home support services), day training and habilitation, homemaker/chore services, respite care (both in-home and out-of-home), and adaptive aids (including home and vehicle modifications), crisis respite, 24-hour emergency assistance, adult day care, supported employment, specialist services, caregiver training and education, housing access coordination, assistive technology, personal care attendant, personal support, transportation, service recipient training and education, and service recipient–directed community supports. Minnesota's "menu" of HCBS is among the most comprehensive in the United States.

Administration of Minnesota's HCBS Waiver Program

The HCBS Waiver program in Minnesota is managed and monitored by the state Department of Human Services. It is administered by the social services agencies of Minnesota's 87 counties.

Allocations of HCBS Waivers to Individuals   The number of individuals allowed to receive HCBS Waivers is managed by the state. Allocations of authority to add service recipients are awarded to counties based on a number of factors including the county size (population and total people with mental retardation and related conditions being served), county efforts to pursue state priorities for its long-term support system (e.g., downsizing large ICFs/MR, closing community ICFs/MR, preventing out-of-home placement of children, serving individuals with elderly parents), the number of people requesting and eligible for HCBS Waivers, historical ICF/MR use, and county plans to develop new resources.

Management of Allocated Funds   Counties are authorized to serve an established number of people within an expenditure limit known as a *unique allowable daily average*. Since FY 1996, state allocations of spending authority to counties have been established by a *waiver allocation structure* that provides one of four substantially different levels of resource allocation to counties for each new HCBS Waiver recipient. The waiver allocation structure is based on an assessment of physical, functional, medical, and behavioral support needs. County spending authority for people receiving HCBS Waivers prior to 1996 was not affected by the introduction of the waiver allocation structure.

HCBS resource allocations are not provided directly to an individual as an individual budget but are allocated to the individual's county to be managed as part of an overall pool of resources for serving all HCBS Waiver recipients within that county. For example, if the resource allocation structure provides a county $150 per day to serve an individual, the county could create a service plan for the individual that would cost substantially more (or less) provided that the amount of spending did not cause the total county spending to exceed the county's allowable limit for supporting all of its HCBS Waiver recipients. Important in this regard, counties do not participate in the HCBS financing, so they have no incentive to underspend their allowable limit, except as a buffer to overspending.

MINNESOTA HCBS WAIVER EVALUATION DESIGN AND METHODS

In 2000, the University of Minnesota was contracted by the Minnesota Department of Human Services to conduct an evaluation of its HCBS (Hewitt, Larson, & Lakin, 2000). The project was guided by an advisory group consisting of major stakeholder groups. Research methodologies used in this study included 1) analyses of existing state data sets on HCBS Waiver recipients, expenditures, and maltreatment reports; 2) direct interviews with individual recipients; 3) written surveys of residential and vocational provider agencies, families, case managers, and direct-support staff; 4) telephone interviews with county HCBS coordinators; and 5) meetings with representatives of stakeholder groups.

Research Questions

Hewitt et al.'s (2000) study examined a number of broad research questions. A subset of these questions is discussed in this chapter, including the following:

- What are the demographic characteristics of HCBS Waiver recipients, and how do their characteristics differ from those of ICF/MR recipients? How do HCBS and ICF/MR service costs differ?

- What are the utilization and costs of specific HCBS and other Medicaid services? How do they differ across service recipient groups?

- How do the total service costs for HCBS Waiver recipients vary? How do costs for various categories of service for HCBS Waiver recipients vary? Are expenditures related to quality-of-life outcomes?

Individual HCBS Waiver Recipient Sample

From a statewide total of 6,548 HCBS Waiver recipients at the time of the study in 1999, a sample was randomly selected that included a controlled oversample of 35 people from racial/ethnic minorities to assure a sufficient sample to permit reasonably reliable estimates of the HCBS experiences of individuals from minority groups. The sampling strategy was controlled to assure proportional representation of HCBS Waiver recipients from the Twin Cities metropolitan (metro) area, non–Twin Cities urban counties with 50,000 or more residents, and "rural" counties with fewer than 50,000 residents. Table 5.1 compares selected characteristics of the 474 people who participated in the study with characteristics of all HCBS Waiver recipients in Minnesota. In general, the sample was statistically equal to the population, with the exception of a higher proportion of females than the HCBS Waiver recipient population (47.9% and 41.9%), and, of course, minority groups, who were overrepresented by design. No statistically significant differences existed between the sample and the population of HCBS Waiver recipients in the average annual amounts allowed to the county for expenditures for HCBS ($47,461 and $48,650, respectively).

State Data Sets

The Minnesota Department of Human Services provided access to three primary data sources for this study: screening document files, administrative reports, and HCBS payment files.

Screening Document Files The Minnesota "screening document" provided demographic, diagnostic, functional, behavioral, health, and service-need information on all 6,548 individuals with intellectual and developmental disabilities receiving HCBS Waivers at the time of the study (including the 474 people in the sample). The files used in this study contained the most recent screening available.

Administrative Reports Information from the Center for Medicare & Medicaid Services (CMS) Form 372 and Form 64 cost reports was used to compare expenditures of HCBS Waiver and ICF/MR recipients, including expenditures for related Medicaid state plan services. A 1999 Report to the Legislature, "Home and Community Based Services for Persons with Mental Retardation and Related Conditions" (Department of Human Services, 1999) provided background on Department of Human Services goals for HCBS and perspectives on trends/challenges in the program.

Table 5.1. Selected demographic characteristics of sample members

Characteristic	HCBS Nonsample		HCBS Sample		χ^2/Sig.
	N	Percent	N	Percent	
Region					1.42
Twin Cities metro	2,930	44.7%	204	43.0%	
Non–Twin Cities urban	1,281	19.6%	88	18.6%	
Rural	2,337	35.7%	182	38.4%	
Level of intellectual disability					6.58
Related condition	213	3.3%	15	3.2%	
Mild	2,189	33.4%	141	29.7%	
Moderate	1,745	26.6%	141	29.7%	
Severe	1,318	20.1%	91	19.2%	
Profound	1,057	16.1%	86	18.1%	
Unspecified	26	0.4%	0	0.0%	
Age group					5.50
Birth–5 years	43	0.7%	4	0.8%	
6–17 years	752	11.5%	64	13.5%	
18–39 years	3,012	46.0%	193	40.7%	
40–64 years	2,320	35.4%	179	37.8%	
65+ years	421	6.4%	34	7.2%	
Gender					6.49*
Male	3,804	58.1%	247	52.1%	
Female	2,744	41.9%	227	47.9%	
Race/ethnicity					10.10*
Black non-Hispanic	157	2.4%	17	3.6%	
American Indian/Alaskan Native	92	1.4%	9	1.9%	
Asian/Pacific Islander	43	0.7%	8	1.7%	
Hispanic	36	0.6%	3	0.6%	
White	6,212	95.0%	437	92.2%	
White/non-white					7.56*
Non-white	328	5.0%	37	7.8%	
White	6,212	95.0%	437	92.2%	

* $p < .05$

HCBS Payment Files   State payment files were used to obtain actual payments for HCBS during FY 1998. The obtained data included total expenditures for each individual, which could be further aggregated by county service provider, resource allocation group, and service procedure code. By merging the obtained data with the screening document data, a wide range of demographic, diagnostic, and other descriptions was integrated into a single comprehensive data file for each individual.

Additional Instrumentation

Several survey instruments and interview protocols were developed or adopted to collect more detailed information about services and outcomes for sample members. The service recipient interview protocol for the study was developed by the Human Services Research Institute with the National Association of State Directors of Developmental Disabilities Services for their "National Core Indicators" Project. The Consumer Interview protocol was piloted by the Human Service Research Institute to establish its reliability and validity (Smith & Ashbaugh, 1998). This protocol was augmented at the recommendation of the Project Advisory Committee to include items of importance to individual HCBS Waiver recipients. Additional survey instruments, developed and tested in previous research at the University of Minnesota, were also employed at the advice of the Project Advisory Committee. These instruments included the Individual Case Manager Survey, General Case Manager Survey, Service Provider Survey (residential and vocational versions), Family Survey (in-home and out-of-home versions), and Direct Support Staff Survey (residential and vocational versions).[1] An interview protocol for county HCBS coordinators was developed based on an instrument being used in a national evaluation of HCBS. This interview protocol was reviewed by Project Advisory Committee members and revised (instruments are available at http://rtc.umn.edu).

Data Collection and Response Rates

Data were gathered through face-to-face interviews, telephone interviews, group discussions, and written surveys. Interviews were completed for 377 of the 405 adult HCBS Waiver recipients who consented to participate (a response rate of 93%). Children were not interviewed. Written surveys were mailed or hand delivered to specific participants. Response rates on written surveys varied by respondent group: family members (50%), provider agencies (60% residential and 50% vocational), case managers (69%), and direct-support staff (24% residential and 23% vocational).

---

[1] All of the surveys are available upon request from K. Charlie Lakin.

FINDINGS

This section summarizes some of the major findings of this study with regard to service costs, use, and outcomes. The full report (236 pp.) is available at the authors' web site at http://rtc.umn.edu/res.

Utilization of HCBS Versus ICF/MR

Table 5.2 presents the distribution and characteristics of Minnesota's ICF/MR and HCBS Waiver recipients, with HCBS Waiver recipients divided

Table 5.2. Distribution of Home and Community-Based Services (HCBS) Waiver program and Intermediate Care Facility for Persons with Mental Retardation (ICF/MR) recipients by residence and selected characteristics, 1999

	Type of residence									
	ICF/MR		HCBS						ICFs/MR and HCBS Total	
			SLS		Non-SLS		HCBS Total			
Characteristic	N	Percent	N	Percent	N	Percent	N	Percent	N	Percent
Age										
Children (0–17 years)	75	8.3%	207	22.9%	623	68.8%	830	91.7%	905	100.0%
Adults (18+ years)	3269	34.6%	5638	59.6%	554	5.9%	6192	65.4%	9461	100.0%
Total	3344	32.3%	5845	56.4%	1177	11.4%	7022	67.7%	10366	100.0%
Level of intellectual disability										
Related condition	29	18.5%	12	7.6%	116	73.9%	128	81.5%	157	100.0%
Mild	613	20.8%	2001	68.0%	329	11.2%	2330	79.2%	2943	100.0%
Moderate	720	27.6%	1500	57.6%	386	14.8%	1886	72.4%	2606	100.0%
Severe	865	38.0%	1190	52.3%	219	9.6%	1409	62.0%	2274	100.0%
Profound	1116	49.4%	1041	46.1%	102	4.5%	1143	50.6%	2259	100.0%
Unspecified	1	3.7%	1	3.7%	25	92.6%	26	96.3%	27	100.0%
Challenging behavior										
Severe property destruction	304	29.3%	585	56.4%	148	14.3%	733	70.7%	1037	100.0%
Severe physical aggression	414	29.7%	778	55.8%	202	14.5%	980	70.3%	1394	100.0%
Race/ethnicity										
White, Non-Hispanic	3204	32.5%	5589	56.7%	1060	10.8%	6649	67.5%	9853	100.0%
Black, Non-Hispanic	69	28.4%	117	48.1%	57	23.5%	174	71.6%	243	100.0%
Native American	36	26.3%	82	59.9%	19	13.9%	101	73.7%	137	100.0%
Asian/Pacific Islander	17	25.0%	29	42.6%	22	32.4%	51	75.0%	68	100.0%
Hispanic	9	18.8%	26	54.2%	13	27.1%	39	81.2%	48	100.0%

into those in Supported Living Services (SLS) settings and those in other "non-SLS" settings. SLS is a service type that includes comprehensive residential supervision, training, and other assistance, almost always (for 87% of recipients) in small-group homes with no more than 4 residents operated by a service-provider agency. Non-SLS settings included family homes, foster family homes, and the service recipient's own home.

Only 8.3% of children (0–17 years) receiving long-term services and supports in Minnesota live in ICFs/MR. A quarter (24.9%) of children receiving HCBS Waiver–financed services live in SLS settings, and the remaining 75.1% live with their own or a foster family. Of the 2,943 Minnesotans with mild mental retardation (28.4% of all recipients of long-term services and supports), only 20.8% were ICF/MR residents; 79.2% were HCBS Waiver recipients. In contrast, of those with profound intellectual disabilities, 49.4% were in ICFs/MR, and 50.6% received HCBS Waivers. Only 1.8% of HCBS Waiver recipients were screened as eligible based on a related condition alone. The vast majority (70.9%) of non-SLS, HCBS Waiver–financed services were delivered in the individual's family home (parents or extended family).

Table 5.3 shows that HCBS Waiver recipients were proportionately more likely than those living in ICFs/MR to exhibit severe property destruction (10.5%) or severe physical aggression (14.0%) than were ICF/MR residents (9.3% and 12.8%, respectively). They were also more likely to display temper outbursts, verbal or gestural aggression, running away, inappropriate sexual behavior, and law-breaking behavior. A higher proportion of ICF/MR residents were reported to engage in serious or very serious self-injurious behavior, to have "other" challenging behavior, and to eat nonnutritive substances. Overall, these data suggest that ICF/MR and HCBS Waiver recipients have similar levels of challenging behavior.

Supports and Services Received

Although HCBS offers a wide variety of services with the potential to support people in many different ways in many different kinds of places, there was notable consistency in the settings and services in the lives of Minnesota's recipients.

Current Residence The most common living arrangement for HCBS Waiver recipients was an SLS setting, licensed as "corporate foster care" with shift staff (65.4% of recipients of all ages and more than 80% of adults 40 years and older). Other HCBS Waiver recipients were living with their immediate family (15.6%), living with live-in caregivers (7.5%),

Table 5.3. Support needs for Home and Community-Based Service (HCBS) Waiver program and Intermediate Care Facility for Persons with Mental Retardation (ICF/MR) recipients (Screening document)

	ICF/MR	HCBS	Total
Number of people	3,344	7,022	10,366
Level of support			
24-hour awake supervision	58.7%	24.2%	34.9%
Independent living skills (Participates only with assistance/Unable to participate)			
Self-care	46.2%	34.0%	37.7%
Leisure skills	52.9%	40.1%	44.1%
Household management	57.9%	45.2%	49.2%
Community-living skills	71.7%	58.3%	62.5%
Money management	83.7%	73.5%	76.8%
Challenging behavior (Severe or very severe)			
Temper outbursts	16.3%	17.4%	17.0%
Physical aggression	12.8%	14.0%	13.6%
Verbal/gestural aggression	11.9%	13.5%	13.0%
Injurious to self	11.8%	10.6%	11.0%
Property destruction	9.3%	10.5%	10.1%
Other challenging behavior	9.9%	9.5%	9.7%
Runs away	4.7%	5.6%	5.3%
Inappropriate sexual behavior	4.9%	5.2%	5.2%
Eats non-nutritive substances	4.6%	3.5%	3.8%
Breaks laws	1.8%	2.1%	2.0%

living with a host foster family (5.6%), living in their own home (4.5%), living with extended family members (0.4%), or living in some other type of residence (0.9%).

HCBS Waiver–Funded Services   The most common HCBS Waiver–funded services were SLS (83.2% of recipients), day training and habilitation (67.8%), and home modifications (40.2%). Other HCBS Waiver–funded services received by between 10% and 20% of HCBS Waiver recipients were in-home family support, specialist services, crisis respite, and assistive technology.

Specific Vocational Services

More than two thirds of HCBS Waiver recipients received day training and habilitation, and/or vocational services financed within the HCBS Waiver program. The primary "other" sources of day/vocation service funding were vocational rehabilitation programs (9.2% of recipients) and non–

HCBS Waiver–financed day training and habilitation services (1.3% of recipients). Although payment files indicated that relatively few HCBS Waiver recipients (1.0%) were receiving supported employment services as a distinct service, the service recipient interviews revealed that many more recipients were actually receiving supported employment and other types of work-related services from day training and habilitation providers. Table 5.4 summarizes the various types of vocational supports provided to adults who were receiving HCBS Waivers and were interviewed for this study.

Overall, 59.5% of all adults interviewed reported working in a center or facility-based program; 35.8% in full or part-time supported employment in community settings; 31.5% in enclaves or work crews in the community; and 23.0% reported receiving nonvocational day training and habilitation supports. (Totals add to more than 100% because individuals could receive more than one type of support.) Overall, 26.8% of adults worked in supported employment, work crew, or enclave settings exclusively; 27.4% worked in both supported employment or work crew/enclave and in facility-based employment; 29.5% worked but only in a center-based program; and 16.3% did not work at all, but instead received supports in a nonvocational day program setting.

There were significant county-type differences in the proportion of HCBS Waiver recipients who received the vocational supports. HCBS Waiver recipients in rural communities were significantly more likely to participate in facility-based work and significantly less likely to participate in supported employment. Enclave and work crew support models were significantly more common for adults in the non–Twin Cities urban counties than in the Twin Cities metro or rural counties. Center-based nonwork was significantly less common in the non–Twin Cities urban counties.

Table 5.4. Type of vocational supports received by adult sample members (consumer interview)

	Region				
Vocational supports	Twin Cities metro $N = 138$	Non–Twin Cities urban $N = 68$	Rural $N = 147$	Total	χ^2
Facility-based work	49.3%	54.4%	71.4%	59.5%	15.40***
Supported employment	45.4%	40.0%	23.3%	35.8%	14.97***
Enclave or work crew	26.5%	46.2%	29.2%	31.5%	8.30*
Nonvocational day program	29.9%	8.1%	23.0%	23.0%	11.37**

Note: One person could receive more than one type of vocational service or support.
*$p < .05$, ** $p < .01$, *** $p < .001$

COSTS OF HCBS

HCBS expenditures were examined generally and for various individual services. Expenditures for different services, service recipients, and county types are summarized next. These summaries are drawn from payments for Minnesota's HCBS Waiver recipients in FY 1998. An explanation of distinctions among three terms, *allowable*, *authorized*, and *paid*, is helpful in understanding analyses of expenditures:

- *Allowable*—The amount of money the state provides the county pool of HCBS funds based on the characteristics of individuals as identified in their screening document.

- *Authorized*—The amount of money authorized by the county to be spent for services that are included in that individual's service plan.

- *Paid*—The amount of money that is actually paid out to service providers for the authorized hours/units of service that they have provided.

HCBS Versus ICF/MR Expenditures

Table 5.5 uses Minnesota's Form 372 report to the federal government on HCBS expenditures and its Form 64 report on ICF/MR billings to compare total Medicaid payments, long-term services and supports, and health services for HCBS Waiver and ICF/MR recipients. In FY 1998, the average annual cost of HCBS for each HCBS Waiver recipient was $47,786. ICF/MR average annual expenditures reported in CMS Form 64 reports were $63,744. In addition to the HCBS and ICF/MR expenditures, the state estimated an additional $5,474.60 per person in expenditures for state plan health services for HCBS Waiver recipients and an additional $4,018.85 in expenditures for state plan services for ICF/MR recipients. The primary difference in health services costs was reported in the "other" category. Among the "other" services was personal care, which was frequently used for HCBS Waiver recipients. For the average Minnesota HCBS Waiver recipient, residential habilitation or SLS made up 69.0% of all health and social services expenditures for the year.

Comparative Expenditures in Minnesota and the United States

In 1999, Minnesota's combined ICF/MR and HCBS utilization rate of 213.6 per 100,000 was 53% more than the national average of 139.5 per 100,000 (Prouty & Lakin, 2000). Because of its high utilization rate for

Table 5.5. Average annual expenditures for Medicaid services for Home and Community-Based Services (HCBS) Waiver program and Intermediate Care Facility for Persons with Mental Retardation (ICF/MR) recipients adjusted for average days of enrollment, 1998

Type of service	ICF/MR	HCBS*
Social services		
Case management		1,416.49
Adult day care/day training and habilitation		8,367.37
Supported employment		9.78
Assistive technology		4.08
Caregiver training and education		1.48
Consumer-directed community support		6.77
Environmental modifications		204.93
Residential habilitation (supported-living service)		36,548.58
Homemaker		24.21
Personal support		104.67
Respite care (including crisis)		1,018.75
Specialist services		75.93
Transportation		0.24
24-hour emergency assistance		3.18
Total social services	$63,744.00**	$47,786.46*
Health services		
Inpatient hospital	249.98	655.74
Physician services	255.81	326.38
Outpatient hospital clinic	168.68	180.62
Laboratory and X-ray service	42.52	46.39
Prescribed drug	1,607.81	1,583.95
Other acute care	*1,628.73*	*2,681.52*
Total health services	*4,018.85**	*5,474.60**
Total social and health services	$67,762.85	$52,961.06

Sources of expenditure data: * Minnesota's CMS 372; ** CMS 64.

Note: Average annual cost for each HCBS recipient by individual service cost was adjusted for average annual days of HCBS enrollment (344). The unadjusted total (i.e., total expenditures divided by unduplicated recipient counts) was $45,037. HCFA 64 expenditures were divided by the average daily ICF/MR recipients as computed by mid-point between first and last day ICF/MR residents in FY 1998.

HCBS and ICFs/MR, Minnesota tends to have higher overall expenditures for ICFs/MR and HCBS than do other states. In FY 1999, Minnesota's combined expenditures equaled $113.88 per state resident as compared with the national average of $65.53. Although Minnesota's overall expenditures were relatively high, its average expenditures for each service recipient were considerably nearer to the national average. In FY 1999, Minnesota had average annual per-recipient expenditures for the combined ICF/MR and HCBS Waiver programs of $53,501, as compared with $47,985 nationwide (Prouty & Lakin, 2000).

Further examination of Minnesota's ICF/MR and HCBS expenditures reveals a substantially different pattern than the nation as a whole. Minnesota's average annual expenditure per ICF/MR resident ($60,600) was substantially less than the national average ($81,830). National HCBS expenditures in FY 1999, however, were $32,750 per recipient, whereas Minnesota expenditures per recipient were $51,545.

Factors Associated with Minnesota Expenditures
Two major factors contribute to the relatively low ICF/MR expenditures in Minnesota. Minnesota has nearly eliminated its state institutions so that ICF/MR resident expenditures are predominately those of private, less costly ICFs/MR. On June 30, 1999, nationally 41% of ICF/MR recipients lived in state institutions, which had an average national cost of $107,550. By the end of FY 1999, Minnesota's dwindling number of state institution residents made up only 2.3% of its ICF/MR residents, but these institutions had an annual average expenditure of $224,500 per person (Prouty & Lakin, 2000).

Another factor accounting for Minnesota's relatively low cost of ICF/MR care is its relatively less-impaired populations residing in ICFs/MR. In 1999, 40.7% of Minnesota's ICF/MR population was made up of people with mild, moderate, or no mental retardation, as compared with 28.6% in ICFs/MR nationally. Among Minnesota's ICF/MR population, only 33.5% were people with profound mental retardation as compared with 48.1% nationally (Karon & Beutel, 2000).

Two other related factors contribute to the relatively high expenditures for HCBS in Minnesota when compared with the United States as a whole. The first relates to the movement of people with severe disabilities out of Minnesota's institutions into community HCBS Waiver–financed settings and the related low rates of placement into ICFs/MR of people with severe disabilities who have recently entered the service system. As Minnesota's state institution populations decreased from over 1,033 residents in June 1992 to 72 residents in June 1999, the HCBS Waiver program was the primary means of financing community services for people who often needed rather high levels of support.

A second factor in Minnesota's relatively high HCBS costs relates to the previously mentioned statistics that showed that relatively few of Minnesota's HCBS Waiver recipients are served in their family homes. In 1999, 15.9% of Minnesota's HCBS Waiver recipients lived with relatives, as compared with 34% nationally. Although no national data are available on cost implications of these differences, obviously the value of the direct support provided by family members is substantial. In Minnesota, for example, the average annual HCBS expenditure in FY 1998 for people living in their family homes was $19,881.69 as compared with $50,209.76 for people living outside the family home.

EXPENDITURE PATTERNS FOR HCBS

This section describes analyses of amounts, variations, and associated factors in expenditures for HCBS in Minnesota.

Allowable, Authorized, and Paid Expenditures

In 1992, the Minnesota legislature required the Department of Human Services to develop plans for implementation of a system of rate setting for HCBS Waivers that "bases funding on assessed need" (Minnesota Legislature, p. 1146). In May 1995, the legislature formally authorized the department's plan for implementing the waiver allocation structure. This methodology was implemented with new HCBS Waiver recipients beginning in FY 1996. Prior to implementation of this methodology, the state added the same amount of funds to each county's pool of resources to provide HCBS Waivers for most people entering the state's HCBS system, irrespective of an individual's degree of support needed. Exceptions were made in certain circumstances to overcome the disincentives for counties to accommodate the state's deinstitutionalization objectives. Thus, a system of "enhanced" and "enriched" funding became based on the placements from which people came rather than what they needed once they entered the community. This system was a source of considerable public criticism.

Beginning in FY 1996, the amounts added to county pools for each new HCBS Waiver recipient were determined by the profile exhibited by the new HCBS Waiver enrollees' screening document (Department of Human Services, 1996). These allocation amounts differ markedly according to the assessed level. Although actual operational definitions are confidential, in general, the levels represent:

- Level 1: Very high self-care needs or mental illness and destructive behavior

- Level 2: High self-care needs or aggressive/destructive behavior

- Level 3: Limited self-care needs but no major behavior problems, or limited self-care needs but aggressive/destructive behavior
- Level 4: Limited self-care needs and no major behavior problems.

The pool of resources managed by counties for people receiving HCBS Waivers prior to implementation of the waiver allocation structure were not recomputed as the waiver allocation structure was implemented.

HCBS Waivers Authorized and Paid

Table 5.6 presents a summary of the average amounts of funding authorized and actually paid by counties for various HCBS in 1998. For each of Minnesota's 23 HCBS, the table presents for children (0–17 years) and adults 1) the average amount of expenditures authorized by counties for HCBS, 2) the average amount paid for each service, 3) the total amount paid for each service in 1998, and 4) the average per-person difference between the amount authorized and the amount paid.

Differences between authorized and paid costs were related to a number of factors. In attempting to maximize their use of HCBS resources, some counties intentionally authorized more expenditures than would be used to avoid the need to change authorization amounts for small adjustments made throughout the year. Another factor was that for certain services in use for longer periods and with established payment histories (e.g., supported living services), counties were able to predict how much could be authorized and still stay within the allowable limit of spending. For some types of services (e.g., respite care), counties authorized expenditures for individuals with more than one service provider for the same number of hours. In this case, the authorization allowed families more flexibility in where they got respite services with the understanding that the number of total hours was not to be exceeded. Finally, there was underspending in some service types due to lack of providers or lack of staff to provide the services.

Authorized Expenditures   In 1998, service plans for HCBS Waiver recipients authorized a total average expenditure of $33,380.44 for 720 children and $52,300.79 for 6,089 adults. By far, the highest average authorized expenditures were for SLS (87% of HCBS Waiver recipients receive SLS in small-group settings). The average annual SLS authorization for the 191 children with SLS authorization was $43,282.30. The average annual authorization for SLS for adults was $40,094.56. Case management was a nearly universally authorized (and generally required) service.

Table 5.6. County authorized and total paid costs for each Home and Community-Based Service (HCBS) Waiver program by service recipient age in FY 1998

HCBS Waiver programs	Average county authorized costs				Average paid costs				Total paid		Average per-person difference, authorized versus paid	
	Service recipient 0–17 years old	N	Service recipient 18 years or older	N	Service recipient 0–17 years old	N	Service recipient 18 years or older	N	Service recipient 0–17 years old	Service recipient 18 years or older	Service recipient 0–17 years old	Service recipient 18 years or older
Home care assessment	0**	0			$146	66	$126	65	$9,604	$8,174	$(146)	$(126)
Assistive technology	$677	42	$562	28	$610	34	$290	20	$20,744	$5,794	$67	$272
Caregiver training and education	$335	32	$468	10	$395	14	$516	8	$5,524	$4,125	$(59)	$(47)
Case management	$2,878	717	$2,641	6,084	$1,694	699	$1,338	5,981	$1,183,889	$7,999,946	$1,185	$1,304
Consumer-directed services	$7,300	5	$7,200	12	$2,330	4	$3,477	10	$9,322	$34,774	$4,969	$3,723
Crisis respite	$10,495	78	$7,321	441	$8,881	73	$5,921	397	$648,299	$2,350,704	$1,614	$1,400
Adult day care	0	0	$7,428	52	0	0	$6,148	50	0	$307,388	0	$1,281
Day training and habilitation	0	0	$13,397	4,478	0	0	$12,241	4,419	0	$54,094,437	0	$1,155
24-hour emergency care	$12,300	1	$1,762	5	$12,255	1	$1,696	5	$12,255	$8,480	$45	$66
Extended transportation	0	0	$220	1	0	0	$160	1	0	$160		$40
Home health aide	$2,942	10	$5,921	25	$2,536	8	$5,495	22	$20,286	$120,900	$406	$426
Homemaker	$2,353	55	$2,577	39	$1,816	47	$1,903	38	$85,334	$72,316	$537	$674
Housing access coordination	0	0	$55	1	0	0	0	1	0	0	0	$55
In-home services	$14,147	446	$12,334	542	$11,557	429	$10,115	498	$4,957,957	$5,037,230	$2,590	$2,220
Environmental modifications	$2,527	153	$2,170	477	$2,692	121	$2,577	388	$325,784	$999,969	$(166)	$(407)
Personal care	$14,911	190	$20,541	132	$9,720	184	$15,382	127	$1,788,530	$1,953,571	$5,191	$5,159
Private duty nurse	$22,405	8	$5,568	3	$19,861	7	$5,789	2	$139,028	$11,579	$2,544	$(221)
Personal support	$11,207	32	$3,360	174	$9,532	27	$2,846	149	$257,359	$424,106	$1,675	$513
Respite care	$4,946	471	$4,661	582	$3,491	414	$3,278	500	$1,445,286	$1,639,080	$1,455	$1,383

(continued)

107

Table 5.6. (continued)

HCBS Waiver programs	Average county authorized costs				Average paid costs				Total paid		Average per-person difference, authorized versus paid	
	Service recipient 0–17 years old	N	Service recipient 18 years or older	N	Service recipient 0–17 years old	N	Service recipient 18 years or older	N	Service recipient 0–17 years old	Service recipient 18 years or older	Service recipient 0–17 years old	Service recipient 18 years or older
Supported living												
Child*	$43,282	191	N/A	N/A	$42,755	187	N/A	N/A	$7,995,222	N/A	$527	N/A
Adult*	N/A	N/A	$40,095	5,584	N/A	N/A	$39,395	5,572	N/A	$219,510,667	N/A	$699
Skilled nursing	$1,247	33	$1,213	80	$869	28	$884	70	$24,332	$61,911	$378	$329
Specialist service	$2,731	89	$2,013	277	$1,992	70	$1,439	240	$139,465	$345,343	$739	$574
Supported employment	0	0	$4,436	18	0	0	$4,549	14	0	$63,691	0	$(113)
Average	$33,380	720	$52,301	6,089	$26,495	720	$48,457	6,089	$19,058,617	$295,046,012	$6,886	$3,844

Note: Expenditures are for an entire year.

*Age is the individual HCBS recipient age on July 1, 1998. As a result, individuals may receive supported living both as a child and as an adult during the year. These amounts have been combined into the category congruent with the age groupings.

**No authorization required. The live-in caregiver category was excluded because there were no authorized or paid costs in FY 1998. N/A = not applicable.

108

Among children, 717 of 720 individuals (99.6%) were authorized to receive HCBS Waiver–financed case management (at an average authorized cost of $2,878.32). Among adults, 6,084 of 6,089 (99.9%) of those with authorized services were authorized to receive HCBS Waiver–financed case management (at an average authorized cost of $2,641.30 per year).

Average Paid Costs Altogether, in 1998, average paid costs for children receiving HCBS Waivers were $26,495 per person. For adults, average paid costs were $48,457 (83% more than for children). Children's expenditures are, of course, typically lower than those of adults because they do not need HCBS Waiver–financed day services because they are in school and because 68.6% of children receiving HCBS Waivers live with family members who share in their care.

The most costly service for both children and adults was SLS ($42,755 and $39,395, respectively). The most common service for which payments were made was case management (97.1% of children and 98.2% of adults received paid case management). The second most common paid service for children was in-home family support (59.6%) with average annual payments of $11,557. Respite care services were received by 57.5% of children at an average annual cost of $3,491. The second most common service for adults was SLS (91.5%) at an average annual cost of $39,395. Day training and habilitation service was received by 72.6% of adult HCBS Waiver recipients, and another 50 people (or 0.8%) received day program services through a licensed adult day care programs. The average annual payment for day training and habilitation was $12,241, and for adult day care, was $6,148.

Differences Between County-Authorized and -Paid Expenditures Notable differences were found between authorized and provided ("paid") HCBS expenditures. Not only did adults have higher service authorizations and expenditures than children, but they also had service expenditures that are much nearer their authorized levels than did children. Specifically, in 1998, adult HCBS Waiver recipients received paid services that were on average $3,844 less than their average authorized expenditures of $52,301, or in other words, they had paid services that equaled 92.7% of authorizations. Expenditures for children's services fell on average $6,886 below authorization and were only 79.3% of the authorized level of expenditures.

In large measure, the differences between adults and children in authorized spending, actual spending, and the differences between authorized and actual spending were attributable to patterns in the use of the SLS service. SLS is by far the most costly of the HCBS, and its recipients were overwhelmingly adults (96.7% of all 5,775 SLS recipients were adults). A notably greater proportion of the authorized spending for SLS was actually spent for services than was the case for other types of HCBS. SLS providers were paid 98.3% of the authorized amounts for their services, whereas services more typically provided to children showed the greatest differences between authorized and reimbursed service costs. For example, average respite care payments for children were 70.6% of the authorized amounts. In-home family support for children payments were 81.7% of authorized amounts. Payments for personal care for children were 65.2% of authorized expenditures.

Authorized and Paid Costs by Age   Table 5.7 shows that children received proportionally less of authorized services than adults. Differences between county-authorized expenses and actual payments increased as service recipient age decreased. HCBS Waiver recipients between the ages of 41 and 70 years had actual expenditures equal to 94.1% of the authorized costs. Children 10 and younger had actual expenditures equal to 72.1% of authorized expenditures.

Expenditures by Age and Level of Intellectual Disability

Table 5.8 presents average HCBS expenditures for HCBS Waiver recipients by age and level of intellectual disability. These data show a consistent

Table 5.7.   Comparison of average costs authorized and costs paid for Home and Community-Based Service (HCBS) Waiver program recipients of different ages

Age group	N	Cost authorized	Costs paid	Percent of authorized costs paid
0–5 years	34	$23,029	$14,509	63.0%
6–10 years	209	$28,599	$21,055	73.6%
11–15 years	337	$36,088	$29,563	81.9%
16–20 years	469	$38,600	$31,991	82.9%
21–25 years	670	$47,161	$42,872	90.9%
26–30 years	770	$51,940	$47,653	91.7%
31–35 years	722	$54,154	$49,897	92.1%
36–40 years	770	$54,756	$51,090	93.3%
41–50 years	1,319	$56,421	$53,030	94.0%
51–60 years	828	$54,646	$51,539	94.3%
61–70 years	420	$50,007	$47,091	94.2%
71+ years	260	$45,751	$42,530	93.0%
Total	6,808	$50,300	$46,135	91.7%

Table 5.8. Average expenditures for Home and Community-Based Services (HCBS) Waiver programs by servicer recipient's age and level of intellectual disability

	Level of intellectual disability								
	Mild		Moderate		Severe		Profound		Related condition	
Age group	Amount paid	N	Amount paid	N	Amount paid	N	Amount paid	N	Amount paid	N
0–10 years	$16,940	50	$20,581	53	$19,500	43	$31,800	18	$22,311	60
11–15 years	$20,530	80	$27,185	107	$33,748	62	$38,386	44	$37,047	44
16–20 years	$28,076	129	$29,746	161	$33,925	95	$45,673	56	$29,116	29
21–25 years	$35,889	205	$38,782	250	$54,096	109	$56,088	79	$49,774	27
26–30 years	$42,196	327	$45,295	203	$53,851	133	$63,336	94	$44,917	13
31–35 years	$43,303	280	$45,991	204	$57,746	129	$65,956	100	$52,539	9
36–40 years	$43,325	279	$45,271	194	$55,570	134	$69,309	150	$48,152	13
41–50 years	$45,083	448	$45,677	285	$53,478	270	$71,487	301	$51,621	15
51–60 years	$43,286	237	$43,811	190	$54,210	215	$67,647	180	$43,357	6
61–70 years	$42,086	157	$43,994	92	$48,377	109	$63,638	60	$15,926	2
71+ years	$40,419	92	$42,122	56	$42,220	78	$50,288	33	$27,869	1
Total	$40,394	2,284	$40,999	1,795	$49,941	1,377	$64,006	1,115	$36,232	219

pattern of increased expenditures in all age categories for people with relatively greater impairments. Although expenditures for people with mild intellectual disabilities were consistently less than those for people with moderate intellectual disabilities, the amount of the difference was very small (about 1.5% in average difference). Costs for people with severe and profound intellectual disabilities differed considerably from those of people with mild and moderate intellectual disabilities. Expenditures for people with severe intellectual disabilities were 21.8% higher than for people with moderate intellectual disabilities. Average expenditures for people with profound intellectual disabilities were 28.2% higher than for people with severe intellectual disabilities and 56.1% higher than for people with moderate intellectual disabilities.

Expenditure information for people with related conditions (e.g., cerebral palsy, spina bifida, autism) but without intellectual disabilities was highly variable by age grouping. This reflects both the significant differences in support needs associated with different types and degrees of impairment and the relatively low number of people who had only related conditions within Minnesota's adult HCBS population. Indeed, it is notable that 61% of all HCBS Waiver recipients who had only related conditions were 20 years or younger, whereas people 20 years and younger, on a whole, made up only 15% of all HCBS Waiver recipients.

Expenditures by Residential Program

Table 5.9 presents the average annual expenditures for HCBS Waiver recipients living in different residential settings, including SLS (87.2% of whom are in small, agency-operated small-group homes), in-home family supports (in the immediate or extended family home), and "other" residential arrangements. The patterns in this table show 1) much higher average costs of SLS as compared with in-family support ($51,501 and $19,882) and 2) consistency of expenditures for SLS and in-family sup-

Table 5.9. Average annual paid costs for Home and Community-Based Services (HCBS) Waiver programs by service recipient's type of living arrangement, age group, and level of intellectual disability

	HCBS residential support services			
	Supported living service	Family (extended or immediate)	Other	Average HCBS amount paid
Level of intellectual disability	Amount paid N	Amount paid N	Amount paid N	Amount paid N
Children (0–17 yrs)				
Related condition	$60,282.40 20	$20,671.79 80	$20,602.65 12	$27,737.64 112
Mild	$47,296.97 35	$14,784.67 112	$11,006.12 17	$21,185.95 164
Moderate	$47,930.46 55	$17,678.47 147	$18,216.50 11	$25,517.80 213
Severe	$51,047.80 37	$21,568.96 93	$14,497.00 7	$29,169.06 137
Profound	$55,824.06 34	$21,016.28 34	$31,537.88 7	$37,777.82 75
Unspecified	N/A 0	$10,330.13 15	$12,863.42 4	$10,863.46 19
Total	$51,292.80 181	$18,261.50 481	$17,386.48 58	$26,494.71 720
Adults (18+ years)				
Related condition	$46,828.28 84	$34,375.59 15	$47,379.91 8	$45,123.80 107
Mild	$44,742.84 1,837	$17,869.67 140	$28,448.93 143	$41,869.12 2,120
Moderate	$46,340.16 1,361	$19,877.72 156	$30,573.60 65	$43,082.91 1,582
Severe	$55,244.13 1,090	$23,396.59 83	$39,020.21 67	$52,235.78 1,240
Profound	$68,374.45 952	$31,156.69 49	$49,095.64 39	$65,897.97 1,040
Unspecified	N/A 0	N/A 0	N/A 0	N/A 0
Total	$51,559.67 5,324	$21,640.87 443	$34,048.46 322	$48,456.92 6,089
All ages				
Related condition	$49,415.54 104	$22,835.55 95	$31,313.55 20	$36,232.25 219
Mild	$44,790.59 1,872	$16,498.56 252	$26,595.63 160	$40,394.45 2,284
Moderate	$46,401.93 1,416	$18,810.76 303	$28,785.07 76	$40,998.58 1,795
Severe	$55,106.36 1,127	$22,430.85 176	$36,700.46 74	$49,940.84 1,377
Profound	$67,941.68 986	$27,002.79 83	$46,423.81 46	$64,006.48 1,115
Unspecified	N/A 0	$10,330.13 15	$12,863.42 4	$10,863.46 19
Total	$51,500.90 5,505	$19,881.69 924	$31,505.31 380	$46,134.59 6,809

N/A = not applicable

ports across the categories of children and adults. People receiving HCBS in non–SLS licensed out-of-home settings were relatively few in number (380), but had relatively modest service costs for both children and adults.

Expenditures by Place of Residence

A breakdown of HCBS expenditures for children and adults according to specific types of residential placement is summarized in Table 5.10. The settings are defined as follows:

1. *Foster family* refers to individuals who are living in the homes of people who are not immediate or extended family members but who are providing services and support to them.

2. *Corporate foster care* is a home of four or fewer people in which services are provided by paid staff in a setting that is under the control of a provider agency (corporate foster care overlaps highly with SLS services).

3. *Own home* refers to a place that is owned or rented by a service recipient or his or her family to serve as the home for the HCBS Waiver recipient.

4. *Family home* refers to a place in which an HCBS Waiver recipient lives with members of the immediate or extended family.

People living in corporate foster care, 71.5% of Minnesota HCBS Waiver recipients in 1998, had by far the most costly HCBS, both for children and adults. Both children and adults living in their own home and their family home have the least expensive services ($21,454 and $19,568, respectively). Although foster family (or "host family") care is considerably

Table 5.10. Home and Community-Based Services (HCBS) Waiver programs expenditures by type of residence and service recipient's age

Type of residence	Children (0–17 years)		Adults (18+ years)		Total	
	Average cost	Recipients	Average cost	Recipients	Average cost	Recipients
Corporate foster	$57,510	19.0%	$54,653	77.7%	$54,733	71.5%
Family home	$17,912	69.2%	$21,329	7.7%	$19,568	14.2%
Foster family	$29,375	7.1%	$31,861	5.2%	$31,518	5.4%
Own home	$7,389	0.1%	$21,499	5.2%	$21,454	4.7%
Other/no record	$20,490	4.5%	$36,997	4.1%	$35,085	4.2%

less expensive to the state than corporate foster care ($31,518 and $54,733 per year respectively), foster family residents made up only 5.4% of HCBS Waiver recipients in 1998.

Expenditures by Type of Residence and Level of Service Needs

Table 5.11 presents a breakdown of expenditures for people in different categories of the waiver allocation structure living in different types of settings. Among foster family, corporate foster, and own family homes, average expenditures were consistently associated with the waiver allocation structure groupings. Within the foster family care settings, people with Level 1 profiles had services that were 56.2% more expensive than those with Level 4 profiles. Among people living in their family homes, those with Level 1 profiles had services that cost on average 68.0% more than those with Level 4 profiles. The difference in average expenditures between people with Level 1 and Level 4 profiles in corporate foster care settings was 84.6%.

Table 5.11.　Home and Community-Based Services (HCBS) Waiver programs expenditures by service recipient's residential situation and allocation profile level of service need

Waiver allo-cation group	Type of residence									
	Foster family		Corporate foster		Own home		Family home		Total	
	Average cost	N	Average cost	N	Average cost	N	Average cost	N	Average cost	N
Level 1 (highest needs)	$30,665	11	$72,224	271	$7,389	1	$21,521	57	$62,189	340
Level 2 (high needs)	$28,301	32	$60,554	489	$16,846	5	$18,655	129	$50,393	655
Level 3 (moderate needs)	$26,939	34	$48,238	567	$24,053	24	$14,460	126	$40,834	751
Level 4 (lowest needs)	$19,626	14	$39,121	205	$14,785	31	$12,812	54	$31,068	304
Pre-WAS (enrolled before FY 1996)	$33,076	279	$54,523	3,338	$22,160	257	$21,259	600	$46,865	4,474
Total*	$31,518	370	$54,733	4,870	$21,454	318	$19,568	966	$46,588	6,524

* An additional 275 people lived in settings that were "unrecorded" or recorded as "other."

Note: Service levels are determined from the individual's profile on the Waiver Allocation Structure (WAS) analysis of individual characteristics on the "Screening Document." Service levels include Level 1, "Very high self-care needs or mental illness and destructive behavior"; Level 2, "High self-care needs or aggressive/destructive behavior"; Level 3, "Limited self-care needs, but no major behavior problems"; Level 4, "Limited self-care needs and no major behavior problems." "Pre-WAS" enrollees are people who were enrolled in HCBS prior to FY 1996 and were not profiled for resource allocations.

Accounting for Expenditure Variations

As part of the analysis of expenditures, attention was given to factors that were associated with variations in expenditures among individual service recipients. Such analyses may contribute to the further development of service systems. They may provide guidelines for negotiating reimbursement rates and may assist with overall budget management. Such analyses also may help determine whether the intended effects of cost allocation and management policy are being realized.

Variables   Total expenditures on all HCBS in FY 1998 for each of the 6,620 recipients were analyzed using hierarchical regression, with predictor variables arranged into six blocks that were entered into the analysis sequentially. The six blocks each involved the following types of predictor variables (total number of predictor variables in each block is shown in parentheses):

1. *Days eligible*—The number of days during the year that each service recipient was eligible for HCBS (1 variable)

2. *Services received*—Whether the service recipient used each one of the specific HCBS during the year (21 variables)

3. *HCBS funding level*—State funding profile (WAS) level (1 variable)

4. *Personal characteristics*—Service recipients' functional, behavioral, and medical characteristics (9 variables)

5. *Residential setting*—Whether the service recipient lived in one of the specified types of residential setting (4 variables)

6. *County characteristics*—County unemployment and personal income levels; the fiscal management and size of county services for individuals with intellectual and developmental disabilities (4 variables)

   Provider characteristics were not included because most service recipients had multiple providers.

Results   Overall, the regression equation predicted 65% of the variance in HCBS expenditures in Minnesota. Each of the six blocks contributed significantly to prediction at the .001 level, as shown by the significance of the change in R^2 for each block (see Table 5.12). Given the large number of predictors (40), we set alpha at .001 when evaluating the significance of individual predictor variables. The coefficients for individual predictors shown in Table 5.12 were drawn from the final step of the hierarchical analysis, when all 40 predictor variables were entered into the

Table 5.12. Hierarchical regression of total expenditures for Home and Community-Based Service (HCBS) Waiver program recipients in Minnesota, 1998 (N = 6,620)

Block/variable	Cumulative R^2	R^2 change for block	Individual predictor variables: Coefficients—final step of analysis		
			Beta	t	p
Block 1: Days eligible	.092***	.092***			
Days			.352	43.221	.000[a]
Block 2: Services received	.408***	.316***			
Home care assessment			−.005	−.530	.596
Assistive technology			.003	.334	.738
Caregiver training			−.013	−1.784	.074
Case management			.004	.484	.628
Consumer-directed supports			−.005	−.728	.467
Crisis respite			.076	9.875	.000[a]
Adult day care			−.002	−.212	.832
Day training and habilitation			.173	19.583	.000[a]
24-hour emergency service			.004	.606	.545
Home health aide			−.002	−.315	.752
Homemaker			.001	.070	.944
In-home family support			−.036	−2.970	.003
Environmental modifications			.044	5.796	.000[a]
Personal care			.004	.443	.658
Private duty registered nurse			−.014	−1.903	.057
Personal support			−.016	−2.097	.036
Respite care			−.092	−9.202	.000[a]
Skilled nursing			.005	.619	.536
Specialist service			.005	.641	.522
Supported employment			.005	.707	.480
Supported living (SLS)			.149	8.261	.000[a]
Block 3: HCBS funding level	.440***	.031***			
State funding profile (WAS) level			−.045	−5.347	.000
Block 4: Personal characteristics	.592***	.153***			
Adaptive behavior			.226	17.721	.000[a]
Challenging behavior			.212	24.254	.000[a]
Adult or child			.025	2.458	.014
Seizures			.022	2.739	.006
Specialized medical needs			.092	10.470	.000[a]
Level of mental retardation			.044	4.286	.000[a]
Needs physical therapy			.029	3.195	.001[a]
Needs mental health services			.032	3.714	.000[a]
Guardianship status			.022	2.714	.007

Block/variable	Cumulative R^2	R^2 change for block	Individual predictor variables: Coefficients—final step of analysis		
			Beta	t	p
Block 5: Residential setting	.631***	.038***			
Foster family			−.036	−3.157	.002
Corporate foster			.204	11.367	.000[a]
Own home			−.035	−3.133	.002
Family home			−.021	−1.046	.296
Block 6: County characteristics	.647***	.016***			
Unemployment rate			−.011	−1.099	.272
Per-capita income 1998			.086	5.940	.000[a]
Percentage of funding used			.060	6.640	.000[a]
Number of consumers			−.001	−.104	.917

[a]Significant predictor variable with alpha = .001
*** $p < .001$; WAS = Waiver allocation structure

regression analysis *simultaneously*. Therefore, the significance of individual predictors is not dependent on the order of entry into the analysis because all were entered at the same time.

Block 1, or days of service, recognized that some individuals were eligible for HCBS expenditures for fewer than 365 days because they entered or left the program during the year. Obviously, and as predicted, the number of days using HCBS predicted variance (9%) in the expenditure for individuals. As expected, those with more days of service had significantly higher expenditures.

Block 2, or services received, examined specific social services used and explained an additional 32% of variance. Five of the 21 HCBS examined were significant predictors ($p < .001$) of total expenditures. Users of crisis respite, day training and habilitation, environmental modifications, and SLS had significantly *higher* expenditures than individuals who did not use each of these services. People who used in-home family support ($p < .003$) and respite care ($p < .001$) had significantly *lower* expenditures than nonusers of each service. Lower cost may have been related to living in the family home. Only 6.5% of service recipients living in the family home received neither in-home support nor respite, whereas 93.0% of individuals living outside the family home did not utilize either service.

Block 3, or state funding level, for individual HCBS Waiver recipients, although significant, only accounted for 3.1% of variance in expenditures. This weak relation between the score that determined the level of HCBS funding provided to counties for HCBS Waiver recipients entering the system after FY 1996 may seem surprising given the substantially different funding allocations across the range from Level 1 ($222.87 per day in FY 2002) to Level 4 ($126.74 per day in FY 2002). The primary reasons why the state funding profile level did not exert stronger influence on expenditures were 1) the resulting funding was added to a county pool and not allocated directly to the individual, and 2) 68.7% of sample members were enrolled in HCBS *before* this funding system was implemented in FY 1996 and continued to be allocated the uniform "base rate" funding. The hierarchical regression was recomputed after omitting all individuals on base rate funding. All six blocks were still significant at $p < .001$, with $R^2 = .084$ for Block 3. As expected, the relationship between profile level and expenditure was stronger for this subsample than for the sample as a whole, suggesting that state HCBS funding allocation policy was having some effect in directing more financial resources to individuals with greater support needs. Even so, 8.4% of variance represents only a medium effect size, suggesting that such policy initiatives may only have a moderate impact on complex funding and service systems.

Block 4, or personal characteristics, accounted for an additional 15% of variance. Adaptive behavior and challenging behavior were the strongest predictors, but 6 of the 9 personal characteristics were significant predictors at the .001 level. Individuals had *higher* expenditures if they had fewer adaptive skills, exhibited more severe challenging behavior, experienced more frequent specialized medical needs, had more severe intellectual disabilities, needed physical therapy, and required mental health services. Personal characteristics associated with higher support needs were consistently associated with higher expenditures.

Block 5, or residential setting, accounted for an additional 4% of variance. Individuals in corporate foster settings (almost always small shift-staff group homes of 4 or fewer residents) had significantly higher expenditures than residents of other settings.

Block 6, or county characteristics, explained a further 2% of variance. Individuals who lived in counties with higher per-capita income had higher expenditures, likely because of the higher cost of doing business (higher staff costs, property taxes, and so forth). People whose county of financial responsibility expended a higher overall percentage of their authorized HCBS expenditures also had significantly higher expenditures.

When examining these findings, certain considerations should be noted. First, provider characteristics were not included because most HCBS Waiver recipients had multiple providers. Second, the amount of variance accounted for by each block (change in R^2) depends, in part, on the order in which it is entered into the regression equation. The order used in this analysis seemed logical, but other orderings would be possible. The fact that all six blocks were significant when entered simultaneously (on the final step of the hierarchical analysis) suggests that each would be significant regardless of order of entry.

Despite these limitations, the findings still are supportive of HCBS expenditures in Minnesota being "rational" in that they are related in expected ways to service recipients' support needs. Evidence exists that needs-based funding allocation policies have influenced expenditure to be somewhat more related to individual support needs. Still, expenditures were strongly tied to service utilization, with users of expensive, fully staffed corporate foster care group homes having more costly services than residents of other settings. Furthermore, per-capita income and county management of HCBS funds were significantly related to expenditures. Overall, these findings show that Minnesota's HCBS expenditures were multiply determined, and the influences on them were complex.

Expenditures and Individual Quality-of-Life Outcomes

The final analysis was an examination of the relationship between expenditures and the quality of services. Service recipients' personal characteristics are related to both outcomes and service expenditures. As Felce and Emerson (Chapter 3) note, it is important to control for personal characteristics when examining the association between costs and outcomes. This control was implemented by including important personal characteristics (adaptive behavior, challenging behavior, level of mental retardation, and medical status) as covariates in our analyses. Likewise, there are differences between service models in both costs and outcomes (e.g., Chapter 6). This was addressed by restricting analyses to recipients of adult SLS in corporate foster care group homes.

Measures Quality was measured using several different surveys (described in Larson, Hewitt, & Lakin, in press). Three outcome measures were developed based on county case manager surveys: overall quality of life (one item scored as poor to excellent); a quality-of-life scale (9 items), and the quality of residential services (one item scored as poor to excellent). Family opinions about quality of residential services for family members in supported living settings were also examined. Five different scales were used, including the following:

- Overall satisfaction with residential services (1 item)

- Family satisfaction with information and communication with the residence (6 items)

- Family satisfaction with residential outcomes, such as the person being healthy and safe (8 items)

- Family satisfaction with residential choices, such as involvement in choosing which organization and which home supported the family member (6 items)

- Family satisfaction with direct support professionals in the residential setting (3 items).

The cost variable examined was the daily paid total expenditures for adult SLS in corporate foster care group homes. *Daily* expenditures (annual expenditures divided by service days) eliminated variation associated with part-year service use.

Case Manager Ratings of Quality
Case manager ratings of quality had no significant association with any of the covariates/independent variables under multivariate analysis. The only significant association under univariate analysis was the quality of residential services scale and medical status. Individuals needing more intensive medical services were rated as receiving higher-quality residential services ($p < .05$). No associations occurred between daily costs of SLS for adults and quality of life or quality of residential services as rated by case managers. Findings for the univariate analyses are shown in Table 5.13.

Family Ratings of Quality
In a multivariate analysis of four dependent variables (family ratings of information and communication, residential outcomes, choices of residential providers, and satisfaction with the residential services staff), challenging behavior was the only variable that was significantly related ($p = .02$) to family satisfaction scores. Families of people with less challenging behavior reported being more satisfied with the quality of residential services. In subsequent univariate analyses, family ratings of the quality of residential outcomes and of residential staff were significantly associated with challenging behavior ($p = .04$ and $p = .001$ respectively). Families of people with less challenging behavior rated their satisfaction higher in both cases. Average daily costs of SLS for adults were *not* associated with family satisfaction with those services. Under univariate analysis, the daily costs of SLS for adults were not associated with

Table 5.13.   Univariate analyses of covariance for variables associated with case manager assessment of quality (N = 284)

Variables	Quality of life scale		Quality of life item		Quality of residential services scale	
	B	t	B	t	B	t
Personal characteristics						
Adaptive behavior	0.0059	1.00	0.0057	0.81	−0.0027	−0.35
Challenging behavior	−0.0005	−0.10	−0.0075	−1.10	−0.0051	−0.67
Level of intellectual disability	−0.0146	−0.40	−0.0435	−1.00	0.0079	0.16
Medical status	0.0708	1.39	−0.0028	−0.05	0.1360	2.02*
Costs						
Daily cost of supported-living services for adults	0.0002	0.21	0.0001	0.12	0.0004	0.40
R^2	.02		.01		.02	
Adjusted R^2	.00		−.01		.00	

*$p < .05$

family satisfaction for any of the four quality of residential services variables (see Table 5.14).

CONCLUSION

The HCBS Waiver program in Minnesota has continued to expand since its beginning years. It greatly exceeds the size of the ICF/MR program (more than 5 times the number of recipients in 2002) and provides supports to individuals at a cost lower than that of the ICF/MR program ($52,961 versus $67,763 per year, per person in 1998). The implementation of the waiver allocation structure was intended to authorize appropriate levels of spending by counties meeting the specific supports needs of individuals entering the HCBS Waiver program. One of the primary reasons for doing so was to expand access to HCBS Waivers for people with more substantial and costly support needs. The introduction of the waiver allocation structure was associated with a modest increase in the proportion of individuals with profound intellectual disabilities receiving HCBS Waivers (15.5% for people entering the HCBS Waiver program prior to July 1995 to 18.3% for people entering in the subsequent 3 years).

Medicaid HCBS Waivers in Minnesota support people with the full range of characteristics and needs, from people with significant medical needs, serious challenging behavior, and substantial support needs, to people living independently. Minnesota has used HCBS Waiver–financed

Table 5.14. Univariate analyses of covariance for variables associated with family satisfaction with the quality of residential services for adults in supported living settings ($N = 107$)

	Quality of residential services							
	Information and communication		Residential outcomes		Choice of residential providers		Residential staff	
Variables	B	t	B	t	B	t	B	t
Personal characteristics								
Adaptive behavior	0.0032	0.48	−0.0064	−1.11	0.0232	2.37*	−0.0014	−0.23
Challenging behavior	−0.0114	−1.70	−0.0119	−2.04*	−0.0030	−0.31	−0.0216	−3.27***
Level of intellectual disability	−0.0139	−0.34	−0.0083	−0.23	−0.0889	−1.46	−0.0117	−0.29
Medical status	−0.0009	−0.02	0.0672	1.39	0.0234	0.29	0.0196	0.36
Costs								
Daily cost of supported-living services for adults	−.0002	−0.23	0.0000	0.01	−0.0021	−1.58	−0.0011	1.23
R^2	.04		.08		.07		.10	
Adjusted R^2	−.01		.04		.02		.05	

* $p < .05$, *** $p < .001$

supports to close its state institutions and to substantially decrease ICF/MR use (24% reduction between 1998 and 2002). Unlike the ICF/MR program, Minnesota's HCBS Waiver program supports families with children (including adult children) in the family home. Ninety-two percent of children who receive Medicaid long-term services and supports in Minnesota in 1998 received HCBS Waivers. By June 2002, 3,820 people were receiving HCBS Waivers while living in the family home, an increase from 1,005 in June 1998. The growing focus on in-home supports may also be related to growing enrollments of individuals who are Asian/Pacific Islander, black, Hispanic, or Native American. The more flexible options of HCBS can be tailored more readily to support people with diverse cultural and ethnic backgrounds, often including the greater focus on family and extended family involvement.

Minnesota continues to make extensive use of small agency-operated group homes (corporate foster care) in providing HCBS. In 1998, the average cost of all HCBS for people living in such settings was $54,733 annually, as compared with $24,420 for all other HCBS Waiver recipients. Given that the majority of HCBS Waiver recipients receive this high cost "package," Minnesota's HCBS costs per recipient tend to be relatively high (only 12 states are higher). Still, including all long-term services and supports and medical expenditures, Minnesota provided HCBS at about 78% of the cost of ICFs/MR in 1998. In considering the differences between HCBS and ICFs/MR, two factors should be recognized. First, only 2.2% of ICF/MR residents were children and youth, and 11.8% of HCBS Waiver recipients were children and youth. The average annual costs of HCBS in 1998 for children were about 55% of that for adults, so the higher proportion of children receiving HCBS Waivers accounted for about 6% of the difference between HCBS and ICF/MR expenditures.

Although it is not known what would be the total costs of ICF/MR services to these children and youth if there were no HCBS Waiver alternative, children's HCBS expenditures are lower because their primary day activity is funded by their school districts and most children live in the homes of family members, who provide much of their needed support. In addition, ICF/MR residents are more likely than HCBS Waiver recipients to have more substantial support needs (e.g., 59% and 36%, respectively, had severe or profound intellectual disabilities). The average cost in 1998 of HCBS for people with mild and moderate intellectual disabilities was only 72% of that for people with severe and profound intellectual disabilities ($40,660 and $56,234, respectively).

In sum, if all of the individual factors associated with expenditures were equal for people receiving HCBS Waivers and those living in ICFs/MR, the cost differences would be substantially less. The primary reason for this is the reliance on small HCBS Waiver–financed group homes (corporate foster care) as the primary approach to HCBS service delivery. This is the most costly approach to providing HCBS in Minnesota, and the approach that most closely resembles the ICF/MR. Both are agency-managed group homes with shift-staff. Investments in training, technical assistance, increased flexibility, and opportunities to learn about other forms of support for individuals, families, and local governments may be needed as a stimulus for more personalized approaches to services.

The discrepancy between services that were authorized and services that were actually received and paid for was much greater for family support services, such as respite and in-home supports, than for out-of-home services, such as SLS (Table 5.6). Interviews with family members indicate that at least in part, this discrepancy was the result of the staff not being available to provide authorized family support services, causing families to get fewer services and the state to pay for fewer hours of service than authorized. These data suggest that family-based services were receiving lower priority in staffing than congregate care services (corporate foster care). Licensing requirements and concern for safety necessitate that providers maintain a sufficient level of staffing in congregate care, even at the expense of not providing authorized family support services when staff are in short supply, as they generally are according to the case manager, service provider, and HCBS coordinator surveys.

But there are major potential ramifications of failing to meet the basic needs of families. The substantial difference between the levels of funding authorized to meet the needs of individual children and adults living at home and the amounts *actually* spent to do so suggests that families are not getting what they need. When, on average, respite care expenditures in 1998 were 70% of the authorized amounts, and in-home family supports expenditures were 83% of authorizations, there should be concern about the impact on demand for much more expensive out-of-home services.

The difficulties faced by families in getting the support they need and want from traditional service providers has been a major factor in support for and rapid growth in Minnesota's Consumer Directed Community Services (CDCS) options. Since its introduction in FY 1998, it has grown to more than 2,000 individual family recipients in FY 2003. With this option, individuals and families receive an authorized spending amount, but they themselves select the people who will provide them with support and what those people will be paid. In doing so, support is available in financial management "employer offered" insurance and other areas from "intermediary" agencies. CDCS allows those who are directing their own supports the flexibility to reduce their number of hours of support in favor of buying higher levels of dependability and convenience in their supports.

Policy makers recognize the substantial cost implication of the current system failing to provide the needed support for people in their homes at relatively low cost. The implication is in the risk of hastening out-of-home placement. Children living with their parents or extended family members had average HCBS expenditures that were 42% of the average HCBS expenditures for children living away from their family home ($17,912 and $43,064, respectively), and adults living with their parents or extended family members had average HCBS expenditures that were 43% of the average HCBS expenditures of adults living away from the family home ($21,641 and $50,561, respectively). Insufficient support of families with children with disabilities, including adult children with disabilities, brings a substantial financial as well as psychological and social cost when it leads to unwanted out-of-home placement. Efforts are needed to fully understand and support the commitment of families, whether through better implementation of traditional family support services or through effective programs of service recipient–directed supports.

An important part of supporting families as well as anticipating future systemwide expenditures is to understand family plans for long-term support of family members with intellectual and developmental disabilities in the family home, the factors that could jeopardize such plans, and the relative likelihood of circumstances that could create unmanageable demands on families as parents age, children grow, or physical/health conditions progress. Although Minnesota has a small proportion of children receiving HCBS Waivers (12%), as these children become adults, based on current expenditure and service-use patterns, the cost for their services will almost double. With almost half (45%) of the HCBS Waiver recipients who are 20 years or younger being between 16 years and 20 years old, the 83% higher costs on average for services to adults than children presents a fairly immediate threat to HCBS budgets without modification of service patterns. Considerable new financial commitments will need to be made unless there is a substantial reduction in the use of SLS services, greater use of other alternatives to group residential settings (including foster/host family), extension of years in family care, and/or proper support of service recipient–directed approaches that allow individuals and families to purchase all of what they need at lower costs than current approaches to support provision.

HCBS Waiver recipients' personal characteristics (including adaptive behavior and challenging behavior) are associated with HCBS expenditures in Minnesota, but the state's waiver allocation structure profile accounts for a small proportion of the variability in cost. Discussion should continue about how resources should be allocated to people with different needs and circumstances. As efforts are made to increase the size, flexibility, and attractiveness of family support through service recipient–directed options, it will be increasingly important that the allocations to individuals fairly but efficiently match the costs of providing the support they need.

The lack of notable association between costs and certain indicators of quality of service outcomes for adult HCBS Waiver recipients in small-group homes has a number of possible explanations. It could mean quality service outcomes are most related to factors not measured in this study (e.g., the skill of the direct support professional providing supports) or the way the money is used (e.g., for salaries or for other expenses), or that quality within a narrowly defined service model is simply not related to cost. It may be that the use of satisfaction surveys with families and case managers who may not see the individual on a daily basis, or even infrequently, may not be sensitive measures of quality. The lack of association between expenditures and quality indicators in this study appears to be consistent with research in the United Kingdom (see Chapter 3).

Noting that, within these analyses, expenditures were not found to be associated with quality is not the same as indicating that expenditures do not affect quality. The system examined in this study provided a substantial amount of expenditure for HCBS Waiver recipients, provided for variation in expenditure based on individual differences, and achieved high overall ratings of quality (82% of the adults in the cost and quality analysis reported they liked where they lived; 82% of case managers of those same individuals reported that they were living in a place the family preferred; 87% of family respondents said they were satisfied with the HCBS Waiver recipient's home). In such a circumstance, the lack of association between cost and quality may be substantially affected by the limited distribution of these variables. In addition, as a whole, the use of variations in cost to achieve similar desired outcomes for individuals with different needs may be working quite well toward that end.

REFERENCES

Department of Human Services. (1996). *Summary report: The HCBS Waiver allocation structure.* St. Paul: Minnesota Department of Human Services.

Department of Human Services. (1999). *Home and Community Based Services for persons with mental retardation and related conditions.* St. Paul: Minnesota Department of Human Services.

Hewitt, A., Larson, S., & Lakin, K.C. (2000). *An independent evaluation of the quality of services and system performance of Minnesota's Medicaid Home and Community Based Services for persons with mental retardation and related conditions.* Minneapolis: University of Minnesota, Research and Training Center on Community Living. Also available on-line at http://rtc.umn.edu

Karon, S.L., & Beutel, P. (2000). *ICF-MR facilities, clients and quality: State profiles, 1999.* Madison: University of Wisconsin, Center for Health Systems Research and Analysis.

Larson, S.A., Hewitt, A.S., & Lakin, K.C. (in press). Multi-perspective analysis of workforce challenges and their effects on consumer and family quality of life. *Journal on Mental Retardation.*

Minnesota Legislature. (1992). Waivered services rate structure. In *Laws of Minnesota for 1992* (Chapter 513, Article 9, Section 38, p. 1146). St. Paul: Author.

Prouty, R., & Lakin, K.C (2000). *Residential services for persons with developmental disabilities: Status and trends through 1999.* Minneapolis: University of Minnesota. Research and Training Center on Community Living. Also available on-line at http://rtc.umn.edu

Prouty, R., Smith, G., & Lakin, K.C. (2003). *Residential services for persons with developmental disabilities: Status and trends through 2002.* Minneapolis: University of Minnesota, Research and Training Center on Community Living. Also available on-line at http://rtc.umn.edu

Smith, G., & Ashbaugh, J. (1998). *Core Indicators Project: Phase I summary and technical reports.* Cambridge, MA: Human Services Research Institute.

CHAPTER 6

Semi-Independent Living and Group Homes in Australia

Roger J. Stancliffe

Since the 1980s, group homes or hostels (larger community-based residences) with 24-hour staffing overwhelmingly have been the dominant types of government-funded community living in Australia for people with intellectual disabilities residing outside of the family home (Van Dam & Cameron-McGill, 1995). Frequently, such settings provided the only available placement for individuals seeking to live in the community, regardless of whether they actually needed 24-hour staff support.

Contemporary Australian data on residential services for people with intellectual or developmental disabilities show that in 2001, group homes made up 70.6% of all community residential services funded under the Commonwealth/State Disability Agreement (Australian Institute of Health and Welfare, 2002; see also Stancliffe, 2002). Data were not available specifically for semi-independent living but were obtained for recipients of *outreach/drop-in services* (including semi-independent living), defined as "individual in-home living support and/or developmental programming services for people with a disability, supplied independently of accommodation" (Black & Eckerman, 1997, p. 45).

The research described in this chapter was funded by New South Wales (NSW) Ageing and Disability Department and conducted with assistance from the NSW Department of Community Services. The views expressed in this report are those of the author and do not necessarily represent the views of the NSW Government, the Minister for Community Services, or the Minister for Disability Services. Likewise, the conclusions drawn in the report do not necessarily represent the policy of either department, and endorsement by either department should not be assumed.

In 2001, outreach/drop-in services constituted 27.8% of all Australian community residential services (Australian Institute of Health and Welfare, 2002). The proportion of these that involved semi-independent living is unknown. Nationally, outreach/drop-in services are growing at a faster rate than group homes, albeit off a much lower base (Stancliffe, 2002). The state of New South Wales (NSW)—where the research presented in this chapter was conducted—had a substantially lower proportion of outreach/drop-in services (17.7%) than any of the other large-population Australian states, so the relative shortage of such services was much more acute in NSW (Australian Institute of Health and Welfare, 2002).

LIMITATIONS OF GROUP HOMES

Although group homes continue to predominate, their limitations have been increasingly recognized, accompanied by a growing perception that, in community living, one size does not fit all. Problems that have been identified with group-home living in Australia include the following (Stancliffe & Whaite, 1997; Van Dam & Cameron-McGill, 1995; Whaite, Stancliffe, & Keane, 1999):

- Incompatibility and conflict among residents

- Inflexibility resulting in inability to respond to residents' changing preferences for living companions and living arrangements

- Constraints on personal choice and individuality in the context of group activities and group decisions, or because of the needs or preferences of other residents

- Rigid routines

- High levels of staff presence and control

There is a growing recognition that a diverse range of community living options is required to meet the needs and preferences of individuals with intellectual disabilities. Some people are much happier living alone (Whaite et al., 1999). Others find constant staff presence intrusive and strongly prefer to receive staff assistance only on a drop-in basis for specific aspects of life (e.g., money management, health care, resolving interpersonal problems).

DIFFERENCES FROM U.S. COMMUNITY LIVING SERVICES

The group homes (Medicaid funded) and semi-independent living services (state funded) I am familiar with in Minnesota differ from one another markedly in resident numbers per household, staffing levels, funding source, resident eligibility requirements, and regulations. In Australia, eligibility for disability services and government funding under the Commonwealth/State Disability Agreement does not differ according to the type of accommodation support service utilized, so residents' characteristics, such as adaptive and challenging behavior, from these two types of settings differ on average, but do overlap.

Australian services are not as readily classified into mutually exclusive categories of semi-independent living or group homes as U.S. services are. In Australia, both household size and amount of staff support vary along a continuum. For example, I have visited Australian households of 4 residents living in an ordinary home that looks like a group home but has drop-in staffing totaling less than 30 hours per week, which indicates that residents were actually living semi-independently. Similarly, I am aware of several individuals who live alone but have either 24-hour staff support or full-time staff support during waking hours (see Whaite et al., 1999). The Australian system may have an important advantage in that a continuum of support levels and a single government-funding source makes it easier to meet an individual's varying support needs without the necessity of changing support agencies or funding arrangements.

Because the features of group homes and semi-independent settings also overlap, for research purposes it is necessary to develop adequate definitions of each to ensure that examples can be identified unambiguously. The following definitions are used in this chapter.

- *Semi-independent living*—household of 1–5 people living together with regular *part-time* support by paid staff from an accommodation support agency for people with disabilities. There is no regularly scheduled overnight staff support (including no sleepovers). On average, the household is *without* paid staff support for at least 28 *waking* hours per week when residents are at home.

- *Group home*—household of 3–7 people with *full-time* support (at least during waking hours) by paid staff from an accommodation support agency for people with disabilities. There may be times on weekdays when all residents are away from the house attending their day programs and no staff are on duty. Night support may be provided by awake shift staff or sleepover staffing, or there may be no staff present when residents are asleep. Staff are present at all other times.

PREVIOUS AUSTRALIAN RESEARCH ON GROUP HOMES AND SEMI-INDEPENDENT LIVING

Several studies undertaken with colleagues in Australia led me to the view that semi-independent living was underutilized in NSW, seemingly less costly than group homes, and at least equally as beneficial in terms of lifestyle outcomes (Stancliffe 1995, 1997; Stancliffe & Parmenter, 1999; Stancliffe & Whaite, 1997; Whaite et al., 1999). We found that people living semi-independently, with fewer living companions and fewer hours of staff presence, exercised more choice and greater control over their lives than their counterparts in group homes (a finding also confirmed in the U.S. context in research with colleagues in Minnesota—see Stancliffe, Abery, & Smith, 2000).

Choice was the only outcome assessed formally in this previous work, so it was important to evaluate many more lifestyle outcomes in the current study, including basic living conditions, health, personal safety, and individuals' subjective views about their lifestyle. Public policy and individual decisions about living arrangements needed to be informed by data about a wide range of outcomes.

In our previous choice research, we noted that semi-independent living service (SILS) staff's contact with service recipients frequently differed from group homes. The amount of staff support was dramatically less in SILS, even after taking into account the larger resident numbers in group homes. The SILS staff often worked by visiting the service recipient's home at a prearranged time for a particular purpose (e.g., budgeting, cooking) and for a specified period, after which they would leave. During that time, staff-to-service recipient contact was extensive and focused on the tasks at hand. This interaction contrasts with group homes because research indicates that group home staff spend substantial amounts of time in the home not working directly with residents (Felce, Jones, & Lowe, 2002). It was also notable that SILS settings provided opportunities to live with preferred living companions and to avoid residing with nonpreferred individuals. For example, there were several (married) couples living in their own home with drop-in support.

Our evaluation of the closure of a large private institution led us to examine these issues further (Stancliffe & Whaite 1997; Whaite et al.,

1999). Initially, all 80 former institution residents moved into 4-person group homes with 24-hour staffing; however, there were such serious incompatibility problems in one household—characterized by arguments, threats, and verbal and physical abuse among residents—that this group home was closed, and its funding was used to establish a SILS. At the time of the evaluation, this service offered regular drop-in support to 10 former group home residents living semi-independently. The fact that the same amount of funding that had previously supported 4 people in a group home could now be used to support 10 people in a SILS strongly suggested that, in this instance, SILS was substantially less costly per person than group homes. Whether this finding was true more generally remained to be seen.

Given the likely cost advantages of SILS, it is perhaps surprising that group homes have remained so dominant in NSW. Perceptions of safety and risk may have been important influences on this situation. The constant presence of staff in group homes could be seen to minimize risks to resident safety, health, and welfare, whereas the intermittent staff presence in semi-independent settings may be regarded as increasing risk. In addition, fellow residents and staff form important parts of group home residents' social networks (Robertson et al., 2001), so the smaller resident numbers and lower staff presence in SILS might be perceived as reducing social networks and making residents more susceptible to loneliness. Therefore, it was important for us to include matters such as safety, health care, domestic management, personal care, money management, social network, and loneliness when evaluating lifestyle outcomes. If significant differences were found for these domains, they might be expected to favor group-home residents because of the greater amount of staff support they received to assist with the basic health, safety, and welfare outcomes mentioned previously.

These issues mostly involve essential living standards, so they were assessed *without regard to independence*. For instance, for the basic personal care task of teeth cleaning, the most fundamental issue is whether the person's teeth were cleaned regularly, irrespective of whether the task is completed independently. A group home resident who has his or her teeth cleaned with staff assistance enjoys better personal care than a person living semi-independently who does not brush his or her teeth at all.

OVERVIEW OF THE CURRENT STUDY

The study presented in this chapter represents the only known Australian comparison of costs and outcomes in semi-independent living and group homes. Previous analyses of findings for a matched subsample from this study appeared in Stancliffe and Keane (2000). This chapter provides an extension and elaboration of Stancliffe and Keane's study in that it reports data for the full 90-person sample rather than the 54-person matched subsample used by Stancliffe and Keane. This larger sample enabled more detailed regression-based analyses of factors associated with service costs to be completed, together with an examination of issues such as needs-based funding and economies of scale.

The current study used *statistical control* (covariance, multiple regression) rather than matching to control for the differences in residents' personal characteristics between residence types, shown in Table 6.1. It is essential to control for differences in characteristics such as adaptive and challenging behavior because they are known to be strongly related to lifestyle outcomes (Stancliffe & Lakin, 1998). Otherwise, differences in outcomes by residence type could be attributed to differences in personal characteristics rather than to different living arrangements.

Personal Characteristics of Participants by Living Arrangement

Of the 90 participants, 56 lived semi-independently, and 34 lived in group homes. There were equal numbers of men and women, and sex was not significantly related to community-living type. Participants' personal characteristics by community-living type are shown in Table 6.1, together with the results of *t*-test comparisons of each characteristic for between-group differences. There were no significant differences by age, but semi-independent participants had significantly better-developed adaptive behavior and less problematic challenging behavior.

Most participants had little or no challenging behavior, and none had very serious challenging behavior. Seventy-four percent had Inventory for Client and Agency Planning (ICAP) (Bruininks, Hill, Weatherman, & Woodcock, 1986) service scores of 70 or above, indicating that most, if not all, participants had *intermittent* or *limited* support needs.

Table 6.1. Personal characteristics by community living arrangement

Personal characteristic	Group home (n = 34)			Semi-independent (n = 56)			
	Mean	SD	Range	Mean	SD	Range	t
Age	44.2	15.7	21.1 to 76.0	38.8	11.4	19.7 to 71.3	1.88
Adaptive behavior	485.1	24.3	429 to 530	508.2	25.5	455 to 554	4.24***
Challenging behavior	−9.50	7.7	−31 to 0	−4.9	5.2	−19 to 0	3.10**

** $p < .01$, *** $p < .001$

Data were obtained about whether participants had any of the following diagnoses: autism, blindness, cerebral palsy, chronic health problem requiring medical care by a doctor or nurse, deafness, epilepsy, formal psychiatric diagnosis, and other diagnosis. The group-home and semi-independent living groups did not differ on any of these characteristics except chronic health problems and formal psychiatric diagnosis. Significantly more group-home residents (27%) had psychiatric diagnoses than semi-independent residents (9%), $\chi^2(1, N = 90) = 8.53, p < .01$. Likewise, significantly more group-home residents (24%) had chronic health problems than semi-independent residents (4%), $\chi^2(1, N = 90) = 4.96, p < .05$.

Settings

Participants were drawn from 13 different community living agencies (9 nongovernment/nonprofit, 4 government services) and 58 different community residential settings. Household size (total number of service recipients living in the household) was greater for participants living in group homes ($M = 4.21, SD = 1.20$) than in semi-independent settings ($M = 2.25, SD = 1.08$), $t(88) = 7.97, p < .001$.

Staff Presence   Expressed as hours per week for the *household*, there were significantly and substantially more staff in group homes ($M = 156.00, SD = 46.81$) than in semi-independent settings ($M = 18.73, SD = 15.70$), $t(37.55) = 16.54, p < .001$; however, it was possible that more staff hours were provided in group homes simply because there were more residents to support. Weekly staff hours *per person* were calculated by dividing weekly household staff hours by the number of service recipients. Once again, there were significantly more staff hours per person for group-home residents ($M = 40.35, SD = 17.49$) than for semi-independent residents ($M = 8.60, SD = 6.07$), $t(37.88) = 10.22, p < .001$.

As specified in the residence type definitions discussed previously, all 56 semi-independent participants had no overnight staffing, whereas only 4 (12%) of the 34 group home residents were without night staff.

LIFESTYLE OUTCOMES

Details of the instruments used to assess lifestyle outcomes are set out in Stancliffe and Keane (2000), and the outcomes examined are listed in Tables 6.2 and 6.3. Information was obtained from resident interviews and from staff who completed written checklists. Table 6.2 presents categori-

Table 6.2. Number of participants with friends and an advocate

Item	Group home Yes	Group home No	Semi-independent Yes	Semi-independent No	χ^2 ($df = 1$)
Has friends (other than family, paid staff, or fellow residents)	26	8	45	11	0.19
Has someone who provides advocacy/ personal support (not paid staff)	20	14	35	21	0.12

cal data for two outcomes—having versus not having outside friends or an advocate. There were no significant differences by living arrangement. Table 6.3 shows mean raw scores on 26 lifestyle outcomes by living arrangement, the results of analysis of covariance with adaptive and challenging behavior as covariates, as well as an estimate of effect size, partial eta squared (η_p^2), for living arrangement. Table 6.3 reveals that there were no significant differences for 20 outcomes, with a nonsignificant trend toward better results for semi-independent settings for 3 outcomes (social dissatisfaction, social belonging, frequency of use of community places) and significantly better results for semi-independent settings for 3 outcomes (empowerment, number of community places used without staff support, domestic participation).

The three variables with significant differences were the *only* outcomes for which *independent* participation yielded higher scores (see Table 6.3). For example, domestic participation was assessed using the Index of Participation in Domestic Life (IPDL) (Raynes, Sumpton, & Pettipher, 1989), which assigns a higher score if the person completes a domestic task, such as ironing, with no staff help. All other outcome measures did *not* assess independence, and the only criterion was that the outcome was achieved. For example, a maximum score on money management was attained if the participant had encountered no money problems (e.g., failure to pay utility bills), regardless of whether participants or staff managed the finances.

Why did the semi-independent participants perform better on outcomes favoring independent participation even though differences in adaptive and challenging behavior had been controlled statistically using covariance? This finding may well have been due to differences in *staff presence* between group homes and semi-independent settings. Arguably, the frequent absence of staff in semi-independent settings facilitated independent performance, whereas group-home staff were always available to help. Semi-independent participants probably completed domestic tasks,

Table 6.3. Mean outcome raw scores and results of ANCOVA

Outcome	Possible range for scale[c]	Scale direction[d]	Group home		Semi-independent		ANCOVA	
			Mean	SD	Mean	SD	F	η_p^2
Participant interview								
Loneliness								
Aloneness	0–12	–	3.91	3.05	4.57	3.28	0.26	–
Social dissatisfaction	0–12	–	1.90	1.94	1.07	1.78	3.68[#]	.04
Safety								
Safety[b]	0–16	+	14.44	2.20	14.40	1.65	1.20	–
Quality of Life Questionnaire								
QOL-Q Satisfaction[b]	10–30	+	22.88	4.15	22.93	3.99	0.53	–
QOL-Q Competence/ Productivity[b]	10–30	+	16.96	7.81	19.99	7.42	0.14	–
QOL-Q Empowerment[a]	10–30	+	21.97	3.04	24.83	2.73	10.51***	.11
QOL-Q Social belonging	10–30	+	20.09	3.03	21.66	3.78	3.29[#]	.04
QOL-Q Total score[b]	40–120	+	82.19	11.73	89.88	11.12	1.92	–
Staff questionnaire								
Personal care[b]	0–16	+	13.45	2.29	13.89	2.21	0.00	–
Domestic management	0–16	+	13.59	2.11	13.43	2.48	0.11	–
Health care	0–36	+	30.37	3.79	31.28	4.13	1.17	–
Money management	0–12	+	11.03	1.39	10.25	2.50	1.99	–
Number of friends contacted in last 3 months[b]	0–	+	4.26	6.33	4.87	6.07	0.00	–
Frequency of contact with friends[b]	0–	+	11.18	16.86	20.70	26.37	2.44	–
Number of family members contacted in last 3 months	0–	+	2.29	1.57	2.57	1.96	0.12	–
Frequency of contact with family[b]	0–	+	8.76	15.93	18.74	49.55	1.41	–
Number of mainstream community services ever used	0–10	+	4.32	1.85	4.93	1.76	0.59	–
Number of mainstream community services used last 3 months	0–10	+	2.35	1.28	2.29	1.19	0.28	–
Frequency of mainstream community service use	0–	+	8.76	10.43	9.89	13.24	0.62	–
Number of community places used	0–18	+	11.65	2.58	11.61	2.31	0.01	–
Frequency of use of community places	0–	+	123.15	62.29	146.63	68.40	3.08[#]	.04
Number of community places used without staff support[a]	0–18	+	3.88	3.50	7.68	3.23	12.83***	.13
Domestic participation[a]	0–26	+	16.26	4.91	20.54	3.47	8.07**	.09
Number of changes of address (adjusted for reporting period) [a]	0–	–	1.60	1.88	1.15	1.41	0.55	–

(continued)

Table 6.3.   *(continued)*

Outcome	Possible range for scale[c]	Scale direction[d]	Group home Mean	Group home SD	Semi-independent Mean	Semi-independent SD	ANCOVA F	ANCOVA η_p^2
Living companion turnover (adjusted for reporting period)	0–	–	3.19	3.32	2.28	3.39	0.28	–
Natural support hours per week	0–	+	0.75	2.02	1.19	3.18	0.04	–

Note: Adaptive and challenging behavior were used as covariates for all analyses.
[a]Variable has higher scores for independent participation.
[b]Data not available for between one and four participants.
[c]A possible range of 0– indicates an open-ended measure with no specified upper limit.
[d]In this column + indicates that *higher* scores denote better outcomes; – indicates that *lower* scores denote better outcomes.
QOL-Q = Quality of Life Questionnaire (Schalock & Keith, 1993).
[#] $p < .10$, [*] $p < .05$, [**] $p < .01$, [***] $p < .001$

such as washing up, more independently because there were no staff on hand to assist. The semi-independent living environment not only provided *opportunities* for independent participation, but it also *demanded* independent participation (Stancliffe, 1997; Stancliffe & Keane, 2000).

Extended periods without staff presence appear to have a facilitative effect on independent participation; however, there are important limits to the applicability of this conclusion. Study participants had intermittent to limited support needs and were able to initiate and carry through a number of activities without help. Research on the importance of active support by staff to assist service recipients to participate in activities has shown that although such support is crucial for individuals with more extensive support needs, staff support is not related to participation among those with more limited support needs (Felce et al., 2002). Such findings also imply the converse—that the facilitative effect on independent participation of extended periods *without* staff presence likely is confined to people with more limited support needs. Many individuals with more extensive support needs clearly need 24-hour support. It is not suggested that those individuals could achieve satisfactory outcomes or greater independence by living semi-independently.

None of the outcomes significantly favored group home residents, even though a number of variables involving basic care and essential living standards might have been expected by some to yield worse results for people living semi-independently because of their much lower level of staff support. That is, the problems that some might anticipate for semi-independent living (e.g., loneliness, problems with safety or personal care) did not differ from group homes. A small number of participants did experience some unsatisfactory outcomes (e.g., had money or possessions stolen, no friends outside the residential setting), but these problems were not exclusive to a particular accommodation type. Overall, SILS residents enjoyed lifestyle outcomes that were as good as their counterparts in group homes, and in the case of outcomes favoring independent participation, SILS residents did better.

COST OF COMMUNITY LIVING SERVICES

Stancliffe and Keane (2000) provided a detailed account of the way that service cost data were gathered. This process is described briefly in Table 6.4. For the sake of simplicity of presentation, only per-person direct-support staff costs are analyzed.

Costs of Semi-Independent Living and Group Homes

Per-person direct-support staff costs were compared for semi-independent living and group homes with adaptive and challenging behavior as covariates. This analysis revealed that the raw cost in Australian dollars ($Au) of group home placements (M = $Au51,853, SD = $Au29,185) was substantially and significantly higher than semi-independent living (M = $Au10,056, SD = $Au7,066), $F(1,86) = 69.08$, $p < .001$. Neither adaptive nor challenging behavior were significant covariates, showing that direct-

Table 6.4. Methods for collection and calculation of annual per-person expenditure data

Collecting annual per-person expenditure data
Agency management and administrators supplied information on the *per-person* recurrent (noncapital) annual expenditure on
a. Direct-support staff to the participant's *household**
b. Administrative costs, including the proportion of the cost of administrative staff attributable to that household*
c. Other costs of running the household, such as recurrent expenditure on housing (e.g., rent) and equipment*
d. Additional direct-support staff costs for an *individual* service recipient funded from the participant's *individual funding*#

Calculating total annual expenditure per person
Annual residential *direct-support staff cost* per person = (a + d)†
Annual *total residential cost* per person = (a + b + c + d)†

Note: Cost data did not include capital costs, resident financial contributions, or the cost of nonresidential services. No adjustments were made to residential service costs to take into account the amount of time individuals spent elsewhere, such as at day programs.
* For items a, b, and c, per-person costs were calculated by dividing household costs by the number of service recipients living in the household.
#Any *individual* funding in item d was assigned solely to that specific person.
† For participants with no individual funding (the majority) the value of item (d) was zero.

support staff costs were not significantly related to either characteristic (see subsequent discussion of needs-based expenditure). The difference between the raw means was very large, with the group home costs more than five times higher than for semi-independent settings. An estimate of effect size, partial eta squared (η_p^2), showed that the effect size for residence type was $\eta_p^2 = .45$, indicating that 45% of the total variability of the per-person staff costs was attributable to residence type. This represents a very robust finding.

Given the marked difference in per-person staffing reported previously, these findings are hardly surprising, but they do illustrate the very substantial magnitude of the cost differences, even after variations in participants' adaptive and challenging behavior had been taken into account using covariance.

Other Factors Associated with Staff Costs

The cost of direct-support staff in semi-independent community living was substantially less than in group homes; however, a number of other factors likely were related to the cost of providing community living, such as differences in residents' personal characteristics and features of the community-living service. These variables were analyzed using backward multiple regression.

Backward multiple regression begins by examining all variables and eliminating nonsignificant variables one at a time on statistical grounds. The variables *evaluated but eliminated* during backward regression and shown *not* to have a statistically significant association with direct support staff costs were

- Greater assessed need for staff support (ICAP Service Score based on a weighted combination of ICAP adaptive and challenging behavior scores). When ICAP adaptive and challenging behavior scores were entered separately instead of the composite ICAP service score, both of these variables were also eliminated

- Having a chronic health problem

- Location within or not within the Sydney metropolitan area.

The backward regression analysis revealed that the following variables were independently associated with *higher* direct-support staff costs per resident (the probability that the regression coefficient for each variable differed from zero is shown in parentheses).

Personal characteristics

- Older age ($p < .001$)
- Having a formal psychiatric diagnosis ($p < .05$)

Community living service characteristics

- Living in a group home ($p < .001$)
- Smaller residence size ($p < .001$)
- Residence size by type interaction ($p < .002$)
- Government operated service ($p < .001$)

These six variables accounted for a very substantial 80% of the variability in direct-support staff costs (i.e., $R^2 = .80$). Living in a group home contributed the largest increase in staff costs, followed by smaller residence size, residence size by type interaction, older age, government-operated service, and having a psychiatric diagnosis. There was a minor statistical problem with collinearity among residence type, residence size, and the residence size by type interaction. The backward regression analysis was run again with the residence size by type interaction omitted to check the stability of the results. This action eliminated the collinearity problem and yielded a very similar result, with all five of the other predictor variables remaining in the final model ($R^2 = .77$), although residence size was relatively less important and was of marginal statistical significance ($p = .055$). The interpretation of the residence size by type interaction is discussed more fully in the section Economies of Scale.

Needs-Based Expenditure   If service funding were needs based, it should have been strongly related to support needs; however, need for staff support (as measured by the ICAP service score) failed to act as a significant predictor of costs. This result likely was related to the nature of the service funding system in NSW, although other factors, such as the method for calculating per-person staff costs and the relative homogeneity of the sample, may have contributed to this finding. Services in NSW traditionally have been funded on a facility or agency basis. In the past, there was little attempt to link funding to the support needs of the specific individuals served, so across the residential service system, staffing and expenditure were found to be unrelated to residents' personal characteristics (Department of Community Services, 1996). The level of staffing within a setting was determined by what could be afforded given the available funding. This traditional funding system continues to prevail in most NSW residential services and is not conducive to needs-based funding or staffing.

Toward the end of the 1990s, attempts were made to provide individual funding packages based on assessed support needs. Only two (2%) individuals (both from the same group home) received *all* of their staff support through an individual funding package. Some other study participants (18%) had *some* funding of this kind (6 from group homes, 8 living semi-independently) that provided specific *additional* individual staff support, but in all of these cases, this funding was a *supplement* to the facility/agency funding that provided core staffing in the residence. Because of this low proportion of individual funding, the current study should not be seen as an adequate test of whether such individual funding is needs based. Rather, the findings speak to the degree to which traditional funding is needs based.

In the present study, per-person staff costs were needs based to a very limited degree in that having a formal psychiatric diagnosis was the only personal characteristic, other than age, significantly related to higher per-person staff costs. The major factors associated with staff costs were structural service-related factors, such as residence type, residence size, the size by type interaction, and government or nongovernment operation. Stancliffe and Lakin (1998) reported similar findings in Minnesota; however, other investigators have found the expected relationship between support needs (as defined by adaptive and challenging behavior) and service costs (Campbell & Heal, 1995; Knapp, Cambridge, Thomason, Beecham, Allen, & Darton, 1992; Raynes, Wright, Shiell, & Pettipher, 1994; see also Chapters 5, 7, 8, and 11).

The presence of a psychiatric diagnosis suggested greater need for support and was associated with significantly higher direct-support staff costs. Higher cost was also associated with older age. Some previous research (Campbell & Heal, 1995) has reported the opposite, with higher costs for younger residents, but that study included children who presumably required more staff supervision. Raynes et al. (1994) found that costs for younger and older residents were greater than costs for those in middle age. The present study only involved adults, so higher cost for older residents could be seen to be consistent with these findings in that there were no children to inflate the costs for the younger age group. Older people typically have more chronic conditions that may necessitate more support. In the present study, there was a significant relationship between age and both the presence of deafness and of a formal psychiatric diagnosis. In both cases, those with a diagnosis were significantly older than those with no diagnosis, $t(88) = -2.19$, $p < .05$ (deafness), and $t(88) = -3.44$, $p < .001$ (psychiatric).

Economies of Scale In manufacturing, economies of (large) scale are realized when high-volume production results in costs being distributed over a larger number of units and unit cost being lowered. In community living, the *scale* of the setting equates to the number of residents, and *unit cost* is equivalent to per-person expenditure on the residential service. Economies of scale would, to the extent that they apply, be expected to yield lower per-person cost as the number of residents in a setting increases.

Supporting people with intellectual disabilities is staff intensive and does not lend itself to automation. Staffing is the major cost in residential services. In the United States, staff wages and benefits typically represent 77%–87% of expenditure on services (Ashbaugh & Nerney, 1990; Knobbe, Carey, Rhodes, & Horner, 1995; Schalock & Fredericks, 1990). Consequently, the relationship between residence size and staffing will strongly influence the extent to which economies of scale operate.

Devolution of group homes into more individualized living arrangements provides one interesting insight into the relationship between residence size, staffing, and per-person cost. In Australia, examples exist of such devolutions that have been achieved *without* employing additional financial or staffing resources (Stancliffe & Whaite, 1997; Van Dam & Cameron-McGill, 1995), suggesting that economies of scale did not necessarily apply. In each case, a key element involved supporting the former group-home residents to live *semi-independently*. Staff hours previously used in the group home were redistributed across the multiple semi-independent settings to which former group-home residents moved. Residents likely received as much (or more) *direct* 1:1 support from staff as they did in the group home, but they did not have staff present in their new home at other times when staff were supporting other residents (who now also lived semi-independently in other settings). Thus, there was no necessary difference in the total amount of staff support (and consequently the per-person cost of staffing the service) based on the size of the residence, so there was no economy of scale. It is most unlikely, however, that such devolution could have been achieved within existing staff resources if 24-hour staff support was also provided in the new individual residences.

To dissect this issue further, it is necessary to consider the *nature* of the staff support provided. Activities involving 1:1 support require the same amount of staff time regardless of the size of the setting. Only when staffing is deployed for general supervision or group activities, rather than individual support, can economies of scale be realized in group settings, in that the larger the group of residents under the supervision of a single staff member, the smaller the per-person cost of staffing. The clearest example of this trend is overnight staffing. If residents do not need any specific individual support overnight but staff are on duty just in case, it is more cost effective to employ one staff member to supervise five residents in a single dwelling than it is to employ five staff to provide this supervision in five different settings. People living semi-independently do not have over-night staffing, so this factor does not apply in such settings. Moreover, drop-in staff in semi-independent settings usually support specific individual activities and rarely provide general supervision.

This analysis suggests that, in relation to expenditure on staffing, few economies of scale exist in semi-independent settings, but there may be more evident effects in group homes. Expressed statistically, this finding represents an *interaction* between residence size and type. These notions were evaluated empirically within the current data set and were strongly supported, as shown by the significance of the residence size by type interaction in the regression analysis mentioned previously. Figure 6.1 shows mean per-person direct-support staff raw expenditure by residence size, and Figure 6.2 shows these means further broken down by residence type.

Figure 6.1 shows that for the complete sample (62% semi-independent, 38% group homes), residence size had a decidedly *non*linear relationship to mean staff costs, with the *smallest* settings of 1 or 2 residents being less costly, as all were semi-independent. When residence size was regressed onto staff costs as part of a multiple *linear* regression, the fit was relatively poor, which is indicated by the marginal significance ($p = .055$) of the residence size variable when it was analyzed in the absence of the residence size by type interaction. For the sample as a whole, economies of scale had limited overall influence on per-person staffing costs.

Figure 6.2 shows little variation in mean direct-support staff costs by residence size for semi-independent living (i.e. no evident economy of scale) but substantial differences by size among group homes, with larger settings generally having lower per-person raw costs, as would be expected with economies of scale. As noted, this interaction was found to be highly significant ($p = .002$) under multiple regression. Indeed, except for the variable *residence type*, the interaction term had the strongest bivariate correlation with staff costs ($r = -.57, p < .001$).

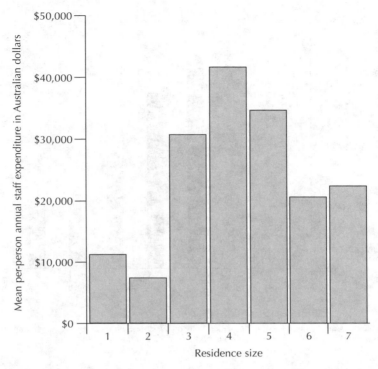

Figure 6.1. Mean per-person raw annual expenditure on direct-support staff by residence size.

For illustrative purposes, these issues were further tested statistically using separate one-way univariate ANOVAs. For semi-independent settings, there was no significant difference in raw per-person staff costs by setting size, $F(3,52) = 0.74$, $p > .50$. In group homes, raw staff costs differed significantly by size, $F(2,31) = 6.73$, $p = .004$, with smaller settings having higher per-person staff costs as expected. Due to small participant numbers for some residence sizes certain cells were collapsed for these analyses. These findings are consistent with the arguments outlined previously and suggest that economies of scale tend to affect per–person staff costs in group homes, but not in semi-independent settings, likely because a significant portion of group home staff time is used for group supervision. That is, whether economies of scale have an effect is *model dependent*.

In relation to semi-independent settings, this finding provides empirical support for Felce's in-principle proposition that

For people whose level of ability allows them to be largely independent and only require episodic support it is possible to keep staff costs per person sim-

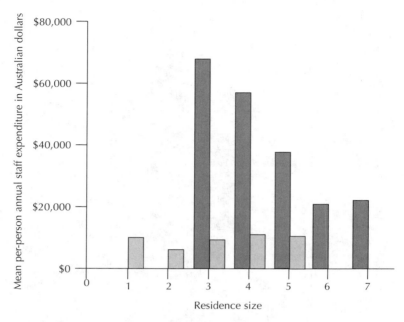

Figure 6.2.   Mean per-person raw annual expenditure on direct-support staff by residence size and type. (Key = ☐ Semi-independent home; ■ Group home)

ilar across different residential sizes. Total service costs need not rise as a function of decreasing size as long as care is taken by the planners of services to keep staff costs in ratio to the number of people served. (1994, p. 502)

The results of the multiple regression mentioned previously show that residence size was significantly related to staff costs in a *multivariate* context, where service recipients' personal characteristics were controlled statistically. However, the *raw* data in Figure 6.2 exaggerate size-related differences in group-home staff costs because a proportion of the cost difference likely is attributable to differences in personal characteristics. Indeed, when service recipients' personal characteristics (age and psychiatric diagnosis) were included in the group-home ANCOVA as covariates, cost differences by residence size were no longer significant, $F(4,29) = 0.95, p > .25$.

POLICY IMPLICATIONS

The current study suggested that some residents of group homes in Australia may achieve similar or better lifestyle outcomes, at lower cost, by

living semi-independently. These individuals should be given the opportunity and support to live semi-independently if they choose. To date, such
opportunities rarely have been available in NSW.

Following the completion and dissemination of the research described
in this chapter, the NSW government announced a Group Homes Devolution Project involving a substantial number of government-operated
group homes housing a total of over 200 people with more limited support
needs. The plan was to offer residents individual funding packages and
the opportunity to negotiate with both government and nongovernment
community-living services to gain access to more individualized semi-
independent living arrangements, followed by the eventual closure of some
of the group homes.

Although some service recipients and advocates welcomed this opportunity, there was substantial opposition from group-home staff and
from many service recipients and their families who did not wish to change
their living arrangements or were unsure about the nature of the alternatives being offered. Perhaps those who were dissatisfied with their current
group-home placement were the ones who embraced the chance to
change. The project may have worked more smoothly if service recipients
and families had been able to decide at the outset if they wanted to participate. Even in the face of research findings revealing the benefits of
change, as was the case for deinstitutionalization, service recipients and
families may initially resist moving to new and unfamiliar living options
(see Larson & Lakin, 1991).

Another important finding was that expenditure on direct-support
staff was not significantly related to fundamental personal characteristics,
such as adaptive and challenging behavior, although expenditure was
higher for people who were older or who had a psychiatric diagnosis.
These findings indicate that, at best, expenditure was needs based to a very
limited degree. If governments and service providers aspire to equity in
provision of community-living services based on individual support needs,
considerable restructuring of existing funding and services appears to be
required. Individual funding packages based on support needs may provide
one method of achieving this, but it should not be assumed that this approach will necessarily result in individualized, needs-based services. In
some instances, consumers with individual funding have moved into existing group homes, and their funding has partially subsidized the overall
operation of the group home, for the benefit of all residents. Few participants in the current study had individual funding packages (only two participants' support was funded fully in this manner), so the data did not

enable evaluation of whether individual funding was associated with needs-based expenditure on staff.

A further key finding concerned the differing applicability of economies of scale to group homes and semi-independent settings. The significant residence size by type interaction and subsequent analyses showed that per-person expenditure on direct-support staff was unrelated to residence size in semi-independent settings, but in group homes with fewer residents, per-person raw costs have been higher. It was argued that this may relate to the different ways in which staff work with residents in these residence types, with 1:1 support not being subject to economies of scale. Future research, however, will need to evaluate this proposition empirically by comparing the proportion of 1:1 support in group homes and SILS.

These findings have significant implications for policy and practice. First, they suggest that, in relation to staff costs, there is no fiscal disincentive for people living semi-independently to live alone or in very small groups (see Felce, 1994). In addition, the results imply that it may be easier to respond to residents' changing preferences for living companions and living arrangements in semi-independent settings. If a resident of a 3-person semi-independent household wished to move out to live alone or with a friend, it may well be feasible for him or her to take a proportionate share of the existing staff support to his or her new home and still leave sufficient support for the two residents who remain. In a group home with 24-hour staffing, if one resident of a 4-person group moves elsewhere and takes an equitable proportion (say 25%) of the funding for staff with him or her, service providers often argue that the remaining 75% of the funds is insufficient to provide 24-hour staffing in a 3-person group home. The current findings on economies of scale were broadly consistent with this view *for group homes*. In NSW, individual funding packages provide portability of funding, so the consumer can take his or her funding and move to another service if desired. Even though individual funding packages were rare in the present study, the findings imply that de-facto portability may be feasible for residents of SILS, regardless of the presence of formally identified individual funding. Of course, this analysis does not take account of other nonstaff costs, notably housing costs.

CONCLUSION

This study found that adults with intellectual disabilities and low to moderate support needs living semi-independently achieved equivalent or better lifestyle outcomes at substantially lower staff cost as compared with peers in group homes. Economies of scale may have operated in group homes, with smaller group homes having somewhat higher per-resident raw staff costs. There were no size-related differences in staff costs for semi-independent settings, indicating that any effects of economies of scale were *model dependent* and were confined to residences with full-time staffing. These findings are consistent with a policy of more widespread availability of semi-independent living.

REFERENCES

Ashbaugh, J., & Nerney, T. (1990). Costs of providing residential and related support services to individuals with mental retardation. *Mental Retardation, 28,* 269–273.

Australian Institute of Health and Welfare. (AIHW). (2002). *Disability support services 2001: National data on services provided under the Commonwealth/State Disability Agreement* (AIHW Cat. No. DIS 25). Canberra, Australia: AIHW (Disability series).

Black, K., & Eckerman, S. (1997). *Disability support services provided under the Commonwealth/State Disability Agreement: First national data, 1995* (AIHW Cat. No. DIS 1). Canberra, Australia: AIHW.

Bruininks, R.H., Hill, B.K., Weatherman, R.F., & Woodcock, R.W. (1986). *Examiner's manual. ICAP Inventory for Client and Agency Planning.* Allen, TX: DLM Teaching Resources.

Campbell, E.M., & Heal, L.W. (1995). Prediction of cost, rates, and staffing by provider and client characteristics. *American Journal on Mental Retardation, 100,* 17–35.

Department of Community Services. (1996). *Community living. Supported accommodation for people with disabilities.* Sydney: Author.

Felce, D. (1994). Costs, quality and staffing in services for people with severe learning disabilities. *Journal of Mental Health, 3,* 495–506.

Felce, D., Jones, E., & Lowe, K. (2002). Active support: Planning daily activities and support for people with severe mental retardation. In S. Holburn & P.M. Vietze (Eds.), *Person-centered planning: Research, practice, and future directions* (pp. 247–269). Baltimore: Paul H. Brookes Publishing Co.

Knapp, M., Cambridge, P., Thomason, C., Beecham, J., Allen, C., & Darton, R. (1992). *Care in the community: Challenge and demonstration.* Aldershot, United Kingdom: Ashgate.

Knobbe, C.A., Carey, S.P., Rhodes, L., & Horner, R.H. (1995). Benefit–cost analysis of community residential versus institutional services for adults with severe mental retardation and challenging behaviors. *American Journal on Mental Retardation, 99,* 533–541.

Larson, S., & Lakin, K.C. (1991). Parent attitudes about residential placement before and after deinstitutionalization: A research synthesis. *Journal of The Association for Persons with Severe Handicaps, 16,* 25–38.

Raynes, N.V., Sumpton, R.C., & Pettipher, C. (1989). *Index of Participation in Domestic Life*. Manchester, United Kingdom: The University Department of Social Policy and Social Work.

Raynes, N.V., Wright, K., Shiell, A., & Pettipher, C. (1994). *The cost and quality of community residential care. An evaluation of the services for adults with learning disabilities*. London: David Fulton Publishers.

Robertson, J., Emerson, E., Gregory, N., Hatton, C., Kessissoglou, S., Hallam, A., & Linehan, C. (2001). Social networks of people with mental retardation in residential settings. *Mental Retardation, 39*, 201–214.

Schalock, M., & Fredericks, H.D.B. (1990). Comparative costs for institutional services and services for selected populations in the community. *Behavioral Residential Treatment, 5*, 271–286.

Schalock, R.L., & Keith, K.D. (1993). *Quality of life questionnaire*. Worthington, OH: IDS Publishing Corporation.

Stancliffe, R.J. (1995). *Choice and decision making and adults with intellectual disability*. Unpublished doctoral thesis, Macquarie University, Sydney.

Stancliffe, R.J. (1997). Community living-unit size, staff presence and resident's choice-making. *Mental Retardation, 35*, 1–9.

Stancliffe, R.J. (2002). Provision of residential services for people with intellectual disability in Australia: An international comparison. *Journal of Intellectual & Developmental Disability, 27*, 117–124.

Stancliffe, R.J., Abery, B.H., & Smith, J. (2000). Personal control and the ecology of community living settings: Beyond living-unit size and type. *American Journal on Mental Retardation, 105*, 431–454.

Stancliffe, R.J., & Keane, S. (2000). Outcomes and costs of community living: A matched comparison of group homes and semi-independent living. *Journal of Intellectual & Developmental Disability, 25*, 281–305.

Stancliffe, R.J., & Lakin, K.C. (1998). Analysis of expenditures and outcomes of residential alternatives for persons with developmental disabilities. *American Journal on Mental Retardation, 102*, 552–568.

Stancliffe, R.J., & Parmenter, T.R. (1999). The Choice Questionnaire: A scale to assess choices exercised by adults with intellectual disability. *Journal of Intellectual & Developmental Disability, 24*, 107–132.

Stancliffe, R.J., & Whaite, A. (1997). *Watagan project evaluation*. Sydney: The University of Sydney, Centre for Developmental Disability Studies.

Van Dam, T., & Cameron-McGill, F. (1995). Beyond group homes. *Interaction, 8*(3), 7–13.

Whaite, E.A., Stancliffe, R.J., & Keane, S. (1999). Compatibility: Living together is hard to do. *Interaction, 13*(1), 24–30.

CHAPTER 7

Costs and Outcomes of Community Residential Supports in England

Eric Emerson, Janet Robertson, Chris Hatton, Martin Knapp,
Patricia Noonan Walsh, and Angela Hallam

The implementation of policies associated with deinstitutionalization has dominated the development of services for people with intellectual disabilities in most, although not all, European countries (Hatton, Emerson, & Kiernan, 1995). In England, for example, the number of people with intellectual disabilities who live in state-operated institutions declined by 93%, from 51,000 in 1976 to just over 3,500 in 2002. This reduction has been accompanied by a corresponding increase in the number of people supported in smaller community-based residential services based on the use of domestic housing (Emerson & Hatton, 1994; Kavanagh & Opit, 1998).

These developments have been accompanied by wide-ranging legislative changes and a significant amount of central policy guidance regarding residential provision (e.g., Department of Health, 1992a, 1992b, 1993, 2001; Office of the Deputy Prime Minister and Department of Health, 2003).

Deinstitutionalization in England has not, however, been a unified policy. There have been, and remain, significant variations over time and across localities in the ways in which these policy changes have been transacted (see Bailey & Cooper, 1997; Emerson & Hatton, 1997, 1998, 2000). Leading up to 1980, deinstitutionalization primarily involved the movement of those individuals with the least severe disabilities to a range of often preexisting services, including hostels, semisupported group homes, family placement schemes, bed and breakfast arrangements, and independent living. Since then, however, attention has switched to the development of community-based housing for people with more severe and complex disabilities. Initially, such services were provided in 20- to 24-resident locally based hospital or community units to serve a defined geographical area (e.g., Felce, Kushlick, & Mansell, 1980). During the mid-1980s, however, these ideas gave way (at least in most areas) to services that provide staff support to people with severe disabilities within smaller domestic-scale dispersed housing schemes (e.g., Felce, 1989; Lowe & de Paiva, 1991). Later, the appropriateness of this model was called into question by advocates of supported-living arrangements (e.g., Kinsella, 1993; Simons, 1995, 1997).

Community-based residential supports are not, of course, the only alternative to traditional forms of institutional care. Other options include intentional or village communities (Cox & Pearson, 1995; Grover, 1995; Jackson, 1996; Segal, 1990) and state-operated residential campuses. Both of these approaches have been vigorously promoted by lobby groups in the United Kingdom as providing viable and cost-effective alternatives to community-based provision (Cox & Pearson, 1995; Jackson, 1996).

A number of intentional or village communities currently exist in the United Kingdom and Ireland. All are operated by charitable organizations and provide support and centralized vocational and leisure services on one or more sites that are clearly segregated from the surrounding community. Although the number of such services is unknown, they are estimated to account for approximately 2% of supported accommodation services for people with intellectual disabilities in England (Department of Health, 1999). The guiding ethos behind these communities is that, by paralleling the operation of rural villages, village communities can provide a relatively self-contained rich and varied life for people with intellectual disabilities in a setting that is to a certain extent physically separate from mainstream society. As such, village communities demonstrate continuity in ideas with romantic notions of village life and the rationale for institutions for people with intellectual disabilities that emerged at the end of the 19th century (Scheerenberger, 1983; Wolfensberger, 1975).

A number of village communities have a clear religious or philosophical foundation. The latter include a number of Camphill communities that are based on life-sharing arrangements between people who do and do not have disabilities (see http://www.camphill.org.uk). As Fulgosi describes,

> As the word "village" implies, each Camphill village centre endeavors to create and maintain an environment where the economic, social and spiritual life of the community complement each other. Villagers [people with intellectual disabilities] and co-workers live and work side-by-side, running their homes, and sharing what needs to be done. Some villages have a village

store, a gift shop, café, and even a post office…. The rhythm of the farming year, the seasons and the celebration of the Christian festivals play an important part in the life of each community. (1990, p. 43)

The vast majority of people who live in intentional or village communities are relatively able and moved there from their family home or from residential special schools for children with intellectual disabilities. As such, the village community movement has developed independently of deinstitutionalization; however, some people have argued that village communities could be created out of state-operated institutions (Brook, 1990). A number of newly built state-operated residential campuses have been developed in the United Kingdom as a direct result of deinstitutionalization. These are operated by National Health Service (NHS) organizations and provide residential support and centralized services on a campus site, typically supporting people with more severe and complex disabilities. None of these share the ideological underpinnings of village communities; rather, they represent a new wave of state-operated institutional provision providing support for up to 100 people housed in living units for 8–12 people.

In a direct response to lobbying from advocacy groups, the English Department of Health (which oversees all health- and social-care services in England) commissioned us to undertake a systematic review of the existing U.K. literature on living arrangements for people with intellectual disabilities. Although no formal evaluations had yet been undertaken of intentional or village communities, this report drew attention to the range of positive outcomes associated with deinstitutionalization. These included 1) increased service recipient satisfaction; 2) increased choice over day-to-day matters; 3) increased participation in community-based activities; 4) increased engagement in ongoing domestic and personal activities; and 5) increased support from care staff (Emerson & Hatton, 1994, 1996a). These results are broadly comparable with those of North American and Australian studies investigating the process of deinstitutionalization (e.g., Kim, Larson, & Lakin, 2001; Larson & Lakin, 1989; Young, Sigafoos, Suttie, Ashman, & Grevell, 1998).

After this review, we were commissioned to undertake a comparative cost–benefit analysis of community-based residential services (including supported-living arrangements), village communities, and NHS campuses. The results of this project have been reported in several project reports[1] and papers (Emerson et al., 1999a, 2000a, 2000b, 2000c, 2001; Gregory,

---

[1]Available online at http://www.lancaster.ac.uk/fss/ihr/publications.htm

Robertson, Kessissoglou, Emerson, & Hatton, 2001; Hallam & Emerson, 1999; Hallam et al., 2002; Robertson et al., 2000a, 2000b, 2001a, 2001b; Walsh et al., 2001). In this chapter, we summarize the main results of the project as they relate to the association between costs and outcomes.

DESIGN, SAMPLING, DEFINITIONS, AND INSTRUMENTATION OF THE STUDY

As full details of the method and instrumentation employed in the study are provided elsewhere (Emerson et al., 2000a, 2000b, 2000c, 2001; Gregory et al., 2001; Hallam & Emerson, 1999; Hallam et al., 2002; Robertson et al., 2000a, 2000b, 2001a, 2001b; Walsh et al., 2001), only the main points are summarized next.

Design and Definitions

The study employed a cross-sectional design. We sought to collect information on a target sample of 540 adults with intellectual disabilities, consisting of 1) three samples of 30 adults randomly selected from the residents of three *village communities*; 2) five samples of 30 adults randomly selected from the residents of five (NHS) *residential campuses*; 3) 10 samples of 30 adults randomly selected from the people supported by 10 different providers of community-based *dispersed housing schemes*, including examples of organizations providing *supported-living* arrangements.

In the category of residential campuses and village communities, we included all forms of long-term residential provision that provided 24-hour support in a campus-style setting. A campus/community was defined as a setting in which housing for people with intellectual disabilities was clustered together on one site and shared some central facilities (e.g., day center, church, shops). In the category of *dispersed housing schemes*, we included all forms of long-term residential supports that provided 24-hour support in dispersed domestic-style housing for no more than eight people. *Supported-living schemes* (a subcategory of *dispersed housing schemes*) were defined as examples of residential supports that satisfied each of the following three criteria: 1) key informants from the provider organization described the arrangements as an example of supported living; 2) the service was not registered under the relevant U.K. legislation as either a Residential Care Home or a Nursing Home; 3) no more than 3 people with intellectual disabilities were living in the same house as co-residents.

Sampling

Potential services were identified through a process of consultation with organizations and advocacy groups representing the interests of parents of people with intellectual disabilities, service providers, and the research and development community. The aim of the consultation was to identify services that were considered by key informants to be examples of "good" or "better" practice within that particular model of residential support.

At the time of completion of data collection, information had been collected on 500 participants across 17 services. These included 86 participants in three *intentional or village communities* (96% of target); 133 participants in five *NHS campuses* (89% of target); and 281 participants in 10 community-based *dispersed housing schemes* (94% of target). Of the latter, 63 people were identified as receiving *supported-living schemes*.

Organizations

The three *village communities* were operated by charities. None of these services had been developed as a direct result of the downsizing and closure of state-operated institutions. All expressed an aim of providing a partially self-contained community for their residents. The number of long-term residents supported on-site ranged from 28 to 179. The mean number of residents per living unit ranged from 7 to 8. In two of the village communities, the majority of living units were freestanding buildings grouped in close proximity to centralized day and leisure facilities. In the third community, 17 of the participants lived in a house for 25 people; the remainder lived in houses for 2–5 people that were clustered around the central facility.

The five *residential campuses* were all operated by NHS organizations. They had all been developed as a direct result of the closure of NHS institutions for people with intellectual disabilities. The number of long-term residents supported on-site ranged from 94 to 144. The mean number of residents per living unit ranged from 7 to 10. In all five residential campuses, the majority of living units were freestanding buildings grouped in close proximity to centralized day and leisure facilities.

The 10 *dispersed housing schemes* provided a mixture of "group homes" or "staffed houses" (e.g., Felce, 1989) and examples of "supported living" (Simons, 1995, 1997). The number of long-term residents supported ranged from 22 to 161. The mean number of residents per living unit ranged from 1 to 8.

Measures

Information was collected by a combination of mailed questionnaires combined with follow-up interviews with a member of the participant's support team, interviews with service recipients, ratings completed by research staff, and a mailed questionnaire distributed to the relatives of service recipients. Full details of the measures used are provided in Emerson et al. (2000a, 2000b, 2000c, 2001), Gregory et al. (2001), Hallam and Emerson (1999), Hallam et al. (2002), Robertson et al. (2000a, 2000b, 2001a, 2001b), and Walsh et al. (2001). A summary of the inputs, processes, and outcomes evaluated is presented in Table 7.1.

A revised version of the Client Service Receipt Inventory (Beecham, 1995; Beecham & Knapp, 1992) was completed for each participant to collect data relating to accommodation arrangements, income and expenditure, and use of services during the previous 3 months. The Residential Services Setting Questionnaire (Emerson, Alborz, Felce, & Lowe, 1995) was used to record information about managing agency arrangements, staffing levels within individual houses, and the physical layout of each site. To allow facility-specific costs to be calculated, additional information was collected from analysis of facility accounts. In order to estimate the long-run marginal (opportunity) costs of building-based services, the cost implications of these buildings were included in the total accommodation facility cost.

All capital costs were annuitized over an expected 60-year life span at a discount rate of 8% (Netten, Dennett, & Knight, 1998). Ten percent of the annual figure was added as an estimate of the replacement of fixtures and fittings. Services received independently of the service recipient's

Table 7.1.   Measures

Inputs	Service processes	Outcomes
Costs	Quality and nature of internal planning procedures	Involvement in leisure and community-based activities
Staffing ratios		Social networks
Staff qualifications	Social climate	Health behaviors (smoking, alcohol use, diet and physical exercise)
Architectural features, size and location of home	Support for self-determination	
Characteristics of participants (age, gender, adaptive and challenging behavior, presence of additional physical and sensory impairments, mental health, autism, residential history)		Risk of exposure to accidents and injuries, abuse and exploitation
		Expressed satisfaction of participants with intellectual disabilities
		Expressed satisfaction of relatives

accommodation arrangements were priced using national unit costs data (Netten et al., 1998). All hospital and community-based services, day centers, and education and training programs in which these services were not included as part of the residential package were priced in this way. At the end of the pricing process, we had defined and priced a service package unique to each study participant: All costs relating to residential services, day activities, and use of all other services were represented as their weekly contribution to the total cost of care. All costs are reported at 1999–2000 price levels and converted to U.S. dollars at a rate of £1 = $1.65.

CHARACTERISTICS OF THE PARTICIPANTS

Information regarding the characteristics of participants is summarized in Table 7.2. There were robust differences between the groups with regard to adaptive behavior, health needs, challenging behavior, age, and residential history. In general, participants living in village communities were significantly more able than participants living in dispersed housing schemes

Table 7.2. Participant characteristics

			Service model			
			Dispersed housing schemes ($n = 281$)			
Participant characteristic	Village communities ($n = 86$)	Residential campuses ($n = 133$)	Overall ($n = 281$)	Large-group homes ($n = 163$)	Small group homes ($n = 55$)	Supported living ($n = 63$)
Age (mean years)	40	48	46	44	54	44
Gender (percent men)	62%	59%	60%	59%	56%	71%
Ethnicity (percent white)	100%	96%	96%	98%	96%	91%
Adaptive behavior (mean ABS Pt1 score)	195	104	150	136	167	175
Challenging behavior (mean ABC score)	18	32	20	19	16	23
Mental health (percent meeting criterion)	23%	24%	24%	22%	16%	33%
Autism (percent reaching DSM-IV criteria)	38%	47%	35%	34%	32%	39%

who, in turn, were significantly more able than participants living in residential campuses (for further details see Emerson et al., 2000c). The latter group showed significantly higher levels of challenging behavior than participants living in either village communities or dispersed housing schemes.

Such differences in the characteristics of participants are not uncommon in research on residential supports. They do, however, represent a significant challenge to interpreting between-model differences given the extensive evidence suggesting that participant ability (or adaptive behavior) may be significantly associated with both the costs and quality of provision (Stancliffe, Emerson, & Lakin, 2004). As a result, two complementary approaches were taken in an attempt to control for the possible confounding effects of these between-group differences. First, under conditions in which dependent variables were significantly associated with either adaptive behavior or challenging behavior, we undertook multivariate analyses in which the potentially confounding variable (e.g., adaptive behavior) was first entered as a covariate. Second, matched subsamples were drawn from the total sample to enable between-model comparisons to be made while controlling for level of adaptive behavior.

COSTS OF SERVICE PROVISION

Full details of the costs of service provision are provided in Emerson et al. (2000b, 2000c, 2001), Hallam and Emerson (1999), and Hallam et al. (2002). A summary of accommodation, nonaccommodation, and total costs per week are provided in Table 7.3. Multivariate analyses indicated that—once costs were adjusted to control for between-model differences in adaptive behavior, challenging behavior, and age—weekly accommodation and total costs were significantly greater in dispersed housing schemes ($1,753) than residential campuses ($1,524), which were in turn significantly greater than in village communities ($1,416) (Emerson et al., 2000c). The results derived from the analyses of the matched samples were broadly consistent with these results in that significantly higher total costs per week were found in dispersed housing schemes (mean weekly cost = $1,903) than residential campuses (mean weekly cost = $1,683), although differences in total costs between dispersed housing schemes (mean weekly cost = $1,511)[2] and village communities (mean

---

[2]The mean values for the dispersed housing schemes differ due to the drawing of two matched samples from this population: one to match with participants living in village communities, and the other to match with participants living in residential campuses.

Table 7.3. Raw service package costs (dollars per week, 1999–2000 prices)

Cost component	Village communities (n = 86)	Residential campuses (n = 133)	Cost			
			Dispersed housing schemes (n = 281)			
			Overall (n = 281)	Large-group homes (n = 163)	Small-group homes (n = 55)	Supported living (n = 63)
Total accommodation cost						
Mean	1,051	1,536	1,486	1,462	1,382	1,689
Range	617–2,980	922–6,159	229–2,994	304–2,060	495–2,540	229–2,994
Standard deviation	518	561	573	396	621	818
Total nonaccommodation cost						
Mean	243	142	227	275	225	116
Range	17–1,100	0–644	0–1,167	0–1,167	0–1,043	1–652
Standard deviation	144	135	202	208	206	133
Total cost						
Mean	1,294	1,680	1,713	1,737	1,606	1,805
Range	662–3,404	945–6,183	350–3,584	471–2,661	571–3,584	350–3,082
Standard deviation	574	563	617	451	739	829

weekly cost = $1,320) did not attain the level of statistical significance (Emerson et al., 2000c). A similar pattern of results was evident for staffing ratios. Further analysis within the dispersed housing sample indicated that there were no statistically significant differences in either raw or adjusted costs between supported-living schemes, small-group homes supporting 1–3 people, and large-group homes supporting 4–6 people (Emerson et al., 2000c).

These results are consistent with the existing U.K. literature that has reliably reported higher costs and higher staffing ratios in community-based services than institutional provision (Emerson & Hatton, 1994). The discrepancy between these results and those reported in the North American literature (institutional costs being higher than community-based provision) is primarily attributable to the general equivalence of pay scales for residential support staff across statutory (government operated) and nonstatutory sectors in the United Kingdom.

Of more interest in the context of this chapter, however, is the ability to explain variation in the costs of service provision within and across service models. As can be seen in Table 7.3, total annual costs ranged from approximately $18,000 to over $322,000. Hallam et al. (2002) reported that 38% of the cost variation in the full sample was accounted for in a multivariate model by 14 variables including participant age, gender, adaptive behavior, severity of challenging behavior, previous accommodation, service model, size, staffing qualifications, and internal working practices. Similarly, they reported that 51% of the cost variation in the *dispersed housing* sample was accounted for in a multivariate model by 10 variables including participant age, adaptive behavior, service model, size, staffing qualifications, and internal working practices.

Additional linear regression analysis was undertaken to determine the extent to which total cost variation could be explained by participant characteristics in the total sample and, separately, for the dispersed housing sample. These analyses cast light on the extent of "rational resourcing" across services (i.e., the extent to which resources appear to be allocated on the basis of need). Variables were entered stepwise in two blocks: 1) participant characteristics associated with need (adaptive behavior, severity of challenging behavior, mental health, autism); and 2) participant characteristics potentially associated with discriminatory practices (age, gender). The results of these analyses are presented in Table 7.4.

In the full sample, 17% of the cost variation was accounted for by adaptive behavior and challenging behavior, and an additional 2% was accounted for by age and gender. In the dispersed housing sample, 22% of the cost variation was accounted for by adaptive behavior, and an additional 3% was accounted for by age and gender. These results are broadly consistent with those reported by Hallam et al. (2002) in suggesting that although resource allocation does appear to reflect individual need, such indicators only account for a minority in the overall variation of costs.

Table 7.4. Predictors of higher total cost

Predictor	beta	Significance
Full sample (Adjusted R^2 = 0.194; F = 29.3; df = 4,466; $p < .001$)		
Adaptive behavior	−0.367	$p < .001$
Challenging behavior	0.100	$p < .05$
Gender	−0.135	$p < .001$
Age	−0.111	$p < .01$
Community sample (Adjusted R^2 = 0.247; F = 29.8; df = 3,261; $p < .001$)		
Adaptive behavior	−0.459	$p < .001$
Gender	−0.119	$p < .05$
Age	−0.116	$p < .05$

NATURE OF THE SUPPORT PROVIDED TO PARTICIPANTS

There were stark differences between models with regard to the types of support provided by dispersed housing schemes, NHS campuses, and village communities (for details see Emerson et al., 2000b, 2000c, and Robertson et al., 2000a). In general, participants in *dispersed housing schemes* were supported in small, homelike noninstitutional settings with high staffing ratios and reasonably well-developed internal planning and management procedures. They were less likely than residents in the other facilities to be prescribed antipsychotic medication, to receive routine health checks, and to have seen a psychologist or psychiatrist. Participants in *village communities* were supported in larger, less homelike settings with moderate levels of institutional climate, low staffing ratios, and well-developed internal planning and management procedures. They were less likely than residents in the other facilities to be prescribed antipsychotic medication or to have seen a psychologist or psychiatrist and were more likely to receive routine health checks, testicular checks, and vision checks. Participants in *residential campuses* were supported in larger, less homelike institutional settings with low levels of staffing ratios and poorly developed internal planning and management procedures. They were most likely to be prescribed antipsychotic medication versus residents in the other facilities.

Comparisons Among Types of Dispersed Housing

There were fewer differences within the dispersed housing sample (Emerson et al., 2000c). When compared with small-group homes, participants in supported-living schemes experienced higher staffing ratios, better internal procedures for allocating staff support on the basis of resident need, and more frequent contact with lawyers, and they were more likely to have had their hearing checked. They also, however, were less likely to have a designated keyworker or an individualized habilitation plan (IHP) and were supported in settings with poorer internal procedures for assessment and teaching. The only significant difference between small- and large-group homes was that large-group homes evidenced greater levels of depersonalization.

ASSOCIATION BETWEEN COSTS AND SIZE OF RESIDENCE

Felce and Emerson (Chapter 3) review the literature on the association between costs, size of residence, and outcomes. In Emerson et al. (2001), we reported a modest association between costs and residence size in the dispersed housing sample once variations in adaptive behavior had been controlled for. In order to explore this more fully, we undertook a series of univariate analyses of variance (with adaptive behavior and severity of challenging behavior as covariates), in which we examined the link between cost and size in village communities, NHS campuses, and (separately for more- and less-able residents) in dispersed housing schemes. Estimated marginal means from these analyses are presented in Figures 7.1 and 7.2. In village communities and NHS campuses, there was no association between size and cost (village communities $F = 0.02$, $df = 2,79$, $p = .98$; NHS Campuses $F = .82$, $df = 2,125$, $p = .44$). In dispersed housing schemes, there was a significant association between size and cost for participants with more severe disabilities (Adaptive Behavior Scale [ABS] Pt 1 score < 140, $F = 6.97$, $df = 5,116$, $p < .001$) but not for participants with less severe disabilities (ABS Pt 1 score $> = 140$, $F = 1.33$, $df = 5,130$, $p = .26$).

OUTCOMES

Data on outcomes are reported in detail elsewhere (Emerson et al., 2000a, 2000b, 2000c 2001; Gregory et al., 2001; Robertson et al., 2000a, 2000b, 2001a, 2001b; Walsh et al., 2001). In summary, participants in dispersed housing schemes experienced relatively greater choice, more extensive social networks with people with intellectual disabilities and local people, and overall, a more physically active life, fewer accidents in their home, and a greater number and variety of leisure activities. They were, however, also more likely to experience exposure to crime and verbal abuse and to have a

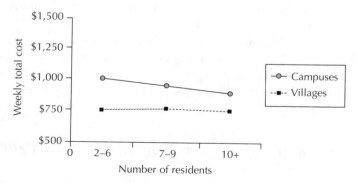

Figure 7.1.   Adjusted total weekly cost by size of residence for village communities and residential campuses.

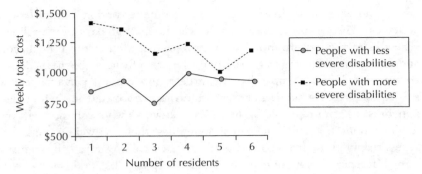

Figure 7.2.   Adjusted total weekly cost by size of residence for people with more and less severe disabilities in dispersed housing schemes.

shorter working week. Participants in village communities experienced relatively more extensive social networks overall, less exposure to crime and verbal abuse, and a longer working week, but they could also expect to experience relatively less choice and a reduced number and variety of leisure activities. Participants in residential campuses experienced relatively less choice, less extensive social networks, a less physically active life, more accidents in their home, a reduced number and variety of leisure activities, greater exposure to crime and verbal abuse, and a shorter working week.

The views of participants in residential campuses were excluded from statistical comparisons due to the very small number of people interviewed in these services. No statistically significant differences were found between the rated satisfaction of participants in village communities and participants in dispersed housing schemes overall or in six of the seven domains assessed. The exception was that participants in village communities tended to express greater satisfaction with their friendships and social relationships (Gregory et al., 2001). No statistically significant between-group differences existed in relatives' ratings of the quality of supports received by participants across the three models (Emerson et al., 2000c; Walsh et al., 2001). There were differences, however, in the extent to which relatives reported support for or opposition to the person's current placement, with the relatives of people living in village communities reporting more support from family and friends and less support from statutory services.

Comparisons Among Types of Dispersed Housing

When compared with small-group homes, participants in supported-living schemes experienced greater choice overall, greater choice over with whom and where they lived, and a greater number of community-based activities. They also, however, had fewer hours and days per week of scheduled activity, were more likely to have had their home vandalized, and were considered at greater risk of exploitation from people in the local community. When compared with large-group homes, participants in small-group homes had larger social networks, more staff in their social networks, and more people in their social networks who were not staff or family and did not have intellectual disabilities; they also were considered at less risk of abuse from co-residents. There were no statistically significant differences in any domain between the rated satisfaction of participants or their relatives in supported-living schemes, small-group homes, and large-group homes (Emerson et al., 2000c, 2001).

RELATIONSHIP BETWEEN COSTS AND OUTCOMES

We used two approaches to exploring the relationship between costs and outcomes. First, given the link between need and resources (mentioned previously), we calculated partial correlations (controlling for the effects of adaptive behavior and challenging behavior) to examine relationships between the total costs of participants' care and the 13 outcomes that discriminated between the service models (Emerson et al., 2000c, 2001). These analyses were undertaken *within* each of the three service models. In village communities, increased costs were only associated with increased performance on 1 of the 13 quality indicators (physical activity, $r_p = 0.33$). In residential campuses, increased costs were associated with increased performance on 3 of the 13 quality indicators (physical activity, $r_p = 0.53$; number of recreational/community activities, $r_p = 0.35$; variety of recreational/community activities, $r_p = 0.23$). In dispersed housing schemes, increased costs were associated with increased performance on 6 of the 13 quality indicators (choice, $r_p = 0.18$; variety of recreational/community activities, $r_p = 0.19$; total size of social network, $r_p = 0.17$; number of "others" in social network, $r_p = 0.15$; number of days, $r_p = 0.27$, and hours of scheduled activity, $r_p = 0.22$; reduced perceived risk of exploitation, $r_p = 0.30$).

Finally, among a subsample of relatively able participants, no significant bivariate associations were found between costs and any domain of service recipient satisfaction (Gregory et al., 2001). In an analysis of supports provided to people with the most severe and complex disabilities (Emerson et al., 2000b), the association between cost and outcome was again explored using partial correlation coefficients, controlling for the effects of levels of adaptive behavior. Increased total costs were associated with poorer procedures for assessment and teaching ($r_p = 0.42$), less block treatment ($r_p = 0.56$), greater variety of community-based activities ($r_p = 0.44$), and greater amounts of praise ($r_p = 0.42$).

Second, in a series of subsequent analyses, we employed more complex multivariate analyses to explore relationships between resource inputs (e.g., cost, staff qualifications, service recipient characteristics), service processes (e.g., internal management arrangements, institutional practices), and selected outcomes (Emerson et al., 1999b, 2000a; Robertson et al., 2000a, 2000b, 2001a, 2001b). The results of these analyses are summarized in Table 7.5.

These data indicate that, across the 12 outcome domains listed, costs were not significantly associated with any outcomes. Staffing ratios were associated with outcomes in four domains for the full sample and just two domains for the community-based sample. Although, in general, increased staffing ratios were associated with better outcomes, lower staffing ratios were associated with increased choice over domestic activities (Robertson et al., 2001a) and an increased probability of the person having a relative in his or her social network (Robertson et al., 2001b).

CONCLUSION

Three methodological limitations need to be kept in mind when considering the results of this study. First, the project did not randomly sample organizations, facilities, or residents. Rather, organizations were identified as exemplars of "good" or "better" practice within their respective fields. Comparison with available national data suggests that study participants: were representative in terms of age (45.1 years in the present study, 45.4 years in the U.K. 1991 Census; Emerson & Hatton, 1996b); contained a slight preponderance of men (60% in the present study, 55% in the U.K. 1991 Census; Emerson & Hatton, 1996b); and were living in slightly smaller living units (6.7 in the present study, 9.1 for voluntary sector provision in England in 1995; Staton, 1996).

Second, relatively few exemplars of each type of model were included within the project (3 village communities, 5 residential campuses, and 10 dispersed housing schemes). Finally, the models were compared on 94 measures of resource inputs (e.g., staffing ratios, buildings), nonresource inputs (e.g., social environment), and process and service recipient outcomes (e.g., choice, activity, social networks, medication usage). Making

Table 7.5. Results of multivariate analyses of costs, other resource inputs, processes, and selected outcomes

Study	Outcome	Association between costs and outcome	Other variables related to outcome
Emerson et al. (1999a)	Family contact	None	*Full sample:* age *Community sample:* age, size of residential setting, staff qualifications, social climate of residence
	Employment	None	*Full sample:* adaptive behavior, staffing ratio, social climate of residence *Community sample:* adaptive behavior, staffing ratio, social climate of residence
	Overall exposure to risk	None	*Full sample:* mental health, architectural features of home, type of current residential setting, staffing qualifications, social climate of residence *Community sample:* adaptive behavior, quality of internal planning procedures
	Frequency of recreational and community-based activities	None	*Full sample:* adaptive behavior, size of residential setting, type of current residential setting, staffing ratio, staffing qualifications, quality of internal planning procedures, social climate of residence *Community sample:* adaptive behavior, size of residential setting, staffing qualifications, quality of internal planning procedures, social climate of residence
Emerson et al. (2000b)	Intervention program for challenging behavior	None	*Full sample:* form of challenging behavior, concurrent use of antipsychotic medication, concurrent use of restraint, quality of internal planning procedures *Community sample:* form of challenging behavior, social climate of residence
Robertson et al. (2000a)	Obesity	None	*Full sample:* adaptive behavior, gender, Down syndrome, staffing ratio, quality of internal planning procedures *Community sample:* adaptive behavior, gender

Study	Outcome	Association between costs and outcome	Other variables related to outcome
	Inactivity	None	*Full sample:* age, adaptive behavior, type of current residential setting *Community sample:* age, adaptive behavior, health staff, staff qualifications
	Smoking	None	*Full sample:* adaptive behavior, gender, type of current residential setting, quality of internal planning procedures *Community sample:* adaptive behavior
	Poor diet	None	*Full sample:* type of current residential setting, quality of internal planning procedures *Community sample:* type of prior residential setting, type of current residential setting
Robertson et al. (2000b)	Receipt of antipsychotic medication	None	*Full sample:* mobility, body mass index, epilepsy, challenging behavior, type of prior residential setting, type of current residential setting, staff qualifications *Community sample:* mobility, staff qualifications
Robertson et al. (2001a)	Opportunity and support for exercising self-determination	None	*Community sample:* adaptive behavior, autism, challenging behavior, mental health, type of prior residential setting, size of residence, staffing ratio, architectural features of setting, implementation of *active support*
Robertson et al. (2001b)	Social networks	None	*Full sample:* age, autism, challenging behavior, type of prior residential setting, type of current residential setting, staffing ratio, social climate of residence, implementation of *active support* *Community sample:* adaptive behavior, age, type of prior residential setting, type of current residential setting, social climate of residence, implementation of *active support*

such a large number of comparisons does, of course, raise the problem of Type 1 error (falsely rejecting the null hypothesis of no difference). Such difficulties are typical of applied research and are only likely to be resolved through replication.

A relatively clear picture emerges from these results. First, across a range of measures of resource inputs (e.g., staffing ratios, buildings), non-resource inputs (e.g., social environment), and process and service recipient outcomes (e.g., choice, activity, social networks, medication usage), residential campuses operated by the NHS offer a significantly poorer quality of care and quality of life than dispersed housing schemes. These deficiencies cannot be accounted for by differences in the characteristics of people supported. It seems plausible to suggest that the additional costs associated with dispersed housing schemes (15% greater than residential campuses) may be justified when considered in light of the substantial benefits noted previously.

Second, a distinct pattern of benefits appear to be associated with dispersed housing schemes (choice, size of social networks, social integration, recreational/leisure activities) and village communities (size of social networks, reduced risk of exposure to verbal abuse and crime, greater number of days and hours per week of scheduled day activities). These patterns are consistent with the ideological bases of these two approaches to providing residential support. The cost differential between the two approaches—the total adjusted costs of dispersed housing schemes being 20% greater than those associated with village communities—is of clear policy relevance given the increasingly unmet needs of people with intellectual disabilities in the United Kingdom for residential support (Office of the Deputy Prime Minister and Department of Health, 2003).

Third, within dispersed housing schemes, a similar pattern of results was evident in that 1) larger group homes were consistently associated with poorer outcomes than either smaller group homes or supported-living schemes, and 2) smaller group homes and supported-living schemes were associated with different patterns of benefit (Emerson et al., 2001). These results were consistent with those reported by Howe, Horner, and Newton (1998) in suggesting that, for similar costs, supported-living schemes may offer distinct benefits in the areas of resident choice and community participation.

Fourth, there were no statistically significant differences in any domain between the rated satisfaction of either participants or their relatives (Gregory et al., 2000; Walsh et al., 2001). In general, and in common with previous research, participants tended to rate their satisfaction highly.

Such high levels of expressed satisfaction are also common among studies that have solicited the views of relatives. This finding is consistent with previous research in the United Kingdom and elsewhere that indicates that discrimination in the views of service recipients and/or relatives is only likely when it is possible for the service recipients and relatives to make comparative judgments (Stancliffe et al., 2004). Thus, for example, relatives typically rate the quality of care provided within traditional institutions very highly and may often express considerable opposition to deinstitutionalization (Tøssebro, 1996); however, longitudinal studies have repeatedly demonstrated that, following their family member's move to community-based services, relatives rate these services highly and, in retrospect, tend to express preference for the new arrangements (e.g., Conroy, 1996; Tuvesson & Ericsson, 1996; Wing, 1989).

Finally, the results of the project were also consistent in indicating that, in multivariate analyses, the costs of service provision were unrelated to outcomes, though some extremely modest positive associations were found between costs and selected outcomes in dispersed housing schemes. Again, these results are consistent with the existing U.K. literature that suggests that, although costs show moderate associations with indicators of participant need, they are largely unrelated to outcomes (see Chapter 3).

Policy Implications

As noted in the introduction, this project was commissioned in response to pressure from advocacy groups to halt deinstitutionalization and embark on the development of village communities for people with intellectual disabilities. We drew three main policy implications from our results (Emerson et al., 1999c). First, we argued that, as village communities had historically developed in complete independence of deinstitutionalization, this policy should be completed through the continued development of dispersed housing schemes (including supported living). Second, we suggested that, given that dispersed housing schemes and village communities appear to be associated with different patterns of benefit, people with intellectual disabilities should be free to choose between these two options. Finally, given that our sample was comprised of better providers, we made the assumption that many participants experienced relatively poor outcomes in areas such as social inclusion, employment, and self-determination. Thus, we argued that many people with intellectual disabilities in all models of provision were being denied access to an acceptable quality of life.

Of course, judging the impact that any piece of research may have on policy direction is extremely difficult; however, our summary report was circulated by the English Department of Health to all relevant agencies with instruction that agencies must "take account" of our results and recommendations. Subsequently, the English Department of Health announced a commitment to complete deinstitutionalization by April 2004 and to review the situation of all people living in NHS Campuses (Department of Health, 2001). Whether such initiatives will mean that more people with intellectual disabilities in England are afforded a decent quality of life remains to be seen.

REFERENCES

Bailey, N.M., & Cooper, S.A. (1997). The current provision of specialist health services to people with learning disabilities in England and Wales. *Journal of Intellectual Disability Research, 41*, 52–59.

Beecham, J. (1995). Collecting and estimating costs. In M.R.J. Knapp (Ed.), *The economic evaluation of mental health care*. Aldershot: Arena.

Beecham, J., & Knapp, M.R.J. (1992). Costing psychiatric interventions. In G.J. Thornicroft, C.R. Brewin, & J.K. Wing (Eds.), *Measuring mental health needs*. London: Gaskell.

Brook, M. (1990). Evolution from a mental handicap hospital into a village. In S. Segal (Ed.), *The place of special villages and residential communities: The provision of care for people with severe, profound and multiple disabilities* (pp. 29–38). Bicester, United Kingdom: AB Academic Publishers.

Conroy, J.W. (1996). Results of deinstitutionalisation in Connecticut. In J. Mansell & K. Ericsson (Eds.), *Deinstitutionalisation and community living: Intellectual disability services in Britain, Scandinavia and the USA*. London: Chapman & Hall.

Cox, C., & Pearson, M. (1995). *Made to care: The case for residential and village communities for people with a mental handicap*. London: The Rannoch Trust.

Department of Health. (1992a). *Health care for adults with learning disabilities (mental handicap)*. Health Services Guidance (HSG) (92)42. London: Author.

Department of Health. (1992b). Social care for adults with learning disabilities (mental handicap). *Local Authority Circular.* HSG (92)15. London: Department of Health.

Department of Health. (1993). *Services for people with learning disabilities and challenging behaviour or mental health needs*. London: Author.

Department of Health. (1999). *Facing the facts: Services for people with learning disabilities—a policy impact study of social care and health services*. London: Author.

Department of Health. (2001). *Valuing people: A new strategy for learning disability for the 21st century*. (CM 5086). London: The Stationery Office.

Emerson, E., Alborz, A., Felce, D., & Lowe, K. (1995). *Residential Services Setting Questionnaire*. Manchester, United Kingdom: University of Manchester, Hester Adrian Research Centre.

Emerson, E., & Hatton, C. (1994). *Moving out: The impact of relocation from hospital to community on the quality of life of people with learning disabilities.* London: Her Majesty's Stationary Office (HMSO).

Emerson, E., & Hatton, C. (1996a). Deinstitutionalization in the UK: Outcomes for service users. *Journal of Intellectual & Developmental Disability, 21,* 17–37.

Emerson, E., & Hatton, C. (1996b). *Residential provision for people with learning disabilities: An analysis of the 1991 census.* Manchester, United Kingdom: University of Manchester, Hester Adrian Research Centre.

Emerson, E., & Hatton, C. (1997). Regional and local variations in residential provision for people with learning disabilities in England. *Tizard Learning Disability Review, 2,* 43–46.

Emerson, E., & Hatton, C. (1998). Residential provision for people with intellectual disabilities in England, Wales and Scotland. *Journal of Applied Research in Intellectual Disabilities, 11,* 1–14.

Emerson, E., & Hatton, C. (2000). Residential supports for people with learning disabilities in 1997 in England. *Tizard Learning Disability Review, 5,* 41–44.

Emerson, E., Robertson, J., Gregory, N., Hatton, C., Kessissoglou, S., Hallam, A., & Hillery, J. (2000a). The treatment and management of challenging behaviours in residential settings. *Journal of Applied Research in Intellectual Disabilities, 13,* 197–215.

Emerson, E., Robertson, J., Gregory, N., Hatton, C., Kessissoglou, S., Hallam, A., Järbrink, K., Knapp, M., Netten, A., & Walsh, P. (2001). The quality and costs of supported living residences and group homes in the United Kingdom. *American Journal on Mental Retardation, 106,* 401–415.

Emerson, E., Robertson, J., Gregory, N., Hatton, C., Kessissoglou, S., Hallam, A., Knapp, M., Järbrink, K., Netten, A., Walsh, P., Linehan, C., Hillery, J., & Durkan, J. (1999a). *Quality and costs of residential supports for people with learning disabilities: A comparative analysis of quality and costs in village communities, residential campuses and dispersed housing schemes.* Manchester, United Kingdom: University of Manchester, Hester Adrian Research Centre. Also available on-line at http://www.lancs.ac.uk/depts/ihr/research/documents/qc_villages.pdf

Emerson, E., Robertson, J., Gregory, N., Hatton, C., Kessissoglou, S., Hallam, A., Knapp, M., Järbrink, K., Netten, A., Walsh, P., Linehan, C., Hillery, J., & Durkan, J. (1999b). *Quality and costs of residential supports for people with learning disabilities: Predicting variation in outcomes.* Manchester, United Kingdom: University of Manchester, Hester Adrian Research Centre. Also available on-line at http://www.lancs.ac.uk/depts/ihr/research/documents/qc_variation.pdf

Emerson, E., Robertson, J., Gregory, N., Hatton, C., Kessissoglou, S., Hallam, A., Knapp, M., Järbrink, K., Netten, A., Walsh, P., Linehan, C., Hillery, J., & Durkan, J. (1999c). *Quality and costs of residential supports for people with learning disabilities: Summary and implications.* Manchester: University of Manchester, Hester Adrian Research Centre. Also available on-line at http://www.lancs.ac.uk/depts/ihr/research/documents/vc_summary.pdf

Emerson, E., Robertson, J., Gregory, N., Kessissoglou, S., Hatton, C., Hallam, A., Järbrink, K., Knapp, M., Netten, A., & Linehan, C. (2000b). The quality and costs of community-based residential supports and residential campuses for people with severe and complex disabilities. *Journal of Intellectual & Developmental Disabilities, 25,* 263–279.

Emerson, E., Robertson, J., Gregory, N., Kessissoglou, S., Hatton, C., Hallam, A., Knapp, M., Järbrink, K., Walsh, P., & Netten, A. (2000c). The quality and costs of village communities, residential campuses and community-based residential supports in the UK. *American Journal on Mental Retardation, 105,* 81–102.

Felce, D. (1989). *The Andover Project: Staffed housing for adults with severe or profound mental handicaps.* Kidderminster, United Kingdom: British Institute for Mental Handicap.

Felce, D., Kushlick, A., & Mansell, J. (1980). Evaluation of alternative residential facilities for the severely mentally handicapped in Wessex: Client engagement. *Advances in Behaviour Research and Therapy, 3,* 13–18.

Fulgosi, L. (1990). Camphill communities. In S. Segal (Ed.), *The place of special villages and residential communities: The provision of care for people with severe, profound and multiple disabilities* (pp. 39–48). Bicester, United Kingdom: AB Academic Publishers.

Gregory, N., Robertson, J., Kessissoglou, S., Emerson, E., & Hatton, C. (2001). Predictors of expressed satisfaction among people with intellectual disabilities receiving residential supports. *Journal of Intellectual Disability Research, 45,* 279–292.

Grover, R. (1995). *Communities that care: Intentional communities of attachment as a third path in community care.* Brighton, United Kingdom: Pavilion.

Hallam, A., & Emerson, E. (1999). Costs of residential supports for people with learning disabilities. In A. Netten, J. Dennett, & J. Knight (Eds.), *Unit costs of health and social care.* Canterbury, United Kingdom: University of Kent at Canterbury, Personal Social Services Research Unit.

Hallam, A., Knapp, M., Järbrink, K., Netten, A., Emerson, E., Robertson, J., Gregory, N., Hatton, C., Kessissoglou, S., & Durkan, J. (2002). The costs of residential supports for people with intellectual disabilities. *Journal of Intellectual Disability Research, 46,* 394–404.

Hatton, C., Emerson, E., & Kiernan, C. (1995). Trends and milestones: People in institutions in Europe. *Mental Retardation, 33,* 132.

Howe, J., Horner, R.H., & Newton, J.S. (1998). Comparison of supported living and traditional residential services in the State of Oregon. *Mental Retardation, 36,* 1–11.

Jackson, R. (1996). *Bound to care: An anthology.* Stockport: RESCARE.

Kavanagh, S., & Opit, L. (1998). *The cost of caring: The economics of providing for the intellectually disabled.* London: Politeia.

Kim, S., Larson, S.A., & Lakin, K.C. (2001). Behavioural outcomes of deinstitutionalization for people with intellectual disability: A review of US studies conducted between 1980 and 1999. *Journal of Intellectual & Developmental Disabilities, 26,* 35–50.

Kinsella, P. (1993). *Supported living: A new paradigm.* Manchester, United Kingdom: National Development Team.

Larson, S., & Lakin, K.C. (1989). Deinstitutionalization of persons with mental retardation: Behavioral outcomes. *Journal of The Association for Persons with Severe Handicaps, 14,* 324–332.

Lowe, K., & de Paiva, S. (1991). *NIMROD—An Overview.* London: HMSO.

Netten, A., Dennett, J., & Knight, J. (1998). *The unit costs of health and social care.* Canterbury: University of Kent at Canterbury, Personal Social Services Research Unit.

Office of the Deputy Prime Minister and Department of Health. (2003). *Housing and support services for people with learning disabilities.* London: Author.

Robertson, J., Emerson, E., Gregory, N., Hatton, C., Kessissoglou, S., & Hallam, A. (2000a). Receipt of psychotropic medication by people with intellectual disabilities in residential settings. *Journal of Intellectual Disability Research, 44,* 666–676.

Robertson, J., Emerson, E., Gregory, N., Hatton, C., Turner, S., Kessissoglou, S., & Hallam, A. (2000b). Lifestyle related risk factors for poor health in residential settings for people with intellectual disabilities. *Research in Developmental Disabilities, 21,* 469–486.

Robertson, J., Emerson, E., Gregory, N., Hatton, C., Kessissoglou, S., Hallam, A., & Linehan, C. (2001a). Social networks of people with intellectual disabilities in residential settings. *Mental Retardation, 39,* 201–214.

Robertson, J., Emerson, E., Hatton, C., Gregory, N., Kessissoglou, S., Hallam, A., & Walsh, P.N. (2001b). Environmental opportunities for exercising self-determination in residential settings. *Research in Developmental Disabilities, 22,* 487–502.

Scheerenberger, R.C. (1983). *A history of mental retardation.* Baltimore: Paul H. Brookes Publishing.

Segal, S. (1990). *The place of special villages and residential communities.* Bicester, United Kingdom: A B Academic Publishers.

Simons, K. (1995). *My home, my life: Innovative approaches to housing and support for people with learning difficulties.* London: Values Into Action.

Simons, K. (1997). *A foot in the door: The early years of supported living for people with learning difficulties in the UK.* Manchester, United Kingdom: National Development Team.

Stancliffe, R.J., Emerson, E., & Lakin, K.C. (2004). Residential supports. In E. Emerson, C. Hatton, T. Thompson, & T. Parmenter (Eds.), *International handbook of research methods in intellectual disability.* Chichester, United Kingdom: Wiley.

Staton, R. (1996). *Residential accommodation: Detailed statistics on residential care homes and local authority supported residents, England 1995.* London: Department of Health.

Tøssebro, J. (1996). Family attitudes to deinstitutionalisation in Norway. In J. Mansell & K. Ericsson (Eds.), *Deinstitutionalisation and community living: Intellectual disability services in Britain, Scandinavia and the USA.* London: Chapman & Hall.

Tuvesson, B., & Ericsson, K. (1996). Relatives' opinions on institutional closure. In J. Mansell & K. Ericsson (Eds.), *Deinstitutionalisation and community living: Intellectual disability services in Britain, Scandinavia and the USA.* London: Chapman & Hall.

Walsh, P.N., Linehan, C., Hillery, J., Durkan, J., Emerson, E., Hatton, C., Robertson, J., Gregory, N., Kessissoglou, S., Hallam, A., Knapp, M., Jarbrink, K., & Netten, A. (2001). Family views of the quality of residential supports. *Journal of Applied Research in Intellectual Disabilities, 14,* 292–309.

Wing, L. (1989). *Hospital closure and the resettlement of Residents: The case of Darenth Park Mental Handicap Hospital.* Aldershot, United Kingdom: Avebury.

Wolfensberger, W. (1975). *The origin and nature of our institutional models.* Syracuse, NY: Human Policy Press.

Young, I., Sigafoos, J., Suttie, J., Ashman, A., & Grevell, P. (1998). Deinstitutionalisation of persons with intellectual disabilities: A review of Australian studies. *Journal of Intellectual & Developmental Disabilities, 23,* 155–170.

CHAPTER 8

Predictors of Expenditures in Western States

*Edward M. Campbell, Jon R. Fortune, Janice K. Frisch,
Laird W. Heal, Kenneth B. Heinlein, Robert M. Lynch, and
Donald D. Severance*

If all people with disabilities required the same level of support, if all wanted the same kinds of support, if all service providers were equally efficient and effective in the provision of services, and if there were no variations in the cost of living across communities, the costs of serving all people with disabilities might be easily determined. Individuals vary in the nature of their disabilities, and even those with similar disabilities may require different levels and kinds of support, with different costs and configurations. State expenditures for people with developmental disabilities are influenced by these individual cost variations, as well as population size, levels of fiscal commitments, funding sources, mix of institutional and community settings, and service eligibility levels. This complex environment has commonalities of funding sources, especially federal Medicaid reimbursement.

TWO LEVELS OF ADVOCACY, PLANNING, AND FUNDING

Advocacy, planning, and funding of supports and services for people with developmental disabilities are activities that are carried out at two distinct levels: the individual level and the system level.

The views expressed in this chapter are those of the authors and do not necessarily represent the views of the governments of the states of Montana, Nebraska, South Dakota, or Wyoming. Likewise, the conclusions drawn in this chapter do not necessarily represent the policies of any of these states, nor should endorsement by any of these governments be assumed.

Individual Level

At the individual level, advocacy activities, whether conducted by an advocacy organization, individuals themselves, friends, or family, are made on behalf of a given individual. For example, an individual advocate would ask the question, "Is John living in an overly restrictive setting?" Planning for settings, services, and supports involves recommendations and decisions that are made by a team process. The team directs attention and efforts to a single person at a time and, ideally, includes that person. The team should have a good understanding of the wants and needs of each person. Funding decisions involve budgeting funds that typically are allocated by those making system-level decisions.

System Level

At the system level, advocacy activities concentrate on how well the system is doing in meeting the service/support needs of all the people needing those services/supports. For example, a system advocate would ask, "How many people are living in settings that are overly restrictive?" A planning team for an individual relies on knowledge of that individual's needs. A system planner cannot comprehend knowledge of each individual in the entire population, so he or she must rely on data and statistics. Funding decisions at the system level involve allocating resources that the individual planning teams then budget for the individual. The tools presented in this chapter are intended for those who work at the system level.

The lack of good empirical data has typically forced rate-setters to rely on an intuitive synthesis of anecdotal information regarding factors that influence the cost of services. The power of intuition is not to be dismissed lightly, however. As demonstrated in the following analyses, these methods have proven to be relatively effective. The analyses presented here will distill the rational component of those historical processes and produce tools to help administer resources in a fair manner.

BACKGROUND

Four Western U.S. states (Montana, Nebraska, South Dakota, and Wyoming) have pooled their data on individual characteristics, service/supports, and reimbursement rates. The data were pooled to illustrate how research methods and analyses may aid in decision making, and be applied to the administration of these and similar programs. The data are regional, but we are confident that the methods have universal application. The four states use the Inventory for Client and Agency Planning (ICAP) (Bruininks, Hill, Weatherman, & Woodcock, 1986) to collect information on service recipient characteristics; however, these methods can be applied with other reliable and valid instruments.

The four states are geographically adjacent and form a block of states committed to assuring that services and supports are available for a large number of people who need them. The proportion of citizens receiving residential services or supports in 2000 for all four states exceeded the national average. The states ranked from 4th (South Dakota) to 14th (Wyoming) (Prouty, Smith, & Lakin, 2001; Smith, 2001b). All four states also demonstrated a commitment to providing services and supports in the community, which is evident by their proportion of total 1998 expenditures allocated to community services, compared with the national average of 72%. These four states ranged from 71% (Nebraska) to 79% (South Dakota) (Braddock, Hemp, Parish, & Rizzolo, 2000).

This community emphasis is also demonstrated by the states' utilization of Medicaid Home and Community-Based Services (HCBS) Waiver programs. The numbers of HCBS Waiver recipients per 100,000 of the general population in 2000 were higher than the national average, ranking from 3rd (South Dakota) to 23rd (Montana). HCBS Waiver expenditures per 100,000 citizens in 2000 ranked from 4th (Wyoming) to 24th (Montana), but expenditures per recipient reflect the region's conservative sense of fiscal responsibility, ranking from 21st (Wyoming) to 36th (South Dakota) (Prouty et al., 2001; Smith, 2001a). (Note that these comparisons are not from the most recent data available. Because the data we are presenting in this chapter are from 1998, we thought it better to provide findings from a time frame closer to our data.)

This chapter explores the usefulness of having a comprehensive set of empirical data related to expenditures, characteristics of the individuals served, environments, economic measures, funding sources, and individual outcomes. Comparable information was taken from existing state databases. The analyses illustrate how reimbursement amounts can be compared between residential settings and programs.

Previous Studies Explaining Cost Variation

Statistical and quantitative models are used widely to examine cost behaviors in many disciplines, though there has been limited application to developmental disability service costs. A widely applied methodology is correlation analysis. These analyses examine the association among the variables, with an R^2 of 0 indicating no statistical association and an R^2 of 1 indicating a complete association among the variables under study.

In a survey of related literature, the former Health Care Financing Administration (now Centers for Medicare & Medicaid Services) reported the following findings concerning health services. Initial validation studies of the Resource Utilization Groups for skilled nursing facilities reported an R^2 between costs and individual characteristics of .56. This amount means that individual characteristics and services needed accounted for 56% of the variation in costs. Diagnostic related groups are used for reimbursement of acute care and yield R^2s ranging from .26 to .33. A pilot home health care case-mix reimbursement model was established with an R^2 at .32. Lastly, the Health Care Financing Administration's preliminary findings for a home health care reimbursement model reported an R^2 of clinical measures with costs of .20, but this increased to .47 when other measures were added, such as additional services provided (Health Care Financing Administration, 1999).

Holmes and Teresi (1998) reported on personnel costs in nursing-home Special Care Units for people with dementia. Costs for nurse aides showed a relationship to nine measures of individual characteristics of the people served ($R^2 = .37$). None of the costs for five other professional categories demonstrated a significant relationship to individual characteristics. The current approach involves applying similar analytic methods to developmental disability service costs and goes a step further by developing more complex models that explain cost variation more fully.

Benefits of Developing a Model of Cost Variation   A model that satisfactorily explains variation in reimbursement rates can be used to generate individual budget amounts. Chapter 11 provides one example of the application of these methods to develop a statewide system of individual budget allocations. Individual budget amounts have several advantages, including the ability of funds to "follow the individual," thus permitting increased choice of service/support providers. Individual budget amounts are also prerequisites for the establishment of service recipient–directed services/supports and increase the equity or fairness in the allocation of available resources.

A second important benefit of modeling costs is that it enables methods to be developed that can highlight certain individuals who likely are being served inappropriately. For example, they may be living or working in less-independent settings than other, similar people. Such information might convince policy makers to accelerate the development of supports to facilitate more people to move into greater independence. An example of such methods and of how incentives for such system change might be built into an individual budget amount model is presented later in this chapter.

Data

Wyoming, Nebraska, and South Dakota data are from fiscal year 1998. Montana's data are from 1999. Montana reimbursement rates were inflation-adjusted back to 1998 dollars. At the time these data were collected, two of the four states were using the ICAP in their rate-determination process. South Dakota and Wyoming implemented such procedures in 1998, and Nebraska is in the process of doing so. South Dakota's expenditure data were derived from provider cost reports and time studies conducted during fiscal year 1998. The expenditure data from the other states came from their information systems used to generate actual reimbursements in 1998 (1999 for Montana). There were 7,611 individuals with complete data (see Table 8.1). Nebraska accounted for the most (2,711, or 35.6%), and Wyoming, the least, with 1,145 (15.0%). Most (4,610, or 60.6%) were served in community programs and funded by Medicaid HCBS Waiver funds. Only 33 people (0.4%)—all from South Dakota—were served in small, less than 15-bed, Intermediate Care Facilities for Persons with Mental Retardation (ICFs/MR). State funding supported 2,108 (27.7%) individuals. The remaining 860 (11.3%) individuals lived in state institutions with ICF/MR funding.

Data on individual characteristics were collected with the ICAP, which included information on each person's residential arrangement and daytime program. Information on funding sources and services and supports provided was gathered from each state's management information system. Because each state has a different structure of services/supports, only the two services that were common to all four states were used: 1) community residential services, including supported living; and 2) community daytime services, including facility-based as well as supported programs. Both of these were further divided into programs for adults and children.

Geographic information included unemployment rate data for each county in which a person received services or supports (Nebraska Department of Labor, 1998; Montana Department of Labor and Industry, 1999; South Dakota Department of Labor, 1998; Wyoming Department of Employment, 1998). The 1998 average per-capita income for the county

Table 8.1. Data sources for analyses, numbers of individuals by states and funding sources

State	Funding source				Total
	State funding	HCBS Waiver	ICF/MR < 15	ICF/MR	
South Dakota	332	1,519	33	257	2,141
Wyoming	196	822	0	127	1,145
Nebraska	719	1,607	0	385	2,711
Montana	861	662	0	91	1,614
Total	**2,108**	**4,610**	**33**	**860**	**7,611**

Note: HCBS Waiver = Medicaid Home and Community-Based Waiver programs
ICF/MR = Intermediate Care Facility for Persons with Mental Retardation, the Medicaid funding program for the states' institutions.
ICF/MR < 15 = ICF/MR for facilities under 15 beds, the Medicaid funding program still being used by South Dakota at the time these data were collected.

where each person was served was also included (Bureau of Economic Analysis, 1998).

PREDICTORS OF REIMBURSEMENT AMOUNTS

Intensity of Service/Support Needs

The ICAP yields a Service Score, which is a composite of all Adaptive Behavior and Problem Behavior items. Figure 8.1 illustrates the relationship between that Service Score and monthly reimbursement rates for community adults. The points on the scatterplot represent the means of each combination of provider agency and funding source. (These means were used simply for clarity of illustration—more than 7,000 individual marks would blot out the figure.) This scatterplot is a "simple" regression, in that there is only one predictor measure: the ICAP Service Score. The diagonal line, or regression line, represents the "best fit" to the points in the figure. The ICAP Service Score ranges from 0 to 99. The higher the Service Score, the lower the level of services or supports needed. The direction of this relationship is what would be expected—as Service Scores increase, costs decrease.

This line explains 65% of all the variation of the mean costs in Figure 8.1; however, accounting for variation in provider means is of little use in determining individual reimbursement amounts. Using the individual scores rather than provider/funding means, the Service Score accounts for only 27% of the rate variation (i.e., an R^2 statistic of .27). The advantage of a simple regression is that it is easy to view on a two-dimensional surface. The disadvantage is the rather small R^2. Although rate-setting appli-

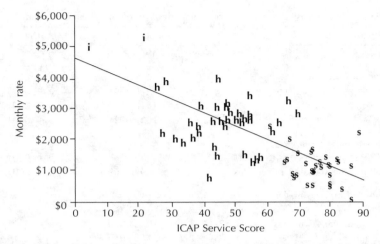

Figure 8.1. Simple regression of monthly rates on ICAP service scores for community adults. *(Key:* i = ICF/MR; h = HCBS Waiver; s = State funding)
Note: This plot shows means for state/funding/provider combinations. To produce a simpler figure, we dropped 89 observations with the highest monthly rate (> $8,000) before figuring means for the plot.

cations in other health-related fields may rely on the relationship with similarly small R^2 statistics, the more variation in reimbursement that can be explained by the model, the better.

Multiple Regression

To explain more of the variation in reimbursement rates, a more complex model using multiple regression was applied. In this analysis, several pre-dictor variables are considered instead of the ICAP Service Score alone. These predictor variables arise from the following clusters: geographic factors, ICAP individual characteristic and environment measures, service and support measures, and funding source. Because we have a large num-ber of variables that can be entered into this regression analysis, many of which will make little difference to the end result, we set the regression analysis such that only those variables that make a significant contribution to the analysis would be included (stepwise regression). For our purpose, we set the significance at the $p < .01$ level. Because many of these variables measure related concepts, and to avoid including those that measure almost the same thing, we set a tolerance level greater than .20 (to minimize mul-ticollinearity) to stay in the model. The seven clusters of variables (geo-graphic measures, ICAP scores, other ICAP measures, residential arrange-ments, daytime activities, community supports, and funding sources) in Table 8.2 are the results of these decisions.

Table 8.2. Summary of stepwise regression analysis on monthly reimbursement rates

Predictor variable	Parameter estimate	Statistical significance
Intercept	1,494.69500	$p < .0001$
Geographic measures		
1997 per-capita income	0.01545	$p = .0013$
Wyoming?	1,181.22836	$p < .0001$
Montana?	182.20928	$p < .0001$
ICAP—Summary scores		
ICAP Broad Independence Index	−3.61984	$p < .0001$
ICAP General Maladaptive Index	−9.85869	$p < .0001$
ICAP—Other Measures		
Age	−7.22349	$p = .0001$
Communicates with gestures? (ICAP A7)	199.78950	$p = .0001$
Communicates with signs? (ICAP A7)	311.70916	$p = .0010$
Diagnosis = autism?	391.53601	$p < .0001$
Diagnosis = brain/neurological damage?	180.28517	$p = .0048$
Diagnosis = mental illness (psychosis)?	265.03476	$p < .0001$
Need for doctor or nurse care (ICAP C6)	77.77476	$p < .0001$
Mobility (ICAP C9)	167.72190	$p = .0072$
Occasional mobility assistance needed?	227.17725	$p < .0001$
Always needs mobility help?	629.19664	$p < .0001$
ICAP—Residential arrangements		
Lives with family?	−378.94699	$p < .0001$
Supported living or foster care*	0.00000*	
Semi-independent unit with staff?	501.57550	$p < .0001$
Group residence?	1,139.99949	$p < .0001$
State institution?	6,227.92266	$p < .0001$
ICAP—Daytime activities		
Day activity center?	123.13472	$p = .0094$
Work activity center or sheltered work?*	0.00000*	
Supported employment?	−181.16749	$p = .0001$
Community services/supports provided		
Adult residential services/supports?	753.22663	$p < .0001$
Child residential services/supports?	617.72463	$p < .0001$
Adult daytime services/supports?	690.00303	$p < .0001$
Child daytime services/supports?	1,297.94863	$p < .0001$
Funding source		
State funding?	−335.69223	$p < .0001$

Note: Entry level = .50; stay level = .01; N = 7610; Adjusted R^2 = 0.7105; $F_{(26,7583)}$ = 890.83; $p < .0001$; C(p) = 25.35. Predictors with a question mark (?) are binary measures (i.e., 1 = yes, 0 = no).
*Reference categories—Not part of model, so parameter estimate is zero.
ICAP = Inventory for Client and Agency Planning (Bruininks, Hill, Weatherman, & Woodcock, 1986)

Overall, this analysis explained 71% ($R^2 = .71$) of the variation in individual costs, a significant improvement over the simple regression presented previously (27%) and a respectable figure for analyses in the social sciences. To gain an understanding of the relative contribution of each grouping of new predictors to explaining individual reimbursement rates, the analysis was repeated introducing each group in a blockwise fashion. The blocks of predictors were added from the least controllable to the most controllable and are illustrated clockwise starting from "noon" in Figure 8.2. The geographic measures explained 4%, the ICAP summary scores (Broad Independence and General Maladaptive Index) added another 28% to the geographic measures, the other ICAP measures contributed another 5%, ICAP environments (residence and day program) added an additional 32%, and services and funding contributed a final 2%.

The remaining 29% of variation in reimbursement rates was not explained by the model (i.e., error). In statistical terminology, *error* is not synonymous with *mistake*; it is closer to *unknown*. In Figure 8.2, error is split into three components. This split is for illustrative purposes only, and the percentage split (10%–10%–9%) is arbitrary. This arrangment was just done to introduce three categories in which sources of error can be considered. The portion not explained is a result of "statistical error," that

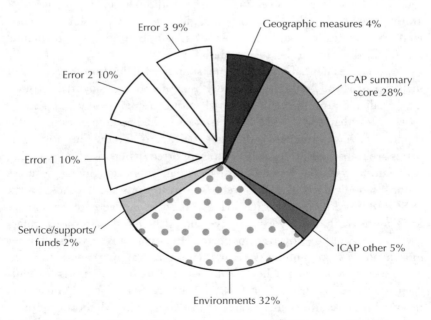

Figure 8.2. "Blockwise" hierarchical regression—predictors added clockwise from 12 o'clock.

is, factors not captured in the model. These factors may be 1) important variables excluded from the model, 2) errors in measurement of some factors, or 3) error caused by impacts unknown to the investigators.

Predictor Measures The detailed results of the multiple regression analysis of individual reimbursement rates are shown in Table 8.2. The parameter estimates in Table 8.2 provide information on the relative importance of each variable and whether it increases or decreases costs. The parameters show that higher per-capita income is associated with higher reimbursement rates because the sign of this parameter (regression coefficient) is positive. Also, Wyoming has much higher reimbursement rates than the other three states, and Montana has slightly higher rates than Nebraska and South Dakota. It might be speculated that this is attributable to Wyoming's involvement in, and resolution of, a lawsuit in the 1990s (see Chapter 11).

People with lower ICAP independence and maladaptive behavior scores receive higher payments, as would be expected. The signs of both parameter estimates are negative. The maladaptive index is a negative scale; for example, -5 represents minor behavior problems, and -20 represents more severe behaviors. As with the independence index, the lower the score, the greater the need for services. Additional ICAP measures that are independently related to costs include age (older people's care costs less); communication skills; diagnosis of autism, brain damage, or mental illness; need for medical care; and mobility factors.

Among residential arrangements, supported living/foster care is not included. It is the "reference category" for the other residential settings. The predicted rates of each residential setting are defined by being either more or less than supported living/foster care. The parameter estimate for supported living/foster care is thus essentially zero, and the four other estimates are to be interpreted relative to supported living/foster care. Living with family costs $379 per month less than supported living, whereas group-home living is $1,140 more. State institutions are the most costly, at $6,228 more than supported living. Likewise, day activity centers are $123 more costly than work activity centers/sheltered workshops (reference category at $0); however, supported employment is $181 cheaper per month. Providing community residential services/supports adds to rates, more so for adults than children, but daytime services/supports for children are more expensive than those for adults. State-funded consumers receive lower reimbursement rates than people with Medicaid funding, with rates reduced by $336 per month.

OTHER THINGS BEING EQUAL COMPARISONS

A model that explains most of the variation, like the one in Table 8.2, enhances the ability to answer many questions when comparing states, programs, agencies, and so forth with "other things being equal" (OTBE). For example, state officials might wish to know if provider agencies' reimbursement rates differ significantly, adjusting for differences in individual characteristics or other predictor measures. With these predictor variables as covariates, an analysis of covariance (ANCOVA) can statistically control for the effects of measures, such as individual characteristics. Table 8.3 illustrates an example of such an OTBE comparison. The top half of Table 8.3 is an analysis of variance, comparing actual (raw) reimbursement rates of each of the four states, and three funding sources—state institutions (ICFs/MR), HCBS Waiver programs, and state-only funding (state dollars). All three funding sources are significantly different, with ICF/MR

Table 8.3. Comparison of states and funding sources on monthly rates

	Analysis of variance Means (actual monthly reimbursement rates)			
State	ICF/MR	HCBS Waiver	State dollars	State means
Wyoming	$11,222	$3,202	$981[a]	$3,783
Nebraska	$6,600	$2,595	$1,186[a]	$2,790
South Dakota	$5,934	$2,420	$907[b]	$2,610
Montana	$9,787	$2,882	918[b]	$2,223
Funding means	**$7,421**	**$2,704**	**$1,014**	

	Analysis of covariance* Least squares means (adjusted to control statistically for the effects of the covariates)			
State	ICF/MR	HCBS Waiver	State dollars	State means
Wyoming	$12,212	$2,878	$1,885[a]	$5,658
Nebraska	$7,512	$2,252	$2,027[a]	$3,930
South Dakota	$6,859	$1,779	$1,580[b]	$3,406
Montana	$10,688	$2,020	$1,666[b]	$4,791
Funding means	**$9,318**	**$2,232**	**$1,789**	

*Covariates are all the independent measures in Table 8.2, except Montana, Wyoming, state institution, and state-funding.
[a,b]All differences between states and funding sources are statistically significant except those with the same superscript.
HCBS Waiver = Medicaid Home and Community-Based Waiver programs
ICF/MR = Intermediate care facility for the mentally retarded, the Medicaid funding program for the states' institutions

rates the highest, and state funding the lowest. All four states also differ significantly from each other. Wyoming's rates are the highest, followed by Nebraska, South Dakota, and Montana, respectively.

If no differences existed between the characteristics of the populations and other factors that we call covariates, the costs would be directly comparable; however, the populations do differ, as do other factors (i.e., other things are not equal). As noted previously, these differences can be controlled statistically using analysis of covariance. We used all of the variables listed in Table 8.2 as covariates (except state and funding source). Controlling for differences in the covariates produces least squares mean statistics, which are adjusted for the effects of those covariates. These are presented in the bottom half of Table 8.3. Funding sources are significantly different, but note that the rather large difference between HCBS Waivers and state funding has been greatly diminished by the introduction of the covariates. Also, OTBE, Montana's overall rates are now second highest, rather than lowest.

There are several things that the lower half of Table 8.3 suggests. First, notice that, within each state, the difference between average monthly reimbursement for the state dollars and HCBS Waiver funding is less in the lower half of the table than in the upper half. This finding would suggest that the difference in reimbursement between these two groups is partially explained by differences in the characteristics of each group, rather than by the reimbursement source alone. Perhaps more simply said, people receiving state dollars do not get less money because the states are cheap; rather, the individuals have less severe disabilities. The fact that differences do not entirely disappear, however, suggests that there remain other factors that explain the differences. Interestingly, the opposite seems to be the case within each state, in that the differences between ICF/MR and HCBS Waiver programs are more pronounced when the effects of the covariates are controlled statistically. The data suggest that states pay ICFs/MR more but not because of differences in the populations served.

Cost of Independence

Mean reimbursement rates for people living in each of the seven different residential settings were contrasted, both with and without controls, for the same covariates used in the previous analysis. The results may be seen in Figure 8.3. As shown previously, state institutions, or "developmental centers," cost more than other alternatives, and this difference is even greater when controlling for the effects of the covariates. The same is true

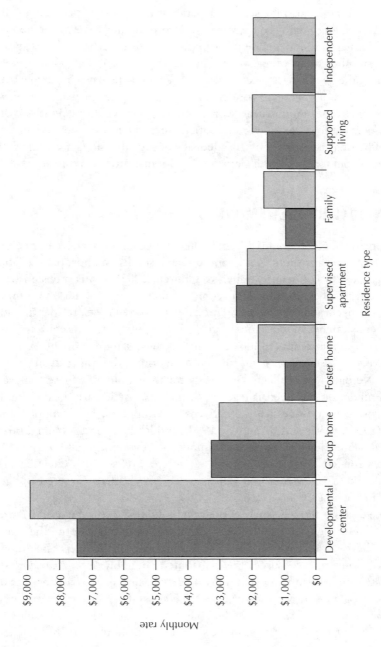

Figure 8.3. 1998 reimbursement rates by residence type: actual means and means adjusted covariates. *Note:* Covariates are most of the predictor variables listed in Table 8.2. (*Key:* ■ = actual; ▢ = adjusted)

when comparing group home rates to the remaining five residential categories. Although rates for semi-independent (supervised apartments) and supported-living settings appear to be slightly higher than foster homes, family homes, and independent settings, these differences were not statistically significant. In other words, any setting more independent than a group home is likewise less expensive. From a taxpayer's perspective, cheaper is always better. From the viewpoint of one receiving services/supports, cheaper might mean worse—but not always. In many cases, the consumer will find life much more satisfying in the more independent setting. The final assessment of the adequacy of such decisions must rest with the individual team, not the statistician, administrator, or rate-setter.

INDIVIDUAL BUDGET AMOUNTS

As reported in Chapters 11–12, individual budget amounts have been cited as prerequisites for service recipient–directed service/support plans (Babin & Fortune, 2001; Fortune, Seiler, & Church, 2002). Using a design with a selected number of individual records, Emerson et al. (2001) presented comprehensive analyses of the relationships between costs, residential settings, consumer characteristics, and quality of outcomes. In contrast, the present design attempts to look at many of these same factors by examining a very large body of data, formed by merging the four existing databases. No data were collected expressly for the conduct of these analyses. The foundation has been laid for such models, particularly in the dominant cost center of residential services and supports, by Campbell and Heal (1995), Lewis and Bruininks (1994), and Rhoades and Altman (2001). Several states have created such models—Wyoming's DOORS (U.S. Centers for Medicare & Medicaid Services, 2001; see also Chapter 11), South Dakota's Service-Based Rates, and Pennsylvania's Targeted Budget Project (Fortune et al., 2002).

Regression models, such as the one in Table 8.2, can be used to produce an individual budget amount. Administrators can identify measures they believe are related to cost and will support their policies. Such models can assure that resources are distributed equitably. *Equitable* suggests that rates are determined by an individual's measured needs for services or supports, or other predictor variables selected, and not by factors captured as error. The *individual* in individual budget amounts means that each service recipient has a budget amount specifically computed for him or her. Because that amount is assigned to that person, administrators can allow those funds to become portable. In other words, service recipients are free to use those funds to secure services/supports from the provider agency of their choice.

An example of such a model is illustrated in Figure 8.4, which was derived from the multiple regression analysis in Table 8.2 and was refined by eliminating 384 (5%) outliers (studentized residuals $> \pm 2.0$). When constructing such models, such outliers should be examined thoroughly to determine why they do not fit the model. This practice may illuminate some important factors that are not addressed by the analysis. Additional predictor measures can then be considered to potentially increase the variation explained by the model. For example, if a specific medical condition were suggested by the outliers, data could then be acquired and included in the analysis. In this exercise, we were not able to do this analysis, so such factors were not added as predictors, and whatever variation they would have accounted for remains part of the error.

The elimination of outliers resulted in a model with an adjusted R^2 of .82. ($N = 7226$, $F_{(23,7202)} = 1414.89$, $p < .0001$). To use the model in Figure 8.4, an individual's measures are entered for each Variable Value, then multiplied by its parameter estimate (regression coefficient). The result is entered in the right-hand column, which is then summed to produce a Predicted Monthly Reimbursement Rate in the small box in the lower right corner.

This hypothetical individual is a verbal 57-year-old with an ICAP Broad Independence score of 454. The person also has moderately serious maladaptive behavior associated with a diagnosis of psychosis, receives residential services in a group home, has day services in an activity center, and has supported employment. The geographic area in which the person lives has a per-capita income of $22,000. Each of these factors becomes part of the calculation for the predicted monthly reimbursement. Notice that the relatively high broad independence score decreases the monthly reimbursement, but the maladaptive score and group home placement increase the amount. Each factor listed has the potential to change the bottom line, but factors with a value of 0 do not add to the monthly amount.

This example is best suited to a reimbursement situation in which a single monthly payment is made to a single entity (provider agency, family, individual, or fiscal intermediary), which covers all services and supports. It is also well suited to a person/family or a fiscal intermediary who manages the funds and arranges all of the services for that person (even if the services are from different providers). The numbers in each row of the right-hand column are summed to produce the payment amount noted at

Column A	Column B	Column C	Column D
Variable	Parameter estimate	Variable value	B x C
Base amount (intercept)	1,694.12328	1	1,694.12
Geographic measure			
Per-capita income	0.01051	**$22,000**	231.20
ICAP Summary Scores			
Broad Independence Index	−3.09680	**454**	−1,405.95
General Maladaptive Index	−6.28330	**−22**	138.23
ICAP—Other measures			
Age	−3.76168	**57**	−214.42
Speaks? (ICAP A7)	−168.92795	**1**	−168.93
Need for doctor/nurse care	43.78951	**1**	43.79
Mobility limitations	199.22918	**0**	0.00
Occasional mobility assistance?	136.51489	**0**	0.00
Always needs mobility help?	586.01795	**0**	0.00
Diagnosis = autism?	295.11821	**0**	0.00
Diagnosis = mental illness (psychosis)?	141.54549	**1**	141.55
ICAP—Environments			
Residential arrangements			
Lives with family?	−289.39317	**0**	0.00
*Foster care/supported living?**	*0.00000*	*0*	*0.00*
Semi-independent unit with staff?	528.96519	**0**	0.00
Group residence?	1,075.33145	**1**	1,075.33
State institution?	5,587.20481	**0**	0.00
Daytime programs			
Day activity center?	64.94696	**1**	64.95
*Work activity center/sheltered workshop?**	*0.00000*	*0*	*0.00*
Supported employment?	−133.60095	**1**	−133.60
Services/supports provided			
Adult residential?	658.21978	**1**	658.22
Child residential?	845.04368	**0**	0.00
Adult daytime services?	652.70797	**1**	652.71
Child daytime services?	1,105.38319	**0**	0.00
Funding			
State funding?	−325.22713	**0**	0.00
Predicted monthly reimbursement rate			**$2,777.20**

Figure 8.4.   Example of spreadsheet to calculate monthly reimbursement rates. *Note:* Variables ending with a question mark (?) are binary measures (i.e., 1 = yes; 0 = no). *Reference categories

the bottom. They are not to be interpreted as the monthly rate for each specific service, such as adult daytime service. Payment systems that require separate payments to different providers from automated reimbursement systems for various services would require some modifications. For example, separate models could be developed for each category of services/supports.

Budget Neutrality

The result generated by this model for a single individual will most likely differ from the current rate by some degree and more for some individuals than for others. Several facts about the model need to be mentioned:

1. The total amount of those differences for which the predicted rates are lower than the current rates will be exactly the same as the differences for which predicted rates are higher.

2. The overall average predicted rate will be exactly the same as the current overall average rate.

3. The total amount of the predicted rates will be exactly the same as the current total amount.

In other words, these methods are budget neutral for the overall amount to be allocated. Inflationary increases can be accomplished by multiplying the predicted rates by the desired inflation percentage. Conversely, such models can also provide a fair basis for allocating scarce resources in times of budget cutting. Yet as some individuals' rates increase and some decrease, total revenues for some providers will increase, and some will decrease. If political exigencies should dictate a "hold-harmless" policy for those that decrease, additional overall funding might become necessary.

Important Points to Consider

Some, but not all, of the following points have been touched on previously. They are all pertinent to anyone considering implementing similar methods.

Funding People Not Facilities   Use of such models does imply a switch to a fee-for-service payment system. Resources will be used to purchase services/supports for people with disabilities, rather than to assure funding of provider agencies. This transition may prove to be challenging for some agencies. Greater resources are assigned to people with greater needs, rather than to facilities with greater costs. Every state's payment scheme is based, at least partially, on an assessment of the needs of the individuals served/supported. These methods do their best to distill whatever logic exists in the system into a payment formula. The methods proposed here are based on correlation, but correlation does not imply causality. Policy makers decide to make the implication that level of need determines costs. Using such regression models to generate individual budget amounts implies that we have made that decision. The amount of money available for services and supports is a legislative decision. The methods proposed do not assure an adequate overall supply of money. They do, however, provide a basis for fairly distributing the funds that are available. In addition, because the models allocate funds precisely, they can be used to equitably increase or decrease funding. They also provide a method to generate an individual estimated resource, which can follow the person and which provides the local teams with a budget for the individual.

Data Driven   The data must be reasonably accurate. These methods are heavily data driven. They depend on objective, empirical measures. The models are mathematical formulas, derived statistically from relationships between actual dependent measures (e.g., staff hours, dollars expended); independent, or "predictor," measures (e.g., intensity of each individual's need for services/supports); and geographic measures (e.g., cost of living, household income, unemployment rate).

Independent measures are selected with the following criteria: 1) their ability to explain, or "predict," variation in the dependent measure (i.e., R^2); 2) their statistical significance, that is, they are not related just by chance (e.g., $p < .01$); 3) their lack of a high correlation with the other predictors to avoid including several variables that measure almost the same thing; and 4) their believed contribution to costs by those who have the responsibility to administer the reimbursements.

Data Integrity   "The more you pay for sicker people, the more sicker people you get." States that have ventured into these methods have found that when individual payments are linked to individual characteristics, ratings tend to drift toward those that yield higher payments (i.e., ICAP scores tend to decrease, indicating less independence, when reimbursement amounts are linked to them). One approach, suggested for this seemingly inevitable data-quality problem, is an "egalitarian" funding idea— equal payments for all individuals. This system should provide an incentive for provider agencies to move as many people as possible into the lower-cost alternatives. This approach seems like an appealing, elegant solution; however, it probably would not work in a system where providers are free to choose whom they do, or do not, serve. With such an egalitarian payment scheme, it would become quite difficult to convince providers to accept and retain those individuals who need particularly intense services/ supports. At this time, we think that individual budget amounts are the best approach to pay for services and supports.

Those states that have implemented individual budget amount payment methods similar to those presented here have found the need to establish some sort of "Data Police" to minimize "gaming" of the system by overstating the degree of disability to obtain more funds. Approaches that have been tried include 1) state personnel monitoring data on individual characteristics as furnished by providers, 2) state agencies generating such data themselves, or 3) hiring independent third parties to complete the assessments.

Many Possible Models   There are a large number of possible models that can be generated with any set of data, many of which will be quite comparable in their ability to explain variation in costs. These methods will look for the best combination of measures that accomplish this task. Most predictors will not be selected—only the best 15–25, depending on the overall number of observations in the data. Some administrators' or providers' favorite measures certainly will not be included. Administrators do have the option of including any measure that they think should be mandatory; however, forcing such measures into the equation adds to the instability of the final model. For example, small variations in seemingly insignificant predictors could have undesirable effects on the reimbursement rates generated. Outliers are those people whose actual reimbursements are widely different from what is predicted by a model. Outliers may be helpful in identifying important factors that are not represented by the present predictors.

No Model Is Perfect   There will always be some error. R^2 rarely approaches 1.00, especially in human services. In physics, an R^2 of .988 might be considered small, whereas in the social sciences, an R^2 of .30 might be thought to be large. Some people will continue to be overpaid and some underpaid, but the total amounts overpaid and underpaid will decrease when a carefully developed model is used. In any event, these methods allow us to decrease the error in determining reimbursement amounts; however, because the model is imperfect, there also needs to be some method of appealing against the amount determined by the model, so that well-informed human judgment can be applied to the unique circumstances of the individual to decide if the amount should be adjusted.

All Models Have Limitations   Do not extrapolate beyond the range of the data used to build the model. For example, if a model uses IQ scores with a range of 30–70 to generate reimbursement amounts, using the model to generate rates for people with IQ scores less than 30 or more than 70 is risky. Obtaining data that reflects as wide a range of dependent (e.g., rates) and independent measures (e.g., ICAP) as possible is important. This practice will produce a model with the best ability to explain variability in the dependent measure.

"Locked in History"   Models based on actual data are relative to the way a state has done business in the past. They are neither conducive to fostering innovation nor to revising the current structures; however, adaptations can be made to these models to make them friendlier to changes in the service/support structures (see the example in Figure 8.5).

Allocation of Funds   These methods allocate resources based solely on individual characteristics of the people served/supported, the services/supports they receive, and the settings in which those services/supports are provided. Micromanaging how providers use funds is difficult. For example, a legislature might appropriate a given percentage increase to be used specifically to raise salaries of direct-care staff. If funds are specified for such purposes, they should be initially *excluded* from the amount to be allo-

Column A	Column B	Column C	Column D
Variable	Parameter estimate	Variable value	B x C
Residential arrangments			
Lives with family?	−289.39317	0	0.00
Foster care*	0.00000	0	0.00
Supported living*	535.00000	0	0.00
Semi-independent unit with staff?	535.00000	0	0.00
Group residence?	535.00000	1	535.00
State institution?	5,587.20481	0	0.00

Figure 8.5.   Example of introduction of incentives—supported living. *Note:* Variables ending with a question mark (?) are binary measures (i.e., 1 = yes; 0 = no). *Reference category from the previous model. In this illustration, supported living has been assigned the average parameter estimate of 535 so that people with supported living would receive an additional $535 per month. The two other categories in the gray box would receive changed amounts relative to the previous model in Figure 8.4.

cated by these models. Later, they can be added separately according to those legislative intentions.

DISCRIMINANT ANALYSIS

Figures 8.3 and 8.4 show that independent settings are less expensive than the restrictive, facility-based settings. For example, group residences cost $1,075 more per month than supported living. Several other chapters in this book demonstrate that supported settings result in better lifestyle outcomes for individuals (see Chapters 6 and 7). Therefore, policy makers may wish to 1) identify those people most in need of increased independence, and 2) devise strategies for implementing system change. To examine the first point, discriminant analysis is applied. The latter point is discussed in the subsequent section. Although this example concentrates on residential settings, the methods are also applicable to many other situations.

Discriminant analysis is a statistical method that can be used to classify individuals based on a set of characteristics. It uses a mathematical model, similar to that shown in Table 8.2, to predict to which group an individual might belong (e.g., in which setting a person might live). Individuals with similar characteristics are assigned to similar settings by the model. The percentage of people that the model correctly classifies is a measure of the model's validity. With predictors similar to those listed in Table 8.2—except for the residential arrangement measures—a stepwise discriminant analysis produced estimates of which of three residential categories a person currently lived in. Table 8.4 shows that 71% of individuals were correctly classified. This result is much better than what one might expect from chance (33%) and points to the model's validity. Also of interest are those people incorrectly classified by the model:

- 958 people (16.4%) were classified into more-independent settings, suggesting that their current residential settings may be unnecessarily restrictive. System planners and service coordinators should pay very close attention to the support plans and plan implementation for these individuals. Systemically, this information may also be useful in indicating that more opportunities need to be developed for people to live in these independent environments.

- 738 people (12.6%) were classified into less-independent settings, suggesting that these individuals could be receiving less support than expected. Close attention might be paid to assure that their health,

Table 8.4. Group classification summary from discriminant analysis of residential settings

Current residence	Predicted residence			
	Developmental center	Group home	Independent	Total
Developmental center	410*	417	34	861
Group home	236	2,429*	507	3,172
Independent	4	498	1,314*	1,816
Total	**650**	**3,344**	**1,855**	**5,849**

*Number of individuals whose current residence was correctly predicted by the discriminant analysis = 4173/5849, or 71%.

safety, welfare, and supervision needs are being adequately met in their current settings. Assuming that these needs, as well as their needs for services/supports, are being well met, program evaluators might find examples among these individuals for commendations for service/support providers, and the provider's approach could become the basis for defining best practices in service/support provision.

Some might find it disturbing that these data imply some sort of mandate that the incorrectly classified people be immediately moved to a different environment, or that correctly classified people be kept where they are, simply on the basis of a statistical analysis. We are not suggesting that such analyses be used to keep people in more restrictive environments or to move them to a different environment simply on the basis of these statistics. Rather, such a statistical tool may be used to help intelligently plan and direct systems of service/support. Like any tool, it may be used productively, or it may be misused.

INTRODUCING INCENTIVES INTO THE MODEL

From the results of a discriminant analysis, as in Table 8.4, a significant number of people might be indicated as being in a more restrictive setting than would be predicted by their individual characteristics, and so they would need a more independent setting. Similar conclusions could also be made from a compilation of current living arrangements contrasted with those recommended in support plans or from comparisons with national per-capita utilization rates. Better lifestyle outcomes and substantial cost savings might be realized by a more independent residential placement for a large number of people, as illustrated in Figure 8.3 and evidenced by the model in Figure 8.4.

For example, consideration of these factors might convince policy makers that the numbers of people currently living in group residences and staffed apartments could and should be reduced, with a commensurate increase in the numbers living in supported situations. The reimbursement model in Figure 8.4, however, is based on the current state of the system and is not necessarily conducive to fostering change. Specifically, reimbursement amounts for those living in group residences are $1,075 per month more than for those living independently with supports. The current incentive for provider agencies, therefore, is to maintain the status quo. The availability of an individual budget amount model, like the one in Figure 8.4, presents a large number of possibilities for reordering these incentives to foster system change.

One possibility would be the somewhat egalitarian approach of leaving the residential arrangements block totally out of the model. This arrangement would provide an incentive for the most people to move to the most independent (and also least expensive) living arrangements. Conversely, as discussed previously, finding and funding settings, services, and supports for people who need higher levels of supervision and attention would become more difficult. One way to limit this impact would be to limit the range of settings selected for this semi-egalitarian approach. One such example is presented in Figure 8.5, which is a modification of the residential block of Figure 8.4. Note the highlighted box, which merges the egalitarian, equal-payments-for-all, payment concept with the individual estimated resource model of Figure 8.4.

This egalitarian approach is limited, however, to the three specific residential arrangements that have been targeted: group residences, semi-independent with staff, and supported living. The parameter estimates for group residences (1,075) and semi-independent with staff (529) were added to that of supported living (0) and divided by three, to yield an average of 535. This average of 535 was then substituted for each of those parameter estimates. The residential component of the rate would be $535 for people living in each of these settings, regardless of the setting in which the consumer was living. For the sake of simplicity, we have used the same variable values as were presented in Figure 8.4. Also, we included only the relevant residential arrangements section in Figure 8.5. Relative to the previous model (Figure 8.4), this method would result in a $535 per month increase for those receiving supported living and a decrease of $540 for those living in group homes.

These amounts are not to be interpreted as the monthly rate for each specific service. Rather, they are increments to the total amount generated by the entire regression model. The parameter estimates in the gray box are not those produced by the regression analysis. They illustrate manipulations to those parameters that policy makers might use to provide incentives for increased independence.

Such an incentive could be applied to all current recipients or only to those who are currently living in group homes and who are identified as likely to benefit from a move to a supported-living setting. Alternatively, to soften the impact, the incentive could be applied only to those people who are new to the system. Note that an incentive system, such as the one illustrated in Figure 8.5, would no longer have the advantage of budget neutrality. It would, however, allow for direct control of the amounts paid for each of the selected residential settings. It could also be adapted to modify an existing model, such as the one shown in Figure 8.4, at a later date. Such modifications to an existing model could be used to implement a reimbursement policy change without needing to go through the process of collecting new data and constructing a totally new model.

Finally, note that the previous discussion centered on which service/support/setting measures could be eliminated or modified to provide incentives for systems change, while leaving the individual characteristic (ICAP) measures intact. This approach leaves the primary emphasis on individual characteristics and needs. An opposite approach might concentrate on eliminating the individual characteristics from the model, leaving just the current services, supports, and settings. This procedure is diametrically opposed to the principles and methods presented in this chapter and puts a major emphasis on provider agencies rather than individuals served or supported. Such methodology might obviate the need for "ICAP Police," but it adds a major obstruction to any possible revamping of the service system to make it more attuned to individual needs. People would tend to stay wherever they were, regardless of their needs or the appropriateness of the setting.

CONCLUSION

This chapter presents data analyses that explain how several factors influence reimbursement amounts for services and supports for individuals with intellectual disabilities in four Western states. Reimbursement rates are highest for those with the most severe levels of disability, as measured by the ICAP. Other ICAP measures were also shown to influence reimbursement rates (e.g., selected diagnoses, mobility limitations). Residential setting also had a major effect on reimbursements, with the most restrictive settings being the most expensive (OTBE). We have also demonstrated methods for translating these analyses into useful tools for policy makers and funding agencies. The results of multiple regression analyses were translated into example models that could be used for generating individual budget amounts. Individual budget amounts allow for the fair and equitable allocation of existing resources, can be portable, and are prerequisites for the establishment of service recipient–directed support plans.

This methodology has the advantages of providing equity in funding along with a rational means of cost containment that is required in these budgetary times. It has appeal for the two primary stakeholders in the use of the money, that is, the consumer and the taxpayer. Other systems do not address the needs of the taxpayers, who provide the funding, to be both fair and prudent. Although some service recipients, or at least their advocates, may believe the individuals should be able to purchase whatever services they want, such methodologies do not supply a means to provide equity or to contain costs. In such cases, the losers are the taxpayers, who have an ever-increasing burden of costs, and the unserved service recipients on waiting lists, who do not then receive services due to a lack of resources.

Also demonstrated was a discriminant analysis to identify individuals who may be most in need of increased independence. Making such information available to policy makers could potentially lead to systems change. We also suggest a possible modification to the reimbursement model that would provide an incentive to promote such systems change.

Many people are engaged in devising indicators to measure the effectiveness of service/support systems and to assess their effectiveness in terms of outcomes. We do not see the ideas presented in this chapter as replacements for those efforts; however, we do envision that the OTBE methodology could provide an enhancement to the assessment of outcomes and that the discriminant analyses could become a useful tool to add to those used to measure overall system performance. These analyses are from four rural Western American states, and findings might be limited to that geographic region; yet, the applicability of these methods is universal. Data analysts in other states are invited to join with us to expand these data to a wider base and to further develop this research.

REFERENCES

Babin, S.L., & Fortune, J. (2001, July 11). *Consumer-centered planning and budgeting.* Paper presented at the workshop "Beyond Olmstead: Community-based services for all people with disabilities," sponsored by the U.S. Department of

Health and Human Services, Agency for Healthcare Research and Quality, Office of Health Care Information, The User Liaison Program, Chicago.

Braddock, D., Hemp. R., Parish, S., & Rizzolo, M.C. (2000). *The state of the states in developmental disabilities: 2000 study summary.* Chicago: University of Illinois at Chicago, Department of Disability and Human Development.

Bruininks, R.H., Hill, B.K., Weatherman, R.F., & Woodcock, R.W. (1986). *Inventory for Client and Agency Planning (ICAP).* Chicago: Riverside.

Bureau of Economic Analysis. (1998). *Regional accounts data, local area personal income.* Available on-line at http://www.bea.gov/bea/regional/reis/drill.cfm

Campbell, E.M., & Heal, L.W. (1995). Prediction of cost, rate, and staffing by provider and client characteristics. *American Journal on Mental Retardation, 100*(1), 17–35.

Emerson, E., Robertson, J., Gregory, N., Hatton, C., Kessissoglou, S., Hallam, A., Jarbrink, K., Knapp, M., Netten, A., & Walsh, P.N. (2001). Quality and costs of supported living residences and group homes in the United Kingdom. *American Journal on Mental Retardation, 106*(5), 401–415.

Fortune, J., Seiler, W., & Church, J. (2002, May). *Individual budgets according to individual need, Wyoming DOORS, South Dakota Service-Based Rates, and Pennsylvania's Targeted Budget Project.* Paper presented at the National Association of Developmental Disabilities Directors Services Mid-Year Meeting. Breckenridge, CO.

Health Care Financing Administration. (1999, October 28). Prospective payment system for home health agencies. *Federal Register, 64*(208), 58179–58182.

Holmes, D., & Teresi, J.A. (1998). Relating personnel costs in special care units and in traditional care units to resident characteristics. *Journal of Mental Health Policy and Economics, 1,* 31–40.

Lewis, D.R., & Bruininks, R.H. (1994). Costs of community-based residential and related services to individuals with mental retardation and other developmental disabilities. In M.F. Hayden & B.H. Abery (Eds.), *Challenges for a service system in transition: Ensuring quality community experiences for persons with developmental disabilities* (pp. 231–263). Baltimore: Paul H. Brookes Publishing Co.

Nebraska Department of Labor. (1998). *Nebraska workforce development information: Labor market information.* Retrieved on-line from http://www.dol.state.ne.us/nwd/center.cfm

Montana Department of Labor and Industry, Montana Research and Analysis Bureau. (1999). *Local area unemployment statistics: 1999 annual average labor force by county.* Retrieved on-line from http://rad.dli.state.mt.us/laus/display.asp

Prouty, R.W., Smith, G., & Lakin, K.C. (2001). *Residential services for persons with developmental disabilities: Status and trends through 2000.* Minneapolis: University of Minnesota, Research and Training Center on Community Living, Institute on Community Integration.

Rhoades, J.A., & Altman, B.M. (2001). Personal characteristics and contextual factors associated with residential expenditures for individuals with mental retardation. *Mental Retardation, 39*(2), 114–129.

Smith, G. (2001a). *Facts and figures—Medicaid long-term services for people with developmental disabilities: 2000 status.* Alexandria, VA: National Association of State Directors of Developmental Disabilities Services.

Smith, G. (2001b). *Facts and figures—Residential services for people with developmental disabilities: 2000 status.* Alexandria, VA: National Association of State Directors of Developmental Disabilities Services.

South Dakota Department of Labor, Labor Market Information Center. (1998). *Labor supply and labor force.* Available on-line at http://www.state.sd.us/dol/lmic/datasearch/laborforce/index.cfm

U.S. Centers for Medicare & Medicaid Services, The MEDSTAT Group. (2001). *Wyoming—Individual budgets for Medicaid Waiver services. Promising practices in Home and Community-Based Services* (Report No. 6). Washington, DC: Author.

Wyoming Department of Employment. (1998). *Wyoming labor market information: Local area unemployment statistics.* Retrieved on-line from http://doe.state.wy.us/lmi/laus/98bmk.htm

CHAPTER 9

Individual Budgets and Freedom from Staff Control

Roger J. Stancliffe and K. Charlie Lakin

In a number of states, initiatives that promote self-determination, funded by the Robert Wood Johnson Foundation, have emphasized funding and service provision features, such as having an individual budget, exercising control over services and decision making, using person-centered planning, having independent support brokerage, and having a fiscal intermediary (Moseley, 2001; see also Chapter 10). As states move toward wider implementation of these notions, not all ideas are being incorporated fully into state service systems. Individual budgets, however, are popular in many state service systems (Moseley, 2001; see also Chapter 12).

WHO HAS AN INDIVIDUAL BUDGET?

Moseley noted that service and funding arrangements, such as individual budgets, "must be . . . open to people with even the most intensive need for support. We can't afford to leave anyone behind" (2001, p. 7). Certain past initiatives that have been characterized by greater service recipient control have not served all people with intellectual disabilities equally. For

The data reported in this chapter were gathered by the Center for Outcome Analysis as part of an evaluation contract with the Michigan Department of Community Health. Through an agreement with the Center for Outcome Analysis, independent analyses of these data were conducted at the University of Minnesota, Research and Training Center on Community Living. The contents of this chapter represent the opinions of the authors and do not necessarily reflect official positions of the Michigan Department of Community Health or the Center for Outcome Analysis.

example, residents of semi-independent living services typically exercise higher levels of choice and personal control than service recipients from traditional community settings with 24-hour staffing (see Chapter 6), but semi-independent living services mostly cater to individuals with milder intellectual disabilities, better developed adaptive behavior, and fewer challenging behaviors (Burchard, Hasazi, Gordon, & Yoe, 1991; Halpern, Close, & Nelson, 1986; Stancliffe, Abery, & Smith, 2000). The Medicaid Community Supported Living Arrangements (CSLA) program tended to serve a similar population (Lakin, Hayden, & Burwell, 1996).

One possible unintended consequence of making individual budgets more available is that they, like some earlier individualized support approaches, will be provided more frequently to individuals with relatively less need of support and who are less costly to serve. Alternatively, service recipients with strong, active support from their families may gain greater access to such initiatives. One purpose of this chapter is to investigate what personal characteristics, levels of family involvement, and service arrangements distinguish people who do and do not have an individual budget.

INCREASED SELF-DETERMINATION

Disturbingly low levels of choice have been reported in community settings (Kishi, Teelucksingh, Zollers, Park-Lee, & Meyer, 1988; Stancliffe & Abery, 1997). Comparisons with community members without disabilities showed that people with intellectual disabilities have fewer choices and exercise less personal control (Kishi et al., 1988; Parsons, McCarn, & Reid, 1993; Sands & Kozleski, 1994; Wehmeyer & Metzler, 1995). In addition, major life decisions about services (e.g., one's residence, living companions, employment) are substantially less available than more routine choices, such as what to eat or what to wear (Emerson & Hatton, 1996; Kishi et al., 1988; Stancliffe, 1995; Stancliffe & Wehmeyer, 1995; Wehmeyer & Metzler, 1995). All too often the price of access to services includes staff/agency dominance of service recipients' lives and choices, especially service-related choices.

Having an individual budget represents one element of the service system increasingly considered to contribute to reduction in staff control of service recipients' lives and greater self-determination, especially regarding control over one's services; however, little published information is available that evaluates the relationship between individual budgets, freedom from staff control, and service recipient choice/personal control.

Research on the impact of service provision on choice has generally been conducted in service settings with traditional funding systems, so the impact of individual budgets could not be examined. Stancliffe et al. (2000) reported that the amount of money a person had available for discretionary spending was positively related to personal control, but this concerned personal expenditure, not control over service funding.

As individual budgets are implemented more widely, there is a risk that they may be seen as a panacea for reducing staff control and increasing self-determination. Dowson and Salisbury commented on the danger that "individualized funding (IF) becomes an end instead of a means, leading to the false assumption that people who receive IF automatically and immediately achieve self-determination" (2001, p. 27). A second purpose of this chapter is to examine the relationship between individual budgets and freedom from staff control, in particular whether people with an individual budget experience a different level of staff control from those without this form of funding.

MAKING VALID COMPARISONS AND DEALING WITH CONFOUNDS

The process of making valid comparisons between groups with and without individual budgets faces several methodological challenges. Important issues relate to potential confounds with 1) adaptive behavior, 2) personal choice and control, and 3) residence type. Individual differences in intellectual functioning and adaptive behavior are related strongly to service recipient choice and personal control, with individuals with milder disabilities typically exercising more choice (Conroy, 1995; Heller, Miller, & Factor, 1999; Schalock & Keith, 1993; Stancliffe, 1997; Stancliffe et al., 2000; Tøssebro, 1995; Wehmeyer, Kelchner, & Richards, 1995). The instrument used in the present study to assess freedom from staff control (the Decision Control Inventory [DCI], Conroy, 1997a) has a strong positive correlation with adaptive behavior ($r = .71$; Conroy, 1995). In addition, smaller, more individualized and/or (semi-) independent living arrangements are associated with greater service recipient choice and personal control of one's life (Burchard et al., 1991; Schalock & Keith, 1993; Stancliffe, 1997; Stancliffe et al., 2000; Stancliffe & Keane, 2000; Tøssebro, 1995; Wehmeyer & Bolding, 1999; Wehmeyer et al., 1995; see also Chapter 6).

If differences in level of staff control by individual budget status were observed, it could be difficult to determine whether the differences were associated with the size and type of settings in which people lived, the characteristics of the people who received an individual budget, the effect of an individual budget itself, or some combination of these factors. To control for such potentially confounded relationships among the variables, we used statistical controls through analysis of covariance with adaptive behavior as the covariate and residential setting size as a factor in the analysis.

DATA SOURCE AND SAMPLING

The Center for Outcome Analysis conducted an independent evaluation of the Robert Wood Johnson Foundation–funded Self-Determination Initiative in Michigan and gathered the data examined in this chapter. Cross-sectional data from the Michigan evaluation, gathered in late 1997 and early 1998 at the beginning of Michigan's Self-Determination Initiative, were subjected to independent secondary analysis at the University of Minnesota.

The sample involved all participants in the Michigan Self-Determination Initiative (including some waiting to enter active involvement in the initiative) who were willing to be involved in the evaluation. Clearly, the sample cannot be considered representative of service recipients in Michigan, nor does it reflect the broader availability of individual budgets in that state.

Participants

We selected participants with intellectual disabilities who had valid data about having an individual budget and about adaptive and challenging behavior. Participants lived in settings with 1–15 residents with disabilities. We excluded those from larger settings because the focus was on the role of individual budgets in community services, not institutions. There were 501 participants, and their personal characteristics are shown in Table 9.1 (categorical variables) and Table 9.2 (continuous variables) by individual budget status.

Settings

Participants lived in one of the following five types of residential settings: 1) own home, 2) family home, 3) group home, 4) foster home, and 5) other (see Table 9.1).

Table 9.1. Personal characteristics and environmental variables (categorical) by individual budget status

Variable	N^a	Level	Individual budget No	Individual budget Yes	Percent with an individual budget
Personal characteristics					
Gender	499	Male	197	71	26.5%
		Female	182	49	24.0%
Ethnic group	501	Caucasian	303	108	26.3%
		African	62	8	11.4%
		Other	15	5	25.0%
Level of intellectual disability	501	Mild	76	10	11.6%
		Moderate	104	32	23.5%
		Severe	178	65	26.7%
		Profound	10	3	23.1%
		Unspecified	12	11	47.8%
Environmental variables					
Residence type	501	Own home	75	87	53.7%
		Family home	70	12	14.6%
		Group home	163	10	5.8%
		Foster home	41	1	2.4%
		Other	31	11	26.2%
Family contact in past year	447	None	47	9	16.1%
		Less than monthly	88	20	18.5%
		Monthly	93	22	19.1%
		Weekly	88	41	31.8%
		Daily	17	22	56.4%
Guardianship status	500	No guardian or conservator	119	46	27.9%
		Has guardian or conservator	260	75	22.4%

^{a}Overall $N = 501$, so $N < 501$ indicates missing data for the variable in question.

Table 9.2. Personal characteristics and environmental variables (continuous) by individual budget status

| | | Individual budget | | | |
| | | No n = 380 | | Yes n = 121 | |
Variable	N[a]	Mean	SD	Mean	SD
Personal characteristics					
Adaptive behavior	501	58.79	19.90	63.56	22.23
Challenging behavior	501	91.05	10.38	92.74	7.08
Age	497	42.44	12.89	42.67	13.38
Environmental variables					
Residence size (number of residents with disabilities)	501	4.02	2.97	2.08	1.37

[a]Overall N = 501, so N < 501 indicates missing data for the variable in question.

INSTRUMENTS

The instruments described next were used to gather information about individual budget status, choice and control, adaptive and challenging behavior, other personal characteristics, and environmental variables. Each of these instruments formed part of the Personal Life Quality Protocol (Conroy, 1997b) used by the Center for Outcome Analysis to evaluate Michigan's Self-Determination Initiative.

Individual Budget Information

The Individual Budget Information questionnaire contains 10 items about the details of the person's individual budget. Individual budget status was assessed using the question: "Does this person have an individual CMH [Community Mental Health] budget (public funds)?" This question identified people with an individual budget prior to implementation of Michigan's Self-Determination Initiative and may also have captured some who were among the first to receive an individual budget under that initiative.

Decision Control Inventory

The DCI (Conroy, 1997a) evaluates who makes choices and exercises control in the lives of people with intellectual disabilities in relation to 35 items about everyday life and services, such as the use of personal money, choice of foods, choice of home, choice of case managers, and whether to have pets. On each item, respondents are asked to rate decision making on an 11-point scale, with 0 meaning that decisions are made entirely by paid staff and 10 meaning that decisions are made entirely by the individual and/or unpaid loved ones. Total scores are recoded into a scale of 0–100. Lower scores represent greater control by paid staff, and higher scores indicate greater freedom from staff control. In our view, DCI scores are appropriately interpreted as *freedom from staff control*. A given level of control concerning the service recipient's life exercised by other family members *or* by the individual him- or herself will yield the same DCI score because the level of *staff* control in both situations is the same.

The DCI's internal consistency (Cronbach's alpha) was .95; test–retest reliability was .98; combined test–retest and interrater reliability was .86; and correlation with adaptive behavior was .71 (Conroy, 1995).

Adaptive and Challenging Behavior

Adaptive behavior was evaluated using the 14-item Current Abilities scale, containing items drawn or adapted from a previous 32-item scale, that, in turn, was derived from the American Association on Mental Retardation Adaptive Behavior Scale. The 32-item version has been found to be highly reliable, with interrater and test–retest reliabilities of $r = .95$ and $r = .96$ (Devlin, 1989), and $r = .99$ and $r = .99$ (Fullerton, Douglass, & Dodder, 1999).

Challenging behavior was measured with the Adjustment and Challenges Scale (Center for Outcome Analysis, 1997), a 20-item scale that examines the severity of behaviors, such as self-injury, assault, property destruction, inappropriate sexuality, substance abuse, and theft, as well as the severity of psychiatric symptoms, including eating disorders, depressive symptoms, hallucinations, anxiety/panic, and suicidal actions/thoughts. No psychometric data were available for this specific scale. Fullerton et al. (1999) examined the reliability of severity ratings of challenging behavior items closely related to eight of the items in the current scale. Their data provide evidence of satisfactory test–retest and interrater reliability for these items.

Total scores on both scales were computed so that they could range from 0 to 100 points, with the higher scores being more favorable in each case. Thus, for challenging behavior, higher scores indicated *less* challenging behavior.

Personal Characteristics

Information about each participant's gender, primary ethnicity, level of intellectual disability, age, guardianship status, and a number of other personal characteristics was gathered from records and/or by interviewing the person who knows the service recipient best on a day-to-day basis.

Environmental Variables

Family contact was evaluated using the number of contacts by all relatives via telephone, mail, visits, outings, individual planning meetings, or consent for medical care. For our analyses, frequency of family contact in the past year was classified into five categories: 1) none, 2) less than monthly (1–11 contacts), 3) monthly (12–51), 4) weekly (52–364), and 5) daily (365+). *Residence size* was measured in response to the question: "How many people with disabilities (including this person) live in this home?"

FINDINGS

Findings about individual budget status are followed by the results for freedom from staff control and for effect size.

Individual Budget Status

All of the personal characteristics and environmental variables reported in Tables 9.1 and 9.2, except gender, guardianship status, and age, were significantly related to individual budget status under *univariate* analysis; however, univariate analyses are inappropriate and potentially misleading because there are significant associations among the various personal characteristics and environmental variables. Therefore, the observed univariate differences may not be the result of the *unique* influence of the variable under examination but instead may be due to other variables to which it was related. For example, a significant relationship existed between ethnic group and residence type. The lower overall proportion of African Americans with individual budgets may have been due to the unequal allocation of this group by residence type (e.g., 21.4% of foster home residents were African Americans, whereas 8.6% of own home residents were from this ethnic group), rather than ethnicity per se.

A better way to evaluate the association of various predictor variables with individual budget status is to use a *multivariate* statistic, such as backward logistic regression, that evaluates the *unique* contribution of each variable, while holding all other predictors constant. Backward logistic regression begins by examining all predictor variables and eliminating nonsignificant variables one at a time on statistical grounds. Variables that remain in the model at the end of this process are the best independent predictors.

Table 9.3 shows that individual budget availability was significantly associated with features of the person's living environment (residence type and residence size) but was not related to service recipients' personal characteristics, family contact, or guardianship status. The eight predictor variables examined but eliminated are listed in the table notes for Table 9.3. Importantly, personal characteristics such as gender, ethnic group, level of intellectual disability, adaptive behavior, challenging behavior, and age were not significant predictors of individual budget status under multivariate analysis, which suggests that individual budgets were generally distributed equitably, regardless of service recipients' personal characteristics. The final logistic regression model, involving residence type and residence size, was highly significant (χ^2 [5, $N = 441$] = 136.65, $p < .001$) and correctly classified 78.5% of cases with respect to individual budget status.

Compared with group-home residents (the reference category), the odds that people who lived in their own home or "other" homes had an individual budget were significantly greater. Residents of foster homes were less likely, and residents of family homes were more likely, to have an individual budget than group-home residents, but neither of these comparisons attained statistical significance. For categorical variables, odds ratios should be interpreted in relationship to the reference category. By definition, the reference category has an odds ratio of 1. The odds ratio of 11.43 for people living in their own home means that their odds of having an individual budget were more than 11 times the odds for group-home residents (the reference category).

Table 9.3. Variables remaining in the final logistic regression model ($N = 441$)

	B	SE	Wald	df	p	Odds ratio
Residence type			47.91	4	.000	
Group home (reference category)						1.00
Family home	.32	.65	.24	1	.627	1.37
Own home	2.44	.48	26.07	1	.000	11.43
Foster home	−.88	1.07	.67	1	.413	0.42
Other home	1.46	.52	7.80	1	.005	4.29
Residence size (number of residents with disabilities)	−.20	.10	4.30	1	.038	0.82

Note: Predictor variables tested but omitted during backward logistic regression were: adaptive behavior, challenging behavior, ethnic group, sex, age, level of intellectual disability, guardianship status, and family contact.
SE = Standard error.
Wald = The Wald statistic can be calculated as $(B/SE)^2$ if df = 1. It is used to test whether the coefficient B is significant. The column headed p shows the significance of the Wald statistic.

For continuous independent variables, such as residence size, the odds ratio refers to the odds of having an individual budget if the independent variable increases by one unit. The odds ratio of 0.82 for this variable means that, for each additional resident with disabilities, the odds of having an individual budget *decreased* by 18%.

Given the cross-sectional nature of the present study, it cannot be determined why residence type and residence size were related to individual budget status. Different possibilities for these associations can be offered, and quite possibly each occurred, although to different, unknown degrees. For example, having access to the individual budget option may have enabled some people living in traditional congregate community living settings, such as group homes, to move to homes of their own. If so, our finding that the odds of having an individual budget were higher in *own home* settings would have been because people with individual budgets had *moved* to those settings with the assistance of the individual budget prior to the data collection for the present study.

Another hypothesis for the association between residence type and individual budget status could be that it is simpler to identify and allocate an individual budget to people *already* receiving individualized services in their *own home* rather than to figure out how to disaggregate the budget for a group facility into a number of individual budgets. That is, there could have been an administrative convenience factor. Of course, it could also be hypothesized that people who had already committed to controlling and maintaining their own homes would be more likely to make the commitment to control and maintain their own budgets. Likely for some of the reasons noted, there might be a tendency to select individual budgeting to support a more individualized approach to services (living in one's own home) and traditional budgeting to support a more traditional placement, such as a group home. But the validity and relative contributions of these possibilities can only be tested in longitudinal research that tracks changes in living arrangements, self-determination, and relevant personal and environmental characteristics before and after an individual budget becomes available.

Freedom from Staff Control

As previously noted, higher DCI scores can arise because of control exercised by other family members or by the individual him/herself. This issue could affect DCI scores in any type of residential setting, but it likely was most prominent for individuals living in the family home. Analysis across residence types revealed that the DCI mean for participants living in the family home (86.02) was very high (the scale maximum is 100) and was significantly higher than every other setting type, $F(4, 494) = 100.71$, $p < .001$. Therefore, for the analysis of DCI scores by individual budget status, we omitted the 82 participants living in the family home because we considered that the higher DCI scores reported for these participants were substantially inflated by the role the family played in daily decision making.

We used an analysis of covariance (ANCOVA) to determine whether those with an individual budget had differing freedom from staff control from those without an individual budget. DCI scores were strongly related to adaptive behavior in the present study ($r = .54$, $p < .001$), so we used adaptive behavior as a covariate. Likewise, choice making is related to residence size (number of residents with a disability), but this relationship has been found to be *nonlinear* across the 1–15 person size range (Tøssebro, 1995), so we included residence size as a factor in the ANCOVA analysis, rather than as a covariate. Based on previous research (Stancliffe, 1997; Tøssebro, 1995), we formed four residence-size groups (1, 2, 3–4, and 5–15 residents with disabilities). This decision resulted in a 2 (individual budget: yes/no) by 4 (residence-size) factorial analysis with adaptive behavior as a covariate. Estimated mean DCI scores adjusted for the effect of adaptive behavior as a covariate are shown in Table 9.4.

Adaptive behavior was a significant covariate, $F(1, 409) = 89.91$, $p < .001$. Overall, there was a significant difference in freedom from staff control by individual budget status, $F(1, 409) = 6.78$, $p < .01$, with those with an individual budget having significantly higher DCI scores that averaged 5.6 points higher than those without. Adaptive behavior was held constant using covariance, and residence size was controlled by using this variable as a factor in the analysis. This cross-sectional finding is consistent with

Table 9.4. Decision Control Inventory (Conroy, 1997a) estimated scores by living-setting size and by individual budget status, adjusted for adaptive behavior as a covariate ($N = 418$)

| Residence size (number of residents with a disability) | Individual budget | | | | | |
| | No $n = 309$ | | Yes $n = 109$ | | Total | |
	Mean	SE	Mean	SE	Mean	SE
1 ($n = 78$)	74.63	2.66	80.39	2.53	77.51	1.88
2 ($n = 95$)	70.88	2.29	80.62	2.32	75.75	1.64
3–4 ($n = 80$)	52.37	1.94	59.83	5.00	56.10	2.67
5–15 ($n = 165$)	50.63	1.31	50.14	4.62	50.38	2.42
Total	62.13	1.04	67.75	1.89		

SE = Standard error

the longitudinal evaluations of the Robert Wood Johnson Foundation Self-Determination Initiatives in New Hampshire and Michigan (Conroy & Yuskauskas, 1996; Conroy, 2000; see also Chapter 10), which reported significant increases in DCI scores over time following self-determination interventions. The present finding is also consistent with the very common programmatic practice in Robert Wood Johnson Foundation initiatives across the country of implementing individual budgets (among other practices) with the intention of enhancing self-determination (Moseley, 2001). Our study is silent on the impact of an individual budget on freedom from staff control within the family home, as these participants were omitted from our analysis of this issue.

A significant main effect was found for residence size, $F(3, 409) = 37.54$, $p < .001$. No significant interaction was found between individual budget status and residence size. Simple contrasts showed that residents of very small settings (i.e., with 1–2 resident with disabilities) had significantly and substantially higher DCI scores than those from larger settings. This finding is consistent with previous studies that have reported a strong relationship between living environment size and choice and control exercised by the person with disabilities (Howe, Horner, & Newton, 1998; Stancliffe, 1997; Stancliffe et al., 2000; Stancliffe & Keane, 2000; Tøssebro, 1995; Wehmeyer & Bolding, 1999). For example, Stancliffe (1997) found that people from community-living settings with 1 or 2 residents had significantly higher levels of choice than those from larger settings.

Effect Size

Estimates of effect size were obtained using the partial eta squared (η_p^2) value for each effect. This statistic describes the proportion of total variability attributable to each factor. The largest effect size was associated with residence size ($\eta_p^2 = .216$), with adaptive behavior having a smaller but similar effect size ($\eta_p^2 = .180$) and individual budget status having a substantially smaller effect size ($\eta_p^2 = .016$). Although individual budget status was significantly related to DCI scores, both adaptive behavior and living-setting size had effects that were more than 10 times bigger than the effect size for individual budget status. That is, the proportion of total variability in DCI scores attributable to individual budget status was far exceeded by that associated with adaptive behavior and with living-setting size.

One likely reason for the modest effect size for individual budget availability was that the data came from the early phases of the Robert Wood Johnson Foundation Self-Determination Initiative in Michigan, so individual budgets (and related supports for self-determination) may not have been available for long enough to have their full effect. This proposition is strongly supported by Head and Conroy's (Chapter 10) finding of a substantial *longitudinal* increase from 1998 to 2001 (mean increase = 14 points) on the 100-point DCI scale for participants in Michigan's Self-Determination Initiative. This finding may be compared with the 5.6-point difference between those with and without an individual budget in the present study.

Taking these two findings together appears to provide clear support for the comments by Dowson and Salisbury (2001) quoted previously, that provision of an individual budget in itself does not "automatically" result in large increases in choice and control. Rather, individual budget availability was associated with only modestly higher DCI scores in the present study. The much more substantial effect reported by Head and Conroy presumably relates to the long-term effects of the full array of supports for self-determination used in Michigan, not just provision of an individual budget.

CONCLUSION

Our findings on who receives an individual budget showed that, in Michigan, individual budgets were provided equitably, regardless of service recipients' personal characteristics or family contact. Residence type and residence size were related to individual budget status, but it was not clear whether this was a cause or an effect of having an individual budget. Moseley, Gettings, and Cooper (Chapter 12) noted that some states provide individual budgets only to certain service recipients. This practice suggests that careful monitoring of equity of access to individual budgets will continue to be needed to ensure that this policy innovation is available to all who seek it.

The current cross-sectional analysis does not provide evidence of a causal link between freedom from staff control and individual budget availability, but the findings do provide intriguing signposts toward possible avenues for intervention that could be tested for cause and effect. It seems clear that, when seeking to enhance self-determination, *all* factors need to be considered, not just having an individual budget. Indeed, there may be some synergy between having an individual budget and access to small scale, individualized living arrangements. Using an individual budget (hopefully with control over decision making, person-centered planning, independent support brokerage, and a fiscal intermediary, if desired) may be one effective (and self-determined) way to enable relocation to a very small, individualized living setting. Other explanations of our findings, however, cannot be ruled out at present. For example, more self-determined individuals may have more success at obtaining an individual budget and at gaining access to individualized residential alternatives, such as one's own home, with the result that residents of such settings and those with an individual budget had higher DCI scores.

Longitudinal data are needed on changes in choice over time for individuals with and without individual budgets who continue with the same living and support arrangements compared with those who move to a more individualized residence type. It would be of interest to see whether changes in freedom from staff control and service recipient choice were more strongly associated with individual budget availability, change of residence, or an interaction among these variables. Head and Conroy's (Chapter 10) findings of a substantial longitudinal increase in DCI scores partially addressed these issues, but the authors did not examine the impact of change of residence.

The role of adaptive behavior requires careful analysis. Self-determination is a right, and preventing people from participating in decisions about their own lives because they lack certain skills is inappropriate, but denying people access to skills training that can make self-determination more easily and independently accessible is also inappropriate. The strong association between adaptive behavior and DCI scores suggests that interventions that enhance adaptive behavior may also contribute to greater self-determination. For example, functional communication skills enable individuals to communicate their choices to others and to exercise greater control over activities (e.g., Carr & Durand, 1985). Stancliffe et al. (2000) suggested that *independent* participation in activities likely results in more control over these activities. Someone who can use a telephone or use public transportation independently can contact family and friends whenever desired, but individuals without those skills must rely on a support person.

We examined only one outcome in this chapter—freedom from staff control. Numerous other benefits of self-determination interventions (that include but are not confined to individual budgets) have been reported in evaluation studies of the Robert Wood Johnson Foundation Self- Determination Initiatives. These benefits include greater satisfaction, improved quality of life, increased community membership, and cost reduction (Conroy, 2000; Conroy & Yuskauskas, 1996; Conroy, Yuskauskas, & Spreat, 2001; see also Chapter 10). Therefore, even if our finding of a modest relationship between freedom from staff control and individual budget availability were confirmed by subsequent research, other important benefits may be associated with offering self-determination interventions (including individual budgets) to service recipients.

REFERENCES

Burchard, S.N., Hasazi, J.E., Gordon, L.R., & Yoe, J. (1991). An examination of lifestyle and adjustment in three community residential alternatives. *Research in Developmental Disabilities, 12,* 127–142.

Carr, E.G., & Durand, V.M. (1985). Reducing behavior problems through functional communication training. *Journal of Applied Behavior Analysis, 18,* 111–126.

Center for Outcome Analysis. (1997). *Adjustment and challenges scale.* Ardmore, PA: Author.

Conroy, J. (1995). *Reliability of the personal life quality protocol: Report number 7 of the 5-year Coffelt Quality Tracking Project.* Submitted to the California Department of Developmental Services and California Protection Agency. (Available from the Center for Outcome Analysis, Ardmore, PA)

Conroy, J.W. (1997a). *The Decision Control Inventory.* Ardmore, PA: Center for Outcome Analysis.

Conroy, J.W. (1997b). *Personal Life Quality Protocol: Michigan Version 5.0.* Ardmore, PA: Center for Outcome Analysis.

Conroy, J. (2000, January). *Positive outcomes of self-determination in Michigan after one year.* PowerPoint presentation and document provided to the Michigan Department of Community Health. (Available from the Center for Outcome Analysis, Ardmore, PA)

Conroy, J., & Yuskauskas, A. (1996). *Independent Evaluation of the Monadnock Self-Determination Project.* Ardmore, PA: Center for Outcome Analysis.

Conroy, J., Yuskauskas, A., & Spreat, S. (2001). *Outcomes of self-determination in New Hampshire.* Ardmore, PA: Center for Outcome Analysis.

Devlin, S. (1989). *Reliability assessment of the instruments used to monitor the Pennhurst class members.* Philadelphia: Temple University Developmental Disabilities Center.

Dowson, S., & Salisbury, B. (2001). *Foundations for freedom: International perspectives on self-determination and individualized funding.* Baltimore: TASH.

Emerson, E., & Hatton, C. (1996). Deinstitutionalization in the UK and Ireland: Outcomes for service users. *Journal of Intellectual & Developmental Disability, 21,* 17–37.

Fullerton, A., Douglass, M., & Dodder, R.A. (1999). A reliability study of measures assessing the impact of deinstitutionalization. *Research in Developmental Disabilities, 20,* 387–400.

Halpern, A.S., Close, D.W., & Nelson, D.J. (1986). *On my own: The impact of semi-independent living programs for adults with mental retardation.* Baltimore: Paul H. Brookes Publishing Co.

Heller, T., Miller, A.B., & Factor, A. (1999). Autonomy in residential facilities and community functioning of adults with mental retardation. *Mental Retardation, 37,* 449–457.

Howe, J., Horner, R.H., & Newton, J.S. (1998). Comparison of supported living and traditional residential services in the state of Oregon. *Mental Retardation, 36,* 1–11.

Kishi, G., Teelucksingh, B., Zollers, N., Park-Lee, S., & Meyer, L. (1988). Daily decision-making in community residences: A social comparison of adults with and without mental retardation. *American Journal on Mental Retardation, 92,* 430–435.

Lakin, K.C., Hayden, M., & Burwell, B. (1996). *An evaluation of implementation of the Medicaid Community Supported Living Arrangements (CSLA) program in eight states.* Minneapolis: University of Minnesota, Institute on Community Integration, Research and Training Center on Community Living.

Moseley, C. (2001). Self-determination: From new initiative to business as usual. *Common Sense, 8,* 1–7.

Parsons, M.B., McCarn, J.E., & Reid, D.H. (1993). Evaluating and increasing meal-related choices throughout a service setting for people with severe disabilities. *Journal of The Association for Persons with Severe Handicaps, 18,* 253–260.

Sands, D.J., & Kozleski, E.B. (1994). Quality of life differences between adults with and without disabilities. *Education and Training in Mental Retardation & Developmental Disabilities, 29,* 90–101.

Schalock, R.L., & Keith, K.D. (1993). *Quality of life questionnaire.* Worthington, OH: IDS Publishing.

Stancliffe, R.J. (1995). Assessing opportunities for choice making: A comparison of self- and staff reports. *American Journal on Mental Retardation, 99,* 418–429.

Stancliffe, R.J. (1997). Community living-unit size, staff presence and resident's choice-making. *Mental Retardation, 35,* 1–9.

Stancliffe, R.J., & Abery, B.H. (1997). Longitudinal study of deinstitutionalization and the exercise of choice. *Mental Retardation, 35,* 159–169.

Stancliffe, R.J., Abery, B.H., & Smith, J. (2000). Personal control and the ecology of community living settings: Beyond living-unit size and type. *American Journal on Mental Retardation, 105,* 431–454.

Stancliffe, R.J., & Keane, S. (2000). Outcomes and costs of community living: A matched comparison of group homes and semi-independent living. *Journal of Intellectual & Developmental Disability, 25,* 281–305.

Stancliffe, R.J., & Wehmeyer, M.L. (1995). Variability in the availability of choice to adults with mental retardation. *Journal of Vocational Rehabilitation, 5,* 319–328.

Tøssebro, J. (1995). Impact of size revisited: Relation of number of residents to self-determination and deprivatization. *American Journal on Mental Retardation, 100,* 59–67.

Wehmeyer, M.L., & Bolding, N. (1999). Self-determination across living and working environments: A matched-samples study of adults with mental retardation. *Mental Retardation, 37,* 353–363.

Wehmeyer, M.L., Kelchner, K., & Richards, S. (1995). Individual and environmental factors related to the self-determination of adults with mental retardation. *Journal of Vocational Rehabilitation, 5,* 291–305.

Wehmeyer, M.L., & Metzler, C.A. (1995). How self-determined are people with mental retardation? The national consumer survey. *Mental Retardation, 33,* 111–119.

CHAPTER 10

Outcomes of Self-Determination in Michigan

Quality and Costs

Michael J. Head and James W. Conroy

In 1993, the Robert Wood Johnson Foundation awarded a 3-year grant to Monadnock Developmental Services of Keene, New Hampshire, to assist in answering this central question: "How would a system of supports look if people with disabilities and their circle of friends, or network, were truly in charge of their own services, if they achieved self-determination?" (Nerney, Crowley, & Kappel, 1995, p. 5). The New Hampshire Self-Determination Project was intended to implement and test this premise by increasing the power, authority, and resources of individuals to control their own destinies (Nerney et al., 1995). The project was "an attempt to fundamentally reform both financing mechanisms and basic structural aspects of the current service delivery system" (Nerney & Shumway, 1996, p. 7). In so doing, the Monadnock service organization addressed three fundamental issues: 1) it enabled individuals and their families to control dollars without dealing with cash; 2) it changed the role of case management to that of personal agents and independent brokers of services chosen by the focus person; and 3) it organized a coherent response to a managed-care culture.

The research reported in this chapter was funded from state funding authorized by the Michigan Department of Community Health to support an evaluation of Michigan's Self-Determination Initiative. It was conducted in conjunction with the implementation of Michigan's Initiative, funded through a grant from the Robert Wood Johnson Foundation. The views in this chapter are those of the authors and do not necessarily represent the views or policies of either the Michigan Department of Community Health or the Robert Wood Johnson Foundation.

In order to bring what appeared to be a complex intervention into the realm of scientific verifiability, we distilled the self-determination concept into a testable form. We stated this hypothesis as three propositions:

1. If people gain control,

2. Their lives will improve, and

3. Costs will not increase.

In this hypothesis, gaining control included getting control of resources. It also implied transfer of control from professionals toward the focus people and their freely chosen allies, usually unpaid, in other words, toward circles of friends. Improvement of lives meant measurable enhancements in one or more qualities of life. Decrease in costs referred to changes in the sum total of public dollars expended to support the person.

In the initial New Hampshire work, all three elements of the operational definition of self-determination were supported (Conroy, Yuskauskas, & Spreat, in review). Later, beginning in 1997, the Robert Wood Johnson Foundation funded a national demonstration. Grants were given to 19 states to further test the notion that shifting control of resources could enhance lives at no greater cost. The Center for Outcome Analysis successfully bid for the evaluation contract for this national project.

The first state to become active in collecting quantitative data about its progress toward self-determination was Michigan. The purpose of this chapter is to describe the outcomes experienced by 70 of the participants in Michigan's self-determination efforts. A variety of aspects of their qualities of life were obtained and compared. The initial 1998 costs of supporting the people within a traditional service framework were also collected and were compared with the amounts in their individual budgets in 2001.

MICHIGAN'S SELF-DETERMINATION INITIATIVE

Michigan's Self-Determination Initiative to promote self-determination for people with developmental disabilities was developed through the assistance of a grant funded by the Robert Wood Johnson Foundation in 1997. Michigan introduced this initiative through the Mental Health and Developmental Disabilities Programs Administration of the Michigan Department of Community Health. Michigan's services system for people with developmental disabilities is operated through a network of county-based systems called Community Mental Health Services Programs (CMHSPs). Work began in 1998 at four local project sites: Washtenaw CMHSP;

Midland-Gladwin CMHSP; Wayne Community Living Services, Inc. (a component of the Detroit-Wayne CMHSP); and Allegan CMHSP. The participants in this study were among their services recipients.

At each project site, commitments were made to develop and implement methods for service arrangements that supported the person's pursuit of self-determination. Each local site established a core group of staff and advocates to learn about self-determination and to develop policies and methods allowing interested service recipients with developmental disabilities to control and direct the use of resources that were allotted to support accomplishment of their plan of services. The local CMHSP entity sought to develop a partnership with the person, supporting his or her pursuit of self-determination. This partnership included developing the needed administrative mechanisms and providing guidance, support, and problem-solving assistance to the person's efforts to directly develop and arrange needed services and supports.

Each participant was first engaged in a person-centered planning process[1] intended to develop his or her plan for needed services and supports. Under arrangements that support self-determination, the plan was transposed into an individual budget, which was a mutually agreed-on estimate of the amount of money needed to accomplish the services authorized in the person's plan. The plan and the budget were then compiled in a written self-determination agreement between the person and the authorizing entity. This agreement authorized the person to proceed to select, control, and direct the provider arrangements necessary to accomplish the plan.

Using their individual budgets, service recipients could choose to contract directly with providers and purchase some or all of the necessary services and supports, or they could choose to have the CMHSP entity make contractual arrangements for these services and supports. When service recipients desired to directly control the service-provision arrangements, they used a fiscal intermediary selected by the CMHSP entity to provide financial assistance and support. The fiscal intermediary held the actual funds allotted by the CMHSP for the service recipient's plan but did not provide direct services. Instead, the fiscal intermediary made payments for services properly contracted between the service recipient and qualified providers chosen by the service recipient. (In some instances, the service recipient chose to have a personal representative be the legal party in

---

[1]Michigan law assures that individuals eligible for mental health or developmental disability services may use a person-centered planning process in the determination of their plan of services and supports.

these contractual arrangements.) Upon receipt of a service recipient–approved invoice, the fiscal intermediary would make payment to the provider.

Service recipients could also choose to hire a provider agency to supply home and community supports or select and directly employ the individuals providing direct support services—that is, function as the employer of record of these personal assistant staff. In those situations, the fiscal intermediary functioned as a payroll agent, assisting the service recipient with the administrative tasks of the employment process by writing paychecks and assuring compliance with payroll tax requirements, unemployment compensation, and worker's compensation laws.

Service recipients involved in self-determination could thus control and direct the use of the resources allotted to support accomplishment of their plan of services, obtaining providers that best met their personal preferences and changing providers as and when they deemed it necessary. They could also use a provider arrangement that the CMHSP already had in place, allowing the CMHSP to draw from their individual budgets in making direct payments to these providers. In any case, service recipients were responsible for managing the provision of their services while controlling expenditures in order to remain within the overall amount of their budgets.

The Michigan Department of Community Health finances the public mental health system through the federal Medicaid program, using a special waiver of Medicaid rules that allows the state agency to contract with the local CMHSP using a prepaid health plan arrangement. Central to this waiver is a range of flexible home and community-based service options oriented toward supported independent living and community participation. In the Michigan self-determination initiative, virtually all participants were involved in pursuing independent lives within their community, with an emphasis on supported employment and attaining personal and community relationships.

METHODS

Next, we describe the study's research methods, starting with the Personal Life Quality protocol (PLQ) used to determine choice making, integration, and perceived quality of life. A Personal Interview is also part of the PLQ. Procedures for data collection and the participants of the study are also described.

Instruments

This section describes the background and the contents of the PLQ. The Center for Outcome Analysis offered this package of instruments to the Robert Wood Johnson Foundation grantee states—and each state identified the scales from the PLQ that were most relevant to the state's unique implementation of self-determination. The PLQ is the core of how we measured the impacts of self-determination. It is so central to our methodology that it is described at length. Readers are encouraged to review the material here before reading the Results section. Interpreting results is much easier if one understands what was measured and how it was measured.

The PLQ's components are collected during an in-person visit with the participant and whoever knows the participant best. We always attempt to complete the package with the focus person as the respondent. When that is not possible, the focus person or an ally can specify someone who knows him or her very well to help complete the PLQ.

Over the years of its development, we have consistently worked to be certain that the PLQ truly taps important dimensions of quality, things that really *matter* to people with disabilities and their families. In psychometric terms, these measures are also psychometrically sound. Many of the elements of this PLQ package evolved from the Pennhurst Longitudinal Study (Conroy & Bradley, 1985). The Pennhurst Longitudinal Study continues to be one of the most influential research efforts, primarily because the measures of quality utilized in that work were scientific, reliable, and valid. Over time, other large groups have been added to the database, people from Philadelphia, Oklahoma, California, North Carolina, and Florida, and more than 1,000 people involved in Robert Wood Johnson Foundation–funded self-determination efforts nationwide.

"Outcomes" have sometimes been cast into the broad categories of independence, productivity, integration, and satisfaction (as specified in the Developmental Disabilities Assistance and Bill of Rights Act Amendments of 1987, PL 100-146). Actually, these are qualities of life, not outcomes. *Changes* in those qualities of life over time are outcomes. Within the PL 100-146 qualities, there are levels of detail, and there are other quality areas that are equally important, such as health. Breaking down these areas further, the following are the elements of quality of life that are touched on by the current version of the PLQ:

- Power to make one's own life choices (self-determination)
- Self-care skills and skill development

- Vocational skills and skill development
- Psychological and emotional adjustment
- Challenging behaviors and reduction of such behaviors
- Stability of living and working environments
- Attitudes and experience of primary caregivers
- Health
- Health care utilization patterns
- Health care satisfaction
- Use (versus overuse) of medications
- Earnings
- Hours per week of productive activity
- Individual planning process timeliness
- Individual planning process usefulness
- Individual planning process degree of "person-centeredness"
- Integration at the home
- Integration at the workplace
- Integration during leisure time
- Relationships with neighbors
- Friendships
- Relationships with housemates
- Family contacts and family relationships
- Opportunities for intimate relationships
- Having a financial interest in the home
- Satisfaction with the home
- Satisfaction with work
- Satisfaction with leisure time
- Satisfaction with services rendered (including case management)
- Individual wishes, dreams, hopes, aspirations, and ambitions
- Size of the home environment
- Human characteristics of the home environment (e.g., staffing)

- Physical quality of the home environment
- Individualized treatment in the home environment
- Normalization in the home
- Costs of the service/support elements
- Family/next friend opinions and satisfaction

Some of the data collection instruments and their reliability were described in the Pennhurst reports and subsequent documents (Conroy & Bradley, 1985; Devlin, 1989). Since that time, more detailed and rigorous reliability studies have been prepared (Conroy, 1995; Dodder, Foster, & Bolin, 1999; Fullerton, Douglass, & Dodder, 1999).

The PLQ is not entirely a static document. We continue to learn how to reliably measure new aspects of life that people tell us are important to them. Modifications made to the battery of instruments over the years have been based on the concept of "valued outcomes" (Conroy & Feinstein, 1990; Shea, 1992). Professionals may value some outcomes most highly, such as behavioral development; parents and other relatives may value permanence, safety, and comfort more highly; and people with intellectual disabilities may value having freedom, money, and friends most highly. The components of the PLQ that were included in the analyses for the present study are described in some detail next.

Choice Making (Power) The scale of choice making is called the Decision Control Inventory (DCI) (Conroy, 1998). It is composed of 35 ratings of the extent to which minor and major life decisions are made by paid staff versus the service recipient and/or unpaid friends and relatives. Each rating is given on an 11-point scale, where 0 means the choice is made entirely by paid staff/professionals, 10 means the choice is made entirely by the service recipient (and/or unpaid trusted others), and 5 means the choice is shared equally. This scale is the single most important one in the evaluation of self-determination impacts. It shows whether power has shifted away from paid workers and toward the person and his or her allies. The interrater reliability of the DCI was reported as .86 (Conroy, 1995). The item-by-item content of this scale is shown later in the chapter when mean scores for every item are listed (see Table 10.4 later in this chapter).

Integration The scale used to assess integration was taken from the Harris poll of Americans with and without disabilities (Taylor, Kagay, & Leichenko, 1986). It measured how often people visit with friends, go shopping, go to a place of worship, engage in recreation, and so forth in the presence of citizens without disabilities. If integration is composed of both presence and participation, then the Harris scale reflects only the first part. The scale simply counts the number of "outings" to places where citizens without disabilities might be present. The scale is restricted to the preceding month. Because the scale was developed by Harris and was used nationally with Americans with and without disabilities, we have national data for comparison.

Perceived Quality of Life Changes

The Quality of Life Changes Scale (Conroy, 2000) asks each person to rate his or her quality of life "a year ago" and "now." Ratings are given on 5-point Likert scales and cover 15 dimensions of quality. These dimensions include broad issues such as "happiness" and "health" as well as more specific matters such as "food" and "money." On this scale, we permit surrogates to respond. Surrogates (usually staff persons) were "whoever knew the class member best on a day-to-day basis." On this scale, approximately 85% of the responses are provided by surrogates. The interrater reliability of the Quality of Life Changes Scale was found to be .76. Over many years, we have been able to compare responses on this scale (e.g., "now" in 1998 compared to "now" in 2001). We also compared each year's *perceived* changes in quality (i.e., "then" as remembered, versus "now"). The two approaches have been found to produce highly consistent results.

Personal Interview

One of the central problems in measuring quality of life among people with developmental disabilities has been that many people cannot communicate with interviewers by traditional verbal, or by any nontraditional, means. Hence, many researchers have permitted surrogates to "speak for" the person. We reserve the Personal Interview of the PLQ as the one section in which no surrogates are permitted. This section is intended to capture the person's thoughts and no one else's.

The Personal Interview is primarily designed as 5-point scales, which can be asked as two either–or questions (e.g., "How is the food here? Good? Okay, would you say good, or very good?"). There are also open-ended items throughout the Personal Interview, and answers to these are written down verbatim for qualitative analysis (e.g., "What things are most important for you to be happy?" "If you had one wish, what would you wish for?").

Procedures for Data Collection

In all cases, the data collectors were trained by the Center for Outcome Analysis directly and on site. In each state, Center for Outcome Analysis representatives met directly with project coordinators—and often also with other stakeholders—to explain why the data would be so valuable, how they would be collected, and how they would be utilized later.

Our intent was simple: to visit and collect data face to face with as many participants as possible and as early in the self-determination project as possible. Then, after waiting as long as possible, we would collect data for the same people again (i.e., 1–3 years later) to see whether people's qualities of life, power, and individual planning and budgeting had changed. We would wait till the last possible minute to do the "post" data collection so that there would be the maximum time interval between the two visits. The more time, the more likely that significant effects could be detected.

In Michigan, the general data-collection procedures were augmented by the State Coordinator, who oversaw direct collection of individual expenditure data. Local coordinators were visited frequently, and tracking of individual budgets was mandated. The State Coordinator examined each budget, questioned incomplete data, and required completion of all information.

Participants

In 1998, the Center for Outcome Analysis trained dozens of local case managers to collect the PLQ data. When the initial efforts in the four pilot counties were completed, 786 people had been visited face to face. The entire PLQ package was completed for each.

Three years later, in 2001, a total of 329 people were visited, and the PLQ was collected. Not all of these 329 people were from the 786 baseline participants. Among these 329 people were 196 individuals for whom the Michigan State Coordinator was able to collect valid individual budget data. From the 196 people, there were 70 who had been included in the 1998 PLQ baseline and also in the 2001 follow-up PLQ round.

This chapter is centered on the outcomes for those 70 participants. Hence, the first question must be, "Are the 70 participants in any way different from the larger group of 329?" The following analyses show that these participants were not substantially different. Therefore, what was found for the 70 participants is probably generalizable to the 329 people visited.

For the continuous variables, there were no significant differences between the 70 participants and the remaining 259 people (see Table 10.1). On categorical variables, including gender, ethnicity, legal status, level of intellectual disability, and ambulation, none of the differences were signif-

Table 10.1. Mean personal characteristics of the study participants and the overall sample

Personal characteristic	Study participants n = 70	Remaining sample members n = 259	Significance of t-test
Age (years)	41.8	44.1	0.17
Adaptive Behavior Scale (0–100)	64.1	58.8	0.07
Challenging Behavior Scale (0–100)	93.0	90.1	0.06

Note: None of the significance tests reached the .01 criterion utilized in the present study. Thus, the subgroup of 70 participants appeared quite similar to the rest of the group of participants.

icant at the .01 level by the standard chi-square and phi coefficient tests. Again, the implication was that the results for the 70 would probably have held for the entire group of 329 Michigan participants in self-determination in the year 2001.

For the 70 participants, the average age was 42, with a range from 20 to 74 years. These participants were divided equally into males and females. Ninety percent of the participants characterized themselves as Caucasian. Eight percent labeled themselves African American, and two percent described themselves as other minorities. The levels of mental retardation reported by the participants are shown in Table 10.2.

RESULTS

As stated previously, a simple version of the theory of self-determination is "if people gain control, their lives will improve, and costs will not increase." Table 10.3 shows two measures of service recipients' opportunities to make choices and, therefore, gain control. Personal control included the service recipients' control as well as control by their freely chosen (usually unpaid) allies. The Decision Control Inventory was used as one index of shifting power. A third party who knew the service recipi-

Table 10.2. Participants' reported levels of intellectual disability

Level	Number	Percent
Profound	9	13%
Severe	10	14%
Moderate	14	20%
Mild	24	34%
None	6	9%
Unknown	7	10%
Total	**70**	

Table 10.3. Two measures of opportunities to make choices

Scale	Mean			Number of valid observations	Significance of t-test, 1-tailed
	1998	2001	Change		
Decision Control Inventory	59.79	73.64	13.85	67	0.0001
Personal Interview, choice-making scale	2.82	3.90	1.08	35	0.0000

ent very well usually answered or assisted the service recipient in answering the Decision Control Inventory. The other measure of choice making was the Personal Interview, which contained six items related to choice making, and these items were summed into one overall scale of directly self-reported choice opportunities.

The Decision Control Inventory total score was converted to a 0- to 100-point scale, and the Personal Interview, choice-making scale, varied over a 5-point range. In both cases, higher scores indicate less control by staff and greater control by the person and/or unpaid friends and relatives. For the Personal Interview, there were only 35 valid observations because many of the participants were not able or willing to engage in a verbal or other format interview.

Both of the indicators showed rather large increases in power and control over life decisions. To view more detail, the Decision Control Inventory was broken down into its 35 component items. Each of the 35 items was scored on a 0- to 10-point scale. Table 10.4 shows the items, their 1998 and 2001 means, the amount of change, and the t-test significance of each change. (These t-tests should be interpreted with caution because there were 35 tests, and some of them might have reached statistical significance by chance alone.) Based on the .01 significance level, 14 items showed significant change over time, with a trend toward change evident for a further 13 items ($p < .05$). In all cases except one (i.e., What clothes to wear on weekends), the change was in the direction of greater control by the person and/or unpaid friends and relatives. It was notable that the 8 items for which there was no significant change ($p > .05$) generally had high scores in 1998, indicating that the person and/or unpaid friends and relatives already exercised substantial control in that area prior to the self-determination intervention.

The data in Table 10.4 revealed that the largest changes were in major life areas. The five largest increases in power were in:

1. Hire and fire direct-support staff

2. Choice of agency support person

Table 10.4. Decision Control Inventory: Item-by-item means, sorted by magnitude of change

Choice dimension	Mean item score			Significance of t-test, 1-tailed
	1998	2001	Change	
Hire and fire direct-support staff	3.47	6.86	3.40	0.0000
Choice of agency support person	3.51	6.47	2.97	0.0000
Choice of people to live with	4.65	7.47	2.82	0.0000
Choice of house or apartment	4.89	7.52	2.63	0.0001
Choice of case manager	3.43	6.01	2.58	0.0001
Choice of which service agency works with you	3.00	5.43	2.43	0.0003
Choice of furnishings	5.03	7.22	2.18	0.0003
Type of work or day program	6.21	8.05	1.84	0.0026
When, where, and how to worship	6.79	8.62	1.83	0.0009
Type of transportation to and from day program or job	3.80	5.46	1.67	0.0099
Amount of time spent working or at day program	5.67	7.24	1.56	0.0149
Express affection, including sexual	7.14	8.66	1.52	0.0045
When to get up on weekends	7.25	8.63	1.38	0.0057
How to spend residential funds	3.79	5.14	1.35	0.0213
Who goes with you on outings	5.38	6.73	1.35	0.0068
Choice of places to go	6.06	7.34	1.28	0.0028
Minor vices	7.05	8.30	1.26	0.0162
What to have for dinner	5.49	6.71	1.22	0.0119
When to go to bed on weekdays	7.13	8.32	1.19	0.0115
How to spend day activity funds	5.49	6.68	1.19	0.0610
Choice to decline	7.69	8.87	1.18	0.0158
What to have for breakfast	5.78	6.95	1.17	0.0105
What to do with personal funds	6.36	7.49	1.13	0.0213
When to go to bed on weekends	7.40	8.53	1.13	0.0159
What foods to buy	4.87	5.94	1.07	0.0101
Choosing restaurants	6.60	7.58	0.98	0.0199
Taking naps in evenings	7.79	8.72	0.93	0.0355
Whether to have pet in the home	6.09	6.89	0.80	0.1171
What to do with relaxation time	8.00	8.75	0.75	0.0293
What clothes to buy	6.69	7.40	0.71	0.0559
Time and frequency of bath	5.91	6.59	0.68	0.0888
Who you hang out with	7.51	8.00	0.49	0.1888
What clothes to wear on weekdays	7.51	7.97	0.46	0.1714
Visiting with friends	6.97	7.38	0.41	0.2371
What clothes to wear on weekends	7.91	7.90	−0.01	0.4877

3. Choice of people to live with

4. Choice of house or apartment

5. Choice of case manager

Such major (service-related) decisions have consistently been found to be among the least available to people with intellectual disabilities (Heller, Miller, & Factor, 1999; Wehmeyer & Metzler, 1995). This fact supported an inference that the increased control experienced by the 70 participants and/or unpaid friends and relatives was far from trivial. Given that the fundamental nature of the service system had been changed, the fact that control of these service-related decisions also changed considerably is not surprising. Even so, confirming that the expected shifts in control of services have, in fact, taken place is fundamentally important.

After obtaining evidence that power has indeed shifted, the next principle of self-determination states that lives should "improve." This principle means that it should be possible to detect significant changes in quality-of-life indicators after control has been gained. Table 10.5 shows three of these quality-of-life measures: number of integrative outings per month as reported using the Harris scale (Taylor et al., 1986), the Quality of Life Changes Scale (Conroy, 2000) (which could be answered by surrogates), and the satisfaction scale gathered during the Personal Interview.

The number of integrative activities could range from 0 to any number of outings per month. The average increased from about 25 activities to about 35 activities per month. This scale reached statistical significance beyond the .01 level. The Quality of Life Changes Scale total score was converted to a 0- to 100-point scale. It increased from an average of 69 points to 81 points, and this increase was highly significant. The satisfaction scale from the Personal Interview was composed of a combination of seven items and could range from 1 to 5 points. The small increase of .25 points was significant beyond the .01 level. Together, these three kinds of indicators of life quality—number of integrative activities, a general quality-of-

Table 10.5.   Three measures of quality of life

Measure	Mean			Number of valid observations	Significance t-test, 1-tailed
	1998	2001	Change		
Integrative outings per month	25.28	34.90	9.61	67	0.0038
Quality of Life Changes Scale	68.71	80.65	11.94	64	0.0000
Personal Interview, satisfaction scale	3.68	3.94	0.25	38	0.0037

life scale, and direct self-report—all tended to support the notion that people's lives had improved markedly.

To provide more detail on the kinds of qualities of life that were perceived to have improved, the Quality of Life Changes Scale was broken down into its 15 dimensions. Each item was rated on a scale of 1 (very bad) to 5 (very good) points. Table 10.6 shows means and the changes, sorted by magnitude, from 1998 to 2001.

The three largest observed changes were in happiness, getting out, and overall quality of life, and all were significant at $p < .01$ or better. Health, which had the smallest observed change, appeared to have been unchanged. Once again, the t-test results should be used only as a general index of the strength of the change. Because there were 15 tests, some might have reached statistical significance by chance alone.

The third principle of the operational definition of self-determination is that public costs should not increase when service recipients (and their allies) obtain control over resources. This principle was tested by collecting baseline costs of traditional services and supports in 1998, then comparing those figures to the individual budgets service recipients were using in 2001. These figures were not adjusted for inflation. The results of this analysis were straightforward and are shown in Table 10.7. The total (unadjusted) public dollars expended to support the 70 people decreased, on the average, by about 8%. The correlation between 1998 costs and 2001 costs was .90,

Table 10.6. Changes on the Quality of Life Changes Scale

Quality of Life Changes Scale dimension	Mean			Significance of t-test, 1-tailed
	1998	2001	Change	
Happiness	2.58	3.31	0.72	0.0000
Getting out	2.52	3.20	0.68	0.0000
Overall quality of life	2.76	3.42	0.66	0.0000
Socializing	2.49	3.08	0.59	0.0005
Privacy	2.80	3.34	0.55	0.0000
Food	2.92	3.41	0.48	0.0000
Treatment by staff/attendants	3.00	3.48	0.48	0.0004
What I do all day	2.58	3.03	0.45	0.0020
Comfort	2.83	3.28	0.45	0.0023
Money	3.61	4.05	0.44	0.0090
Run own life	2.67	3.10	0.43	0.0023
Family relationships	2.44	2.85	0.41	0.0285
Safety	2.98	3.37	0.38	0.0039
Health care	3.02	3.33	0.31	0.0028
Health	2.94	3.06	0.12	0.1906

Table 10.7. Change in public costs

	Mean public costs			Significance of t-test, 1-tailed	Percent change
	1998	2001	Change		
Unadjusted	$61,788	$56,778	−$5,010	0.0047	−8%
Adjusted for inflation, using 2001 dollars	$67,322	$56,778	−$10,545	0.0010	−16%

which suggested that these costs were not wildly or randomly varying, but rather were being influenced in some relatively uniform way.

Table 10.7 also provides the same data adjusted for inflation according to the Consumer Price Index. From 1998 to 2001, prices increased approximately 8.96%. By adjusting the 1998 cost upward by that percentage, we obtained another kind of comparison of baseline traditional to 2001 self-determination costs. This figure was more dramatic, at about a 16% reduction.

Costs tended to decrease the most among people who started out with initially high traditional levels of expenditure. This change was shown both by the simple correlation coefficient between the initial cost and the decrease in cost, which was −.39 ($p < .001$), and more graphically, by the scatterplot of initial costs by cost reductions. Figure 10.1 shows a notice-

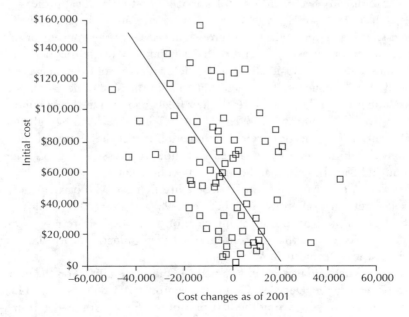

Figure 10.1. Scatterplot of initial cost (1998) by cost changes as of 2001 (unadjusted for inflation).

able tendency for the points to cluster around a line going from the top left to the bottom right. The line of best fit has been inserted into the graph to illustrate this general trend. This trend should be interpreted as a tendency for the people with high initial costs (i.e., the people at the upper left portion of the graph) to show greater cost savings.

The graph also shows something of equal or possibly greater importance: For some of the participants, costs went up. This increase was also observed in the New Hampshire demonstration (Conroy et al., in review). The implication is that individual budgeting within self-determination need not be tied to individual "caps" on expenditures. Rather, the person-centered budget-planning process in Michigan was (and some would argue should be) set according to individual needs. It stands to reason that, in a complex and flawed traditional service system, some people might currently be underserved. Therefore, costs should be permitted to increase if necessary. The *average* cost may stay the same or decrease in the self-determination paradigm.

DISCUSSION

Power and control in the lives of people with developmental disabilities has traditionally been held by professionals—first by medical professionals, and more recently by generic human service professionals, as well as paid staff under the guidance of professionals. Until the concept of self-determination, service recipients with developmental disabilities (and their families and other unpaid allies) had little or no control over their everyday lives. The concept of self-determination in the field of developmental disabilities is simple: If people (and their freely chosen allies) gain control, their lives will improve, and costs will not increase. Another element inherent in the concept of self-determination is that the service-planning teams should be deprofessionalized and should increase the involvement of unpaid friends, family, and community volunteers.

Data were analyzed from 70 people in Michigan who participated in a self-determination project with before (1998) and after (2001) quality-of-life data *and* individual budget information in 2001. The results of this study showed clearly that the concept of self-determination worked well in demonstration projects in Michigan.

The Michigan participants gained 14 points ($p < .0001$) on the measure of power, the Decision Control Inventory (100-point scale). Thus, power did shift, supporting the first part of the theory of self-determination. The Michigan participants also gained 12 points ($p < .0001$) on the

Quality of Life Changes Scale (also computed on a 100-point scale). Interviews with the participants themselves (i.e., those who had the ability and willingness to communicate directly) also revealed greater satisfaction with the participants' lives ($p < .01$), thus providing important firsthand corroboration of the findings just discussed. In addition, a 38% increase existed in socially integrated community activities ($p < .01$). Regardless of the source of the information, or the aspect of life quality evaluated, a consistent pattern emerged of improved quality of life following the introduction of self-determination.

The control gained by individuals involved three main aspects of life. First, some individuals moved from settings that were licensed and regulated to supported independence. Second, individuals were supported and allowed to incorporate more allies into their lives. Allies were freely selected family members and friends. Third, with the support of these allies, individuals were expected to make decisions about the facets of their lives that mattered most to them. These included their jobs and other day activities, as well as other major aspects of how public funds were used. The indicators in the Decision Control Inventory were aimed at specifying and capturing these dimensions of living.

The change in control over service-related choices is a central intended outcome for arrangements that support self-determination. In Michigan, the goal of the Self-Determination Initiative, from a systems-change standpoint, was to infuse values and promote specific methodologies within the local sites that could afford individuals the power and authority to make service-related choices. True person-centered planning objectives were derived from individuals' preferences about which aspects of services they would use. For example, professional interventions were selected by the participants, and the emphasis during the planning process was to provide that service in a manner specifically preferred by the individual. In addition, individuals were able to change provider organizations within their local service system and to control the choice of personnel actually providing their services. Some individuals had specific contractual clauses with provider organizations that required the organization to support and promote choice of staff. Other people actually became the direct employer of their personal assistant support staff. This opportunity to gain and effect direct control over service-delivery staff was deemed to be crucial in the design and implementation phases of work in all local sites and across the involved parties (professionals, services managers, family members, and individuals themselves).

The study also found that unadjusted costs *decreased* for the Michigan participants by an average of $5,010, or about 8%. When adjusted for inflation, this amount became 16%. Some people's costs went up, though these individuals tended to have lower previous costs. This finding may indicate that a number of service recipients with lower 1998 costs under traditional service-provision arrangements were underserved. Analysis also revealed that people who started with the highest costs tended to have the largest percentage decrease in costs through self-determination.

These findings were quite consistent with the results from the original Robert Wood Johnson Foundation's demonstration grant in New Hampshire (Conroy et al., in review) but were generally of greater magnitude. For example, the power shift in New Hampshire had been about 4%, but in Michigan it was 14%. What had been learned from the original efforts in New Hampshire may have informed and accelerated the outcomes in Michigan.

Individual budget determination was based on working through very specific scenarios about the composition, delivery process, and frequency of planned services. Local sites oriented care managers (Supports Coordinators) to conduct planning toward individual budgets using a target amount of funds that was a percentage of, but less than, the calculated costs of previous service arrangements. Regulations precluded applying a predetermined cap on the budget amount, as regulations required plans to be responsive to actual service needs. However, the mix of services and the determination of the amount and frequency of specific services making up a person's plan and budget were affected by how that mix calculated in comparison with the budget target amount.

Use of a target during the planning process was viewed as a major factor in arriving at individual budget amounts that ended up being less (in most but not all cases) than the previous cost of traditional services. The use of a budget target in the planning process also appeared to provide an incentive for conducting a critical examination of planned services and to achieve, in some cases, a more creative approach to providing support at a lower cost. This value-added aspect was crucial to satisfaction both for the consumer involved and for the local sites that participated. It also has much to do with whether the expansion of self-determination as a growing piece of public policy can be supported in the Michigan Public Mental Health System.

The components of reduction of services costs can only be speculated on because this study did not involve a detailed breakdown of each participant's budget; however, anecdotal information suggested several factors. First, individuals were not required by outside parties (i.e., professionals, care planners, and provider agencies) to accept unwanted services. Second, because individuals more directly decided how their service delivery would occur, they chose service and support arrangements that more exactly fit their needs and preferences. For example, individuals could make more independent decisions about when and whether paid staff were in their life and for what purposes. Some participants reportedly expressed relief that they could control their privacy and decide when they did not want anyone with them.

Third, individuals could negotiate prices with providers and shop for lower rates. In some reported instances, the process of negotiation was interlaced with the planning process, so prices were known prior to finalizing the plan and budget. Fourth, by eliminating the middle-man elements of using a provider agency, and instead directly employing personal assistant staff, budgeted costs per service hour could be reduced. Some of the local sites actually produced financial models that could document this, even when the costs of a fiscal intermediary service were included. Costs of staff supervision, administrative costs, and provider profit/overhead that are inherent in an agency-provided support model were gone. In some cases, participants were able to plan toward an increase of the hourly wages for staff, while maintaining overall hourly costs at or below previous gross hourly costs.

These findings from one state's self-determination initiative cannot automatically be generalized to other very different service-delivery systems in other states. It is true that very similar findings have been reported from nine other states' demonstration projects (Conroy, Fullerton, Brown, & Garrow, 2002). This fact would lend support to the notion that shifting control of resources toward people and their allies can occur in any system, and when it does, qualities of life improve, and average costs do not increase. Still, it must be acknowledged that the analyses presented here did not include a control or comparison group, which would have lent greater scientific certainty to the work. Nonparticipants were included in the Michigan data collection process, and their outcomes could be analyzed separately in a later study. The study done in California did include a comparison group of nonparticipants, and the results there were very consistent with the Michigan data (Conroy, Brown, Fullerton, Beamer, Garrow, & Boisot, 2002).

This circumstance would appear to be a "win-win" situation in public policy; however, to implement and/or expand such approaches requires either belief in the research or faith in service recipients and their allies to be inherently fiscally conservative. All of the available data thus far (including the newly emerging studies of Cash & Counseling demonstrations[2]) tend to support either belief structure. This new knowledge may lend support to ongoing efforts to alter the face of Medicaid, which is by nature a system of provider payment.

CONCLUSION

The human service system in America is moving toward the idea of self-determination in all areas of service delivery. Trends in many fields, notably developmental disabilities and aging (via the Cash & Counseling demonstrations), support this movement toward service recipients and their allies having direct control over the money used to support them, as well as the types of service and assistance they can purchase with that money. The results in Michigan show not only that self-determination is a fiscally conservative approach to service delivery but also that participants in self-determination perceive themselves as having more choice, less professional domination, and higher overall quality in their lives.

A more in-depth study would provide further information concerning the extent to which individuals have made life changes over time as a direct result of the opportunity to control and direct funds allotted for their services and supports. In Michigan, all anecdotal information to date has suggested that service recipients, their families, and their allies all highly valued the opportunity to participate in arrangements that support self-determination. This support has resulted in an expanded emphasis on policy development in this direction. To date, Michigan has continued to expand access to self-determination by promulgating a Self-Determination Policy & Practice Guideline. This policy has become a requirement in all contracts between the State and its local CMHSPs. Central to the policy is the promise that adult service recipients may initiate access to arrangements that support self-determination by requesting the opportunity to develop a plan of services and an individual budget. Once agreed to by the CMHSP, this results in the person's individual budget being authorized. This individual budget may be applied by the person to control and direct the delivery of his or her services from directly chosen, preferred providers. This policy applies to individuals with mental illness as well as individuals with developmental disabilities. Many service recipients are eager to begin working in this new paradigm. Working within a Medicaid environment, this new way of thinking and delivering supports is by no means easy, but the enthusiasm appears to be as powerful as the evidence.

---

[2]See the Cash & Counseling web site at http://www.hhp.umd.edu/AGING/CCDemo/

REFERENCES

Conroy, J. (1995). *Reliability of the personal life quality protocol: Report number 7 of the 5-year Coffelt Quality Tracking Project*. Submitted to the California Department of Developmental Services and California Protection and Advocacy. (Available from the Center for Outcome Analysis, Ardmore, PA)

Conroy, J. (1998). *The Decision Control Inventory*. Ardmore, PA: Center for Outcome Analysis.

Conroy, J. (2000). *Quality of Life Changes Scale*. Ardmore, PA: Center for Outcome Analysis.

Conroy, J., & Bradley, V. (1985). *The Pennhurst Longitudinal Study: A report of five years of research and analysis*. Philadelphia: Temple University Developmental Disabilities Center.

Conroy, J., Brown, M., Fullerton, A., Beamer, S., Garrow, J., & Boisot, T. (2002, March). *Independent evaluation of California's Self-Determination Pilot Projects: Final report*. Submitted to Eastern Los Angeles Regional Center and California Department of Developmental Services. (Available from the Center for Outcome Analysis, Ardmore, PA)

Conroy, J., & Feinstein, C. (1990). Measuring quality of life: Where have we been, where are we going? In R. Schalock & M. Begab (Eds.), *Quality of life: Perspectives and issues*. Monograph Number 12. Washington, DC: American Association on Mental Retardation.

Conroy, J., Fullerton, A., Brown, M., & Garrow, J. (2002, December). *Outcomes of the Robert Wood Johnson Foundation's National Initiative on Self-Determination for Persons with Developmental Disabilities: Final report on 3 years of research and analysis*. Submitted to the Robert Wood Johnson Foundation as the impact assessment of the Foundation's national initiative entitled Self-Determination for Persons with Developmental Disabilities. (Available from the Center for Outcome Analysis, Ardmore, PA)

Conroy, J., Yuskauskas, A., & Spreat, S. (in review). Outcomes of self-determination in New Hampshire. *Journal of The Association for Persons with Severe Handicaps*.

Developmental Disabilities Assistance and Bill of Rights Act Amendments of 1987, PL 100-146, 42 U.S.C. §§6000 *et seq.*

Devlin, S. (1989). *Reliability assessment of the instruments used to monitor the Pennhurst class members*. Philadelphia: Temple University Developmental Disabilities Center.

Dodder, R., Foster, L., & Bolin, B. (1999). Measures to monitor developmental disabilities quality assurance: A study of reliability. *Education and Training in Mental Retardation and Developmental Disabilities, 34*(1), 66–76.

Fullerton, A. Douglass, M., & Dodder, R. (1999). A reliability study of measures assessing the impact of deinstitutionalization. *Research in Developmental Disabilities, 20*(6), 387–400.

Heller, T., Miller, A.B., & Factor, A. (1999). Autonomy in residential facilities and community functioning of adults with mental retardation. *Mental Retardation, 37*, 449–457.

Nerney, T., Crowley, R., & Kappel, B. (1995). *An affirmation of community: A revolution of vision and goals. Creating a community to support all people including those with disabilities*. Durham: University of New Hampshire Institute on Disability.

Nerney, T., & Shumway, D. (1996). *Beyond managed care: Self-determination for people with disabilities* (1st ed.). Available from the authors at University of New Hampshire, Institute on Disability, Durham.

Shea, J.R. (1992). From standards to compliance, to good services, to quality lives: Is this how it works? *Mental Retardation, 30,* 143–149.

Taylor, H., Kagay, M., & Leichenko, S. (1986). *The ICD survey of disabled Americans: Bringing disabled Americans into the mainstream.* New York: Louis Harris and Associates.

Wehmeyer, M.L., & Metzler, C.A. (1995). How self-determined are people with mental retardation? The national consumer survey. *Mental Retardation, 33,* 111–119.

CHAPTER 11

Individual Budgets According to Individual Needs

The Wyoming DOORS System

*Jon R. Fortune, Gary A. Smith, Edward M. Campbell,
Robert T. Clabby, II, Kenneth B. Heinlein, Robert M. Lynch,
and Jerry Allen*

Wyoming has pioneered an individual budget model for people with intellectual disabilities who receive services and supports through the state's Medicaid Home and Community-Based Services (HCBS) Waiver programs for adults and children. The DOORS individual budget model allocates dollars to each individual by objectively taking into account each person's support needs. More broadly, this model is the cornerstone of Wyoming's "person-centered system architecture" that positions each individual and his or her team to decide what services will best meet the person's needs and to freely select service providers. This chapter describes the origins, development, implementation, and refinement of the DOORS budget allocation model. The model's outcomes and its implications for people supported in Wyoming and their families, service providers, and the state's developmental disabilities service system are also discussed.

PERSON-CENTERED SYSTEM ARCHITECTURE

The principles of person-centered supports are displacing old service paradigms. These principles call for tailoring services and supports to each individual's needs and aspirations. The principles extend beyond allowing individuals and their allies to make "choices" to giving them the authority to make fundamental decisions about their lives in the community, including how, where, and by whom they will be supported (National

Association of State Directors of Developmental Disabilities Services [NASDDDS], 2000).

In many states, the widespread adoption of the principles of person-centered supports has been stymied by the existing "system architecture"—namely, the constellation of state policies that govern service and spending authorization processes, paying and contracting for services, and support coordination. System architecture has a profound impact on the provision of services and supports. Efforts to promote person-centered supports frequently are thwarted by serious defects in system architecture. For example, funding often is locked into provider agencies or service categories rather than tied directly to each individual. This practice undermines the principle that the person's support plan should drive how dollars are deployed instead of being made to fit what is available. Furthermore, state contracting policies can severely limit choice concerning the sources of paid supports because individuals and families are confined to obtaining services from a few specialized disabilities agencies.

More and more, states are realizing that their system architecture inhibits rather than promotes person-centered supports. Oftentimes, furnishing person-centered supports means having to work around existing policies in cat-and-mouse fashion. Or a state resorts to launching a special initiative aimed at overcoming the obstacles to person-centered supports posed by its own policies and practices.

In order to expand person-centered supports systemwide, states must adopt a new opportunity-enhancing "business model" that: 1) attaches funding in the form of an individual budget to each individual; 2) gives individuals, their families, and their allies the authority to select the services and supports that reflect the person's priorities; 3) affirms uninhibited free selection of service providers; and 4) employs open (rather than slot-based) contracting to foster a marketplace that encourages the free entry of providers. Under this business model, the service recipient's own plan drives the system, not vice versa. Adopting this business model requires that states make fundamental changes to their system architecture.

A major challenge that confronts a state in shifting to a "person-centered system architecture" is developing a solid approach to establishing individual budgets that is fair and equitable. The Wyoming DOORS individual budget model has played a linchpin role in the state's adoption of a person-centered system architecture (Smith, Taub, Heaviland, Bradley, & Cheek, 2001).

EVOLUTION OF WYOMING'S DEVELOPMENTAL DISABILITIES SERVICE SYSTEM

Before 1990, Wyoming's community service system for people with intellectual disabilities (especially adults) was extremely limited in its scope. Most state dollars were earmarked for services at the Wyoming State Training School (WSTS) in Lander, the state's only public institution. Only 200 individuals received state-reimbursed community residential services before 1990. Wyoming stood alone among the states in not using federal Medicaid dollars to underwrite the costs of long-term services and supports for people with intellectual disabilities.

As a result of the 1990 *Weston* lawsuit (*Weston et al. v. Wyoming State Training School et al.*, 1990), state officials agreed to: 1) arrange for community services for WSTS residents who could be appropriately served in the community; 2) obtain intermediate care facilities for people with mental retardation (ICF/MR) certification of WSTS in order to improve conditions there; and 3) expand and enhance the quality and availability of community services and supports. With the strong support of state policy makers, Wyoming moved quickly to downsize WSTS and scale up community services.

To finance the expansion of Wyoming's community service system, the Wyoming Developmental Disabilities Division (DDD) turned to the HCBS Waiver program. In 1991, Wyoming launched a HCBS Waiver program for adults with intellectual disabilities. In 1992, the state started a second HCBS Waiver program for children and youth (until age 21) with intellectual disabilities. Since their beginning, both HCBS Waiver programs have played a vital role in underwriting the community placement of children and adults from WSTS as well as expanding community services for other citizens with intellectual disabilities. Wyoming opted to employ the HCBS Waiver program to finance community services because the program enabled the state to offer a wide, flexible range of services and supports.

Between 1990 and 2002, Wyoming's total spending for intellectual disabilities services almost quadrupled, growing from approximately $30.0 million to $114.4 million. Between 1988 and early 2003, the number of WSTS residents dropped from 374 to 92 (Heinlein & Fortune, 1995). In 2002, 987 individuals participated in the adult HCBS Waiver program at an annual cost of $45.3 million; the children's HCBS Waiver program supported 520 children at a cost of $8.4 million. Wyoming supported more individuals relative to state population through its HCBS Waiver programs than most other states. In 2000, Wyoming ranked 6th among the states in its fiscal effort to support people with intellectual disabilities (Braddock, Hemp, Parish, & Rizzolo, 2000). In addition, Wyoming had an especially vibrant early intervention program. Wyoming's system is vastly different today than it was in 1990 (Fortune, Heinlein, & Fortune, 1995; Smith et al., 2001). The system is firmly rooted in and financially committed to supporting individuals in communities.

MANAGING MONEY IN WYOMING BEFORE DOORS

Employing Medicaid funding to pay for community services required that Wyoming change how it managed community funding. New payment systems had to be implemented. Prior to the development of the DOORS individual budget model, Wyoming managed community funding by employing conventional rate schedules, overall cost caps, and ad-hoc negotiation with provider agencies. Although Wyoming's strategies did not differ appreciably from those in other states, the results were not completely satisfactory. In order to control spending, DDD found itself micromanaging the service system from Cheyenne, Wyoming, by performing close review and approval of participants' service plans to ensure cost effectiveness. This practice, however, was fundamentally at odds with the essential principle that the individual's planning team should have the primary responsibility and authority to develop and manage the person's plan, including selecting the services and strategies that would best meet the individual's needs.

During the early 1990s, when Wyoming was building out its community system, the state followed the practice of negotiating payment rates for community services provider by provider. However, problems with the approach soon emerged. Expenditures started to rise sharply. Ad-hoc negotiation led to variations in payments from provider to provider and individual to individual. In 1995, when faced with climbing HCBS Waiver individual plan of care funding requests, DDD decided to adopt a "level payment" system, modeled after Utah's approach (Wrigley, 1992). Utah had linked its payments for community services to "service scores" derived from the administration of the Inventory for Client and Agency Planning (ICAP) (Bruininks, Hill, Weatherman, & Woodcock, 1986). ICAP service scores range from 1 (total personal care and intense supervision) to 100 (infrequent or no assistance for daily living) and are based on a weighted combination of ICAP adaptive and challenging behavior scores. Utah's approach established five payment levels, with payments for services scaling up based on the intensity of ICAP-measured support needs.

Wyoming dropped its negotiated provider rates and adapted Utah's method. The goal was to substitute a more objective method of determining funding amounts that would be keyed to measured individual service need and, hence, would yield greater consistency in funding decisions across providers and individuals. Many other states have adopted an approach broadly similar to this method, using either the ICAP or another assessment tool of their own design (Arizona Department of Economic Security, 2002).

As can be seen in Table 11.1, this early Wyoming model linked ICAP scores to fixed staffing ratios. Based on the staffing ratios, daily rates were calculated for residential and day services. Payment rates for individuals with the most significant challenges (i.e., ICAP range 1–19) were twice as high as rates for people in the next tier and five times greater than the lowest tier.

This reimbursement model was reviewed by a Federal court and deemed reasonable and fair; however, many stakeholders felt that this approach was too crude and arbitrary. Small differences in ICAP scores could result in major differences in the money available to support service recipients. This approach also caused DDD to continue to be entangled in negotiations about the content of service plans when the plans' costs fell outside the fixed amount, thereby undermining the principle that decisions about services should be made by planning teams rather than managed from afar. Five levels of funding proved not to work well. The need for a new, more individualized model quickly became evident.

Table 11.1. Early Wyoming adult Home and Community-Based Services (HCBS) Waiver habilitation guidelines (1995)

ICAP Service Score range	Daily rate	Staff ratio
Residential habilitation guidelines		
1–19	$165.00	1:1
20–39	$82.00	1:2
40–59	$55.00	1:3
60–79	$41.00	1:4
80–100	$33.00	1:5 or more
Day habilitation guidelines		
1–19	$110.00	1:1
20–39	$55.00	1:2
40–59	$36.00	1:3
60–79	$27.00	1:4
80–100	$22.00	1:5 or more

Note: Special supports by arrangement through State Level of Care Committee. Rates may be modified as necessary to meet the needs of the people served.

THE NEW MODEL

The development of the new DOORS individual budget model was anchored by five core principles:

1. Individual needs take priority over those of the providers, agencies, or groups.

2. Individuals with greater needs should have access to more resources; those with lesser needs should receive less.

3. No two people have the same needs, supports, and priorities.

4. Individuals and their teams—not the state or federal government—know best what services are most important for the person.

5. People should choose providers, not the other way around.

In other words, the new funding system would be keyed to individual need rather than broad groupings of people as previously. It would assign an individual budget allocation to each person. Individuals and their teams would decide the services that would be purchased with these dollars. Funding would not be tied to specific providers so that individuals and their teams would be in a position to select the providers that they would use. In addition, dollars would be "portable"—a person's changing his or her services or selecting a new provider would not affect funding. Lastly, the hope for the new system was that it would at last extricate DDD from intervening in planning team decisions about services that people received.

With these principles in mind, in 1998, Wyoming revamped its method for determining budget limits for people supported through the HCBS Waiver program. The goal was to make these limits as sensitive as possible to objectively measured individual needs and observed costs and to minimize appeals concerning funding amounts (Smith, 1999). The aim was not to reduce overall funding systemwide but instead to make sure that money is distributed equitably and fairly based on measured needs.

BROAD DESIGN OF DOORS

The DOORS individual budget model is designed to establish an overall individual budget amount (IBA) for each person. The model is *not* a provider rate-setting tool. Within this budget amount, teams have free rein in designing the best mix of services. The budget amount is not influenced by which organization(s) or individual(s) currently serve or would serve the person. The IBA is calculated the same way for all individuals (distinguishing only between adults and children), including individuals presently receiving services and people new to the service system. Funding requirements also can be figured for people waiting for services, a facet of the model that has proven very useful in securing additional funding to serve such individuals.

The DOORS individual budget model ties IBAs principally to information about each individual that is extracted from the ICAP but includes other information as well. The model, however, differs substantially from most other systems that key funding to assessment results. Instead of grouping individuals by broad ICAP service need scores (as Wyoming previously had done), the model generates person-by-person budget amounts.

The DOORS model mathematically describes the relationship between observed costs and factors that, from a policy perspective, affect costs. In Wyoming, the policy perspective adopted was that funding should be tied principally to indicators of individual need rather than linked to provider characteristics or service modalities. The aim was to develop a model that essentially would reduce or eliminate funding disparities among individuals that had arisen over the years by keying budgets to a common set of objective factors. The current distribution of resources among HCBS Waiver participants was reasoned to reflect rational decisions and the needs of each individual. Although decision making was carried out more or less consistently over the years, variance had crept into resource allocations. Similarly-situated individuals received different resource allocations. If IBAs were to be determined in an evenhanded fashion, this variance would need to be reduced or removed.

TECHNICAL ELEMENTS OF THE MODEL

In order to develop the model, statistical methods developed by Campbell and Heal (1995) and Rhoades and Altman (2001) were chosen. These studies, reinforced by Lewis and Bruininks (1994), clearly supported the fundamental precept that variations in the costs of community services can be explained by underlying differences in individual support needs and other quantifiable factors.

In a nutshell, the DOORS model treats the IBAs resulting from the previous reimbursement scheme as the dependent variable. Factors that, from a policy perspective, are deemed to be the principal determinants of costs are treated as independent variables. Stepwise, multiple regression methods are employed to identify the extent to which each of these factors explains differences in costs person to person. The model seeks out the factors that contribute the most to explaining observed variance in costs and discards those that do not appear to influence costs. In the end, the model identifies the mix and weight of variables that best fits the array of observed costs across all individuals receiving services. Inserting the values for each variable into the model yields the person's IBA. Individuals with different characteristics and in different situations will have different IBAs.

There are several factors considered as independent variables in the DOORS model. The HCBS services previously authorized for each person are included. Including these services affirms that existing service plans address legitimate needs of program participants. Individual characteristics of each person as measured by and recorded in the ICAP were also included. Here, the aim is to take into account the characteristics that have been found to covary with costs.

Initially, economic factors were included in the model. Such factors included the costs of serving an individual living in one town versus another (e.g., "cost of doing business") and provider characteristics that, from an efficiency standpoint, seemed likely to have a bearing on costs. However, as a matter of policy, these factors were removed from subsequent iterations of the models in order to avoid linking IBAs to specific providers so that IBAs would not change when individuals selected different providers. Decoupling the IBA from specific providers was necessary in order to affirm free choice of provider.

Many factors were not included in the model. In particular, while the broad types of services that a person receives are included, their exact location, type, and intensity are not. The model solely reflects that a person is receiving residential supports, day supports, or other specified types of services. This practice permits planning teams to change support strategies without such changes triggering a change in the IBA. The model contains no adjustment for the individual's using different providers.

Separate DOORS adults' and children's models have been developed. In the first iteration, 25 variables were included. Variables were removed when they did not contribute significantly to forecasting an IBA. The statistical methods used permitted keeping a large number of variables in play in order to continuously weigh the effects of including or excluding one or several variables. This methodology permits the identification of variables that would contribute the most to the regression model. The current adult model contains 22 predictor variables, including 15 items from the ICAP. The regression equations weight each of these variables. The current model explains 75% (i.e., $R^2 = .75$) of the variance in previous reimbursement amounts. A comparison of the provider reimbursement system in 1997 and after the implementation of the current adult HCBS DOORS model is illustrated in Figure 11.1.

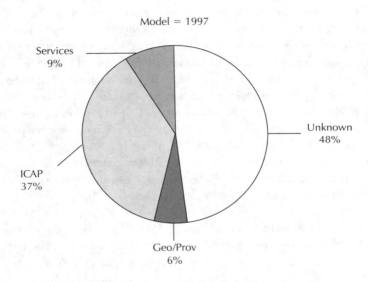

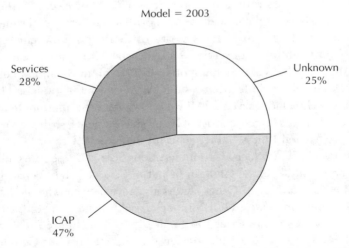

Figure 11.1. Explained variance before the first 1998 DOORS model and after implementation of the 2003 DOORS model. Geo/Prov = geographic economic conditions and providers' efficiencies; ICAP = Inventory for Client and Agency Planning.

As can be seen in the figure, prior to DOORS (when Wyoming was using the "level payment" system described in Table 11.1), about one half of the variance in the reimbursement amounts arose from unknown factors. In other words, rates varied for reasons that were not explainable by differences among individuals in their support needs, by the services they received, or by the day or living-service environments in which they were received. Differences in individual characteristics measured by the ICAP explained only 37% of the variance in rates. Geographic economic conditions, such as the unemployment rates of counties, and providers' efficiencies, such as the economies of scale (measured by the total number of people served by a community provider), were taken into account in the first DOORS model. These types of measures helped explain variance but were abandoned because they interfered with the choice of a service provider by the service recipient. With DOORS, there is a much tighter fit between the dependent variable and individual characteristics/current environments. In 2003, a total of 75% of variance can be explained: 47% by the ICAP measures and 28% by the services/supports provided by Wyoming's Adult HCBS Waiver program.

In both the adults' and children's DOORS models, the best statistical fit is achieved between individual budget allocations and the factors that state officials elected to include in the model. The DOORS models do not identify the causes of cost differences among individuals but instead identify variables that co-vary with these differences. As statisticians are quick to note, "Correlation does not imply causality." For example, the ICAP factors employed in the model are not portrayed as "true" determinants of costs but serve as proxies for severity of disability. Different severities require different mixes of services and, thereby, different costs.

Although the ICAP is an important source of information in developing each model, the influence of the ICAP varies in the models. The children's model includes seven ICAP factors whereas the adult model has 15. The ICAP factors largely consist of ICAP sub-elements, such as "Diagnosis of Severe Mental Illness," "Frequency of Seizures," "Use of Psychotropic Medication," "ICAP Social Communications Score," "Does the Child Live with the Family," "Is the Child in or out of School," and "What Services Do They Use or Need." Other factors also vary between the models.

The current *adult* DOORS model variables and their estimated impact on the IBA are described in Figure 11.2. This figure shows a completed example of IBA calculation for a hypothetical adult. Computation starts with a base amount (4.39005) that is then adjusted up or down depending on the person's individual characteristics and services received.

Column A	Column B	Column C	Column D	Column E
Predictor variable	Parameter estimate	Variable value	B x C	Estimated range of fiscal impact
Base amount (intercept)	4.39005	1	4.39005	
ICAP measures				
ICAP Broad Independence	−0.00279495	404	−1.1291598	$7,487
ICAP General Maladaptive	−0.004806757	−12	0.057681084	$1,887
Age	−0.02205103	32	−0.070563296	$1,124
Diagnosis = autism?	0.088635	0	0	$881
Diagnosis = brain/ neurological damage?	0.045409	0	0	$425
Diagnosis = chemical dependency?	0.11922	0	0	$1,230
Diagnosis = deafness?	0.12074	0	0	$1,248
Level of mental retardation	0.030344	3	0.091032	$1,131
Psychotropic medications?	0.071711	0	0	$653
Lives with family?	−0.14618	0	0	$1,200
Lives independently?	−0.25273	0	0	$1,757
Independent with monitoring?	−0.078247	0	0	$663
Sheltered workshop?	−0.056035	0	0	$489
Supported employment?	−0.092672	0	0	$779
Competitive employment?	−0.14002	0	0	$1,107
Home and community-based services received				
Residential services?	0.24897	1	0.24897	$1,926
Day habilitation?	0.10444	1	0.10444	$878
Nursing?	0.10268	0	0	$943
Personal care?	0.1309	0	0	$1,420
Psychological services?	0.083741	1	0.083741	$800
Second assessment?	0.03118	0	0	$284
In-home services?	0.066377	0	0	$637
Sum: predicted Log₁₀ monthy rate			3.776190988	
Predicted monthly rate	(10 to the	power)	$5,972.98	
Log-adjusted monthly rate (x 1.06096928517)			$6,337.15	
Inflation adjustment (6%)			$6,717.38	

Figure 11.2. Worked example of individual budget amount (IBA) calculation for a hypothetical adult and the estimated range of fiscal impacts. Predictors with a question mark (?) are binary measures (i.e., 1 = yes, 0 = no).

Predictor Variables

The predictor variables are listed in Column A in Figure 11.2, with the ICAP measures in the top half of the column and the home and community-based services provided at the bottom of the column. Variable names ending with a question mark (?) are binary measures (i.e., 1 = yes, 0 = no). Residential and day habilitation services are listed in the bottom (i.e., home and community-based services received) group; however, *where* these services are provided (e.g., lives with family, sheltered workshop) can be found under the "ICAP measures" heading. Day habilitation services may be received in a facility-based setting (i.e., day activity center, work activity center, or sheltered workshop), or in more integrated settings (i.e., supported employment or competitive employment—with minimum supports).

The person whose IBA is presented in Figure 11.2 is receiving day habilitation services under the HCBS Waiver program (note the value of "1" in Column C for this variable). These services, however, are not received in competitive or supported employment setting, nor in a sheltered (> 25% of minimum wage) workshop—all those settings have a "0" in Column C. Therefore, the person is receiving services in either a day or a work activity center (wages, if any, < 25% of minimum wage). These are the only community settings left in which day habilitation is provided.

These two settings become the "reference category" for the three that *are* included in the model. In other words, no amount is deducted from the IBA of an individual serviced in these two settings. If the individual's setting were "upgraded" to sheltered workshop, then .056 (about $486) would be deducted from the individual's monthly rate. If the individual were in competitive employment, .140 (about $1,107) would be deducted. These amounts are rough estimates only. The actual impact for each predictor is relative to the other predictors and would vary depending on the other measured characteristics.

Calculating an Individual Budgeted Amount

To calculate an IBA using Figure 11.2, insert the service recipient's values from the ICAP and from his or her record of services received into the shaded parts of Column C. In each row, multiply the value in Column C by the Parameter Estimate in Column B; then, put the product in Column D. Sum all of the Column D values. (In Figure 11.2, this sum is 3.77619.)

This resulting sum is a relatively small number because the model was constructed using a Log_{10} transformation of the old reimbursement amount. This statistical procedure is often recommended when certain statistics describing the model are not normally distributed. A Log_{10} scale converts the actual dollars to a scale (i.e., $2 = 10^2 = 100; 3 = 10^3 = 1,000$), somewhat like the Richter Scale, which is used to measure earthquakes. Therefore, $1,000 would transform to 3, and $10,000 would transform to 4. To convert the answer from the model back to real dollars, take 10 to the power of the result from the model. In Figure 11.2, 3.77619 yields a predicted monthly rate of $10^{3.77619} = \$5,972.98$.

Such transforming and "untransforming" usually comes up with a predicted amount, *across all adult home and community-based services recipients*, which is less than the starting value (i.e., the total expenditure on adult home and community-based services). To come back to the original amount, simply figure out a factor by which to multiply each value (in this example, 1.06097). This action yields an IBA log-adjusted monthly rate for the adult in Figure 11.2 of $\$5,972.98 \times 1.0609 = \$6,337.15$. Adding these log-adjusted monthly rates *across all adult home and community-based services recipients* would come up with the exact same *total* amount as the *total* of the current rates (the dependent variable in the regression analysis underlying the DOORS model). This amount is what we call *budget neutral*. Finally, the example in the last row of Figure 11.2 shows how an across-the-board 6% inflationary increase could be given: Simply multiply the predicted rate by 1.06 (i.e., $\$6,337.15 \times 1.06 = \$6,717.38$, the amount in the shaded box at the foot of Column D in Figure 11.2).

Impact of Each Predictor Variable The information shown in Column E of Figure 11.2 is not related to the computation of the IBA for our hypothetical adult. Rather, Column E contains estimates of the maximum possible impact that each predictor might have on predicted monthly reimbursement rates, across the full range of possible values for that variable, assuming all other variable values are average and stay unchanged. Roughly, the ICAP Broad Independence Index, comparing the minimum possible value with the maximum, appears to have the largest influence on predicted rates ($7,487), whereas the Second Assessment service has the least ($284).

In July 1998, the DOORS methodology was first implemented to determine IBAs for individuals who participated in the state's HCBS Waiver program for adults with intellectual disabilities. In January 1999, DDD extended the use of IBAs to participants in the state's HCBS Waiver program for children with intellectual disabilities. A revised adult model was developed in 2000 and then again in Summer 2002. A revised child's model was implemented in 2000, and a further revision was completed in

Fall 2003. Each iteration of the model has resulted in altered factors and different factor weightings.

New models are necessary in order to use new dollars from the legislature, to serve new people, and to update changes in the characteristics of the people served. These clinical and behavioral changes are captured in new ICAP assessments that are completed at least every 3 years or new intelligence testing that is completed at least every 5 years. With young children and in cases where there have been significant changes, more frequent assessment is conducted. When a new model changes everyone's IBA, half of the individuals win additional support, and half lose some financial support. In most cases, the changes to individual budgets are small. Although there is always some up or down movement, these adjustments are seldom substantial. In fact, many families recognize that a reduced individual budget indicates that other children or adults have greater needs or that their family member has made progress compared with other state service recipients.

Increasing political pressure urges states to implement models that are harmless to current participants and do not reduce anyone's IBA; however, political and financial pressure also push states to use these types of models with existing appropriated dollars to serve all people who are eligible but on waiting lists. This situation creates competition for service and support dollars among all of the people receiving services. New models help keep the distribution of money as fair and equitable as possible. From the point of view of the service recipients and providers, changes brought by new models are accepted and seldom cause enough negative change to be of concern.

EXCEPTIONS TO THE MODEL

As with any statistically based modeling process, the DOORS IBA model works well for a large portion of the individuals, but the model does over- or underestimate resource requirements for some individuals. Some individuals are clearly "outliers" who have a unique set of characteristics and behaviors that are not captured by the model. Others are not outliers (i.e., they fit a profile reasonably well) but require an additional level of services. In each case, additional funding may be required. For example, the model does not consider unlawful sexual behavior or obsessive compulsive disorders. Individuals with these behaviors require substantially more oversight and supervision and higher funding for additional services.

The DOORS IBA model is a "best fit" model (i.e., it is designed to generate funding levels that fit the majority of individuals). Sometimes, the model does not generate sufficient budget amounts for people who have low-prevalence, high-cost circumstances (e.g., need for 24-hour oxygen), rare degenerative neurological diseases, changing or long-term mental health challenges, and caregiver illness or incapacity. These cases are better handled as exceptions. The implementation of DOORS was accompanied by providing for appeals to be made to a State Level of Care Committee (SLOCC). The SLOCC serves as the safety net to address the shortcomings of the model. Rather than deny important services by rigidly adhering to the calculated IBA, petitioning the SLOCC provides the opportunity to direct additional funds to individuals with unique challenges. DDD reserves a modest fund to address these situations.

The aim for future DOORS models is to be able to formalize and classify the results of SLOCC individual funding decisions and to update procedures in order to improve the fit of individual funding levels. This outcome can be accomplished by the specific coding of behavior, medical, and other low-prevalence characteristics that are not in the ICAP but show up in enough cases to be important, such as the previously mentioned factors of unlawful sexual behavior and obsessive compulsive disorders.

DATA INTEGRITY

The integrity of the DOORS IBA model obviously hinges on the trustworthiness of the ICAP assessment data it employs. Guarding against "gaming" (assessing a person as having more challenges in order to increase funding) is necessary. To prevent gaming, the DDD took two steps. First, individual assessment data were gathered from three respondents rather than one. Second, an independent testing agency, Arbitre Consulting, which specializes in ICAP administration in Wyoming, Alaska, and several other states, was engaged to administer the ICAP.

Each person is administered an ICAP once every 3 years. The exact ICAP factors that DOORS uses to generate IBAs were masked until Arbitre took over the administration of new ICAPs for individuals previously receiving supports. This masking was done to avoid gaming. The factors included in the models are among the more concrete subelements of the ICAP instrument and, thus, the most readily verifiable.

LIMITATIONS OF THE MODEL

The model has limitations. As previously discussed, it is sometimes necessary to override the model in the case of individuals who have low-prevalence, high-cost conditions that will not be registered in a model like DOORS. In addition, the model forecasts budget requirements based on *current* observed costs within the context of overall system funding levels, but current costs may mask serious funding problems.

For example, Wyoming—like nearly every other state—has struggled with the problem of low community worker wages. Low wages caused significant worker turnover and retention problems (Heinlein & Fortune, 2002). The DOORS model generates IBAs within the confines of the overall funding available to pay for community services rather than using ideal funding levels to calculate the amount of funding necessary. Hence, DOORS IBAs are not the same as ideal funding amounts. The DOORS model generates more equitable funding amounts across individuals based on objective measures that are anchored in policy but constrained by available resources. Fortunately, in 2002, the Wyoming legislature appropriated extra dollars to boost Wyoming's direct-service wages from an average of $7.38 an hour to an average of $10.23 per hour. This welcome funding increase has contributed significantly to improved workforce stability and was translated quickly into new DOORS IBAs.

Another potential limitation of the model is that it is tied very closely to the ICAP. The ICAP is designed to measure adaptive and maladaptive behaviors; however, it does not measure other factors that might bear on costs. For example, some health conditions (e.g., diabetes) affect costs. In the DOORS model, these effects are only approximated by employing a proxy—namely the presence or absence of nursing services. Efforts elsewhere (especially in Pennsylvania) to develop DOORS-like models are examining ways to directly include health conditions in their models.

OUTCOMES OF DOORS

Thus far, the results of employing the DOORS IBA model of care are encouraging. There have been no fair-hearing requests. Also, families have given positive verbal and written responses, and teams have accepted the model in forming new plans. The DOORS model appears to enjoy broad stakeholder acceptance. The system is perceived to be fair and equitable. It informs individuals and families of the amount available in clear terms. It has reduced the suspicion that some individuals and families have been treated better than others or that some providers have secured more favorable funding than others. In addition, because DDD was able to simulate the results of applying the DOORS methodology prior to its implementation, it could identify in advance the potential that community-service organizations might face a significant overall decline in payments once DOORS was implemented. DDD alerted the people served, their families, and the provider organization to this potential problem so that they could begin to make necessary operational changes.

The implementation of the model has led to several positive developments in administration. DDD experienced a sharp reduction in the number of instances when it had to become involved in funding/service-plan decisions. To date, there have been no appeals that have led to administrative hearings concerning protests of the budget amounts or state decisions regarding requests to change those amounts.

At this stage, it is still too early to tell what effect the IBAs are having on per capita costs. As previously noted, the implementation of DOORS was not tied to a spending reduction plan; however, lower per capita costs are welcome. Wyoming has been among those states reporting no waiting list for services (Prouty, Smith, & Lakin, 2002); however, Wyoming officials do anticipate a dramatic change in the next few years. Figure 11.3 illustrates a 14-year struggle to get service development ahead of waiting-list growth (Allen, Fortune, & Fortune, 1998) and shows that the routine assessment of all HCBS Waiver applicants and the use of consistent service reimbursement models like DOORS can play an active role in containing the number of eligible people waiting for funded services and supports.

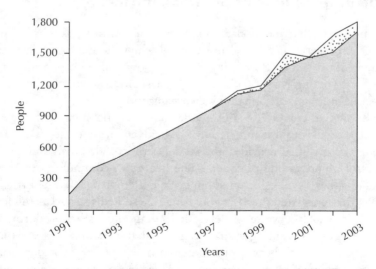

Figure 11.3. People with intellectual disabilities on waiting lists in Wyoming. (Key: ☐ = people being served; ⊡ = people waiting to be served)

DOORS is valuable to the Wyoming legislature and governor's office because it provides them with solid estimates of waiting-list costs. The Governor's Council for Developmental Disabilities has used this information to coordinate the efforts of a wide assortment of the state's active stakeholders. These efforts have generated significant support over the years for the DDD's funding requests to reduce or eliminate the waiting list.

One of the aims of DOORS was to create a framework in which individuals and families would have greater decision-making authority in the service planning process. Individual and family choice is a cornerstone of the Wyoming system. So far, there seem to be differences in the extent of involvement and participation by families with children who take part in the HCBS Waiver program and by families with a member supported by the adult HCBS Waiver. The former appear to be more actively involved in managing services than the latter, possibly as an outgrowth of their involvement in special education programs. Older parents seem less inclined to take an active role. In addition, it is not clear that individuals, family members, and teams understand the opportunities afforded by the IBA funding model with respect to altering services. Wyoming has initiated statewide training efforts to help individuals served and their families to understand and utilize the system to their advantage.

PROMOTING CHOICE OF SERVICE PROVIDERS

The principle that individuals must have the authority to choose their service provider(s) is rapidly undermined when there are only a limited number of providers. Promoting choice in low population-density states such as Wyoming is especially daunting. Usually, low population-density areas can only support one provider organization.

Because the DOORS IBA model does not tie funding to specific provider organizations and because individuals are free to select from among any qualified provider, the model permits individuals and families to shop for and among providers. The history of community services in Wyoming has revolved around nine large Regional Services Providers (RSPs) that pre-dated the *Weston* lawsuit. These RSPs served as the foundation on which Wyoming developed community services during the 1980s. Because Wyoming is sparsely populated, one would expect that it would be difficult to broaden the provider base, but new provider organizations are appearing in Wyoming, and existing providers are extending their operations to other areas of the state. Although many states report difficulty in attracting more providers—and, indeed, the number of providers is sadly shrinking in some states due to provider organization consolidations and mergers—choices have been expanding in Wyoming. At the end of 2002, Wyoming had

- 20 habilitation service providers offering extensive personal care, daytime learning activities, and vocational and residential HCBS services as well as most of the other HCBS services

- An additional 36 provider organizations with two or more employees serving one or two individuals with any of the HCBS services

- Over 1,400 individual service providers supporting individuals with respite care, individually selected service coordination, and a wide assortment of individual therapies.

In part, Wyoming's provider base is becoming more robust because the state's IBAs have been structured so that funding can truly follow the individual. New providers are not shut out of the marketplace. In addition, Wyoming has the capability to approve new individual plans of care quickly and pay individuals to provide services. Qualified providers—organizations or individuals—can enter the marketplace and compete on equal footing with existing organizations.

ADAPTING THE DOORS MODEL

Wyoming was especially well positioned to develop the DOORS model. Overall funding in Wyoming compares favorably to other states. The expansion of the community-service system occurred almost entirely through the HCBS Waiver program. As a result, Wyoming's system is more unified than many other states' systems. In places where multiple funding streams are present, service systems become more fractured, and, hence, per-capita costs vary. When Wyoming's system was built out, state officials used relatively consistent decision-making rules concerning funding. In combination, these factors eased the implementation of DOORS because they did not result in massive reallocation of resources among service recipients.

Development of the DOORS model also was feasible because Wyoming possessed a comprehensive database of service recipient characteristics (demographic and ICAP), as well as information concerning current dollar allocations and service-use patterns on a person-by-person basis. The DOORS model, however, is not ICAP dependent. ICAP data were chosen to provide a reasonably complete picture of service recipient characteristics. The ICAP instrument has known levels of reliability and validity and is normed. Other instruments or sources of information concerning service recipient characteristics can provide the data necessary to construct a DOORS-like model. For example, in 2002, Pennsylvania developed its own set of variables rather than using an existing instrument by working successfully on service-provider reimbursement state models (Pennsylvania Office of Mental Retardation Department of Public Welfare, 2001; Fortune, Seiler, & Church, 2002), and North Carolina used the NC-SNAP and other selected variables (Fortune, 2002).

From a clinical perspective any state wishing to establish a scientifically valid assessment and resource-allocation system should address four separate but related features:

1. Operational definitions for all funding-related qualifying conditions and diagnostic categories and the type/timeliness of the evaluations acceptable to establish them must be available. States that allow eligibility determination at the local level rarely have such basic definitions in place.

2. Operational definitions for adaptive skill scoring and for recording maladaptive behaviors—even when a nationally standardized instrument such as the ICAP is employed—should be present. Without these operational definitions, evaluators will use subjective definitions, and both the reliability and validity of the results will deteriorate accordingly.

3. A centralized clinical-review system must be established for the correction of invalid scoring. The system also must provide feedback to respondents or be able to remove individual ICAP respondents who demonstrate a pattern of producing questionable results.

4. The clinical data must serve as a contributor to funding decisions even in the face of opposition from service-provider companies, guardians, service recipients, and advocacy groups. Each of these groups has legitimate interests and concerns that should be considered apart from clinical practice. Clinical practice should have no self-interest.

CONCLUSION

The DOORS individual budget model has served two purposes in Wyoming. One purpose was to reform the funding of community services to ensure that the allocation of the resources to support individuals would be determined fairly and equitably and would be based on individual service needs. The DOORS model yielded IBAs that were resolutely linked to observable individual characteristics and were based on the costs of meeting the needs of individuals with those characteristics. The model also affirms that planning team decisions concerning services and supports should be given weight in determining IBAs (U.S. Centers for Medicare & Medicaid Services, 2001).

The second purpose was to aid in the adoption of a person-centered architecture for the Wyoming system. The DOORS model could just as easily have been designed to serve as a provider-based payment system. Instead, Wyoming decided that its IBAs would be tied to the individual and would operate in tandem with policies that affirm that planning teams have the authority to make decisions about services and the freedom to select among service providers.

REFERENCES

Allen, J., Fortune, J., & Fortune, B. (1998, May). *Managing the rising tide: The Wyoming waiting list revisited.* Paper presented at the 122nd Annual Meeting of the American Association on Mental Retardation, San Diego.

Arizona Department of Economic Security. (2002). *Use of needs assessment tools across states survey results.* Phoenix, AZ: EP&P Consulting.

Braddock, D., Hemp, R., Parish, S., & Rizzolo, M.C. (2000). *The state of the states in developmental disabilities: 2000 study summary.* Chicago: University of Illinois at Chicago, Department of Disability and Human Development.

Bruininks, R.H., Hill, B.K., Weatherman, R.F., & Woodcock, R.W. (1986). *Inventory for Client and Agency Planning (ICAP).* Chicago: Riverside Publications.

Campbell, E.M., & Heal, L.W. (1995). Prediction of cost, rate, and staffing by provider and client characteristics. *American Journal on Mental Retardation, 100*(1), 17–35.

Fortune, J. (2002, May). *Wyoming DOORS: Individual budgets according to individual need.* Paper presented at the Department of Health, Raleigh, NC.

Fortune, J., Heinlein, K.H., & Fortune, B. (1995). Changing the shape of the service population. *European Journal on Mental Disability, 2*(8), 20–37.

Fortune, J., Seiler, W., & Church, J. (2002, May). *Individual budgets according to individual need: Wyoming DOORS, South Dakota Service-Based Rates, and Pennsylvania's Targeted Budget Project.* Paper presented at the National Association of Developmental Disabilities Directors Services Mid-Year Meeting, Breckenridge, CO.

Heinlein, K.H., & Fortune, J. (1995). Who stays, who goes? Downsizing the institution in America's most rural state. *Research in Developmental Disabilities, 16*(3), 165–177.

Heinlein, K.H., & Fortune, J. (2002). *Non-professional direct care staff: What they make and why they leave.* Paper presented at the 126th Annual Meeting of the American Association on Mental Retardation, Orlando, FL.

Lewis, D.R., & Bruininks, R.H. (1994). Costs of community-based residential and related services to individuals with mental retardation and other developmental disabilities. In M.F. Hayden & B.H. Abery (Eds.), *Challenges for a service system in transition: Ensuring quality community experiences for persons with developmental disabilities* (pp. 231–263). Baltimore: Paul H. Brookes Publishing Co.

National Association of State Directors of Developmental Disabilities Services. (2000). *Person-centered supports—They're for everyone.* Alexandria, VA: Author.

Pennsylvania Office of Mental Retardation Department of Public Welfare. (2001). *Wyoming DOORS developing an individual budgeted amount: A statewide system.* Harrisburg, PA: Author.

Prouty, R.W., Smith, G., & Lakin, K.C. (Eds.). (2002). *Residential services for persons with developmental disabilities: Statistics and trends through 2001.* Minneapolis: University of Minnesota, Institute on Community Integration.

Rhoades, J.A., & Altman, B.M. (2001). Personal characteristics and contextual factors associated with residential expenditures for individuals with mental retardation. *Mental Retardation, 39*(2), 114–129.

Smith, G. (1999). *Wyoming DOORS: Setting Individual Resource Allocations for HCB Services.* [Monograph]. Cambridge, MA: HSRI, National Association of State Directors of Developmental Disabilities Services.

Smith, G., Taub, S., Heaviland, M., Bradley, V., & Cheek, M. (2001). *Making person-centered supports a reality: The equality state's experience.* Cambridge, MA: Human Services Research Institute.

U.S. Centers for Medicare & Medicaid Services, The MEDSTAT Group. (2001). *Wyoming—individual budgets for Medicaid waiver services. Promising practices in Home and Community-Based Services* (Report No. 6). Washington, DC: Author.

Weston, et al. v. Wyoming State Training School, et al. (1990). United States District Court, District of Wyoming. Civil Action C90-0004.

Wrigley, S. (1992). *Using the ICAP for funding levels with a Home and Community Based Utah Waiver for Individuals with Developmental Disabilities.* Paper presented at the 1992 HCF 10th National Conference on Home and Community-Based Waiver, Salt Lake City, UT.

CHAPTER 12

Having it Your Way

A National Study of
Individual Budgeting Practices within the States

Charles R. Moseley, Robert M. Gettings, and Robin E. Cooper

Individuals with developmental disabilities and their families have expressed concern that traditional services do not offer the supports they need to succeed in community settings. In response, state and federal officials are expanding service system capacity to fund more flexible, individualized, self-directed service options. In the mid-1990s, three national initiatives funded by the Robert Wood Johnson Foundation and supported by the Department of Health and Human Services provided funding for state demonstration projects aimed at applying the principles of self-directed services to older adults and to people with developmental disabilities receiving Medicaid-funded long-term care services. Self-direction is a centerpiece of President George W. Bush's New Freedom Initiative, a multifaceted effort to shift the focus of federally funded long-term services away from institutional solutions toward home and community-based services and supports. In 2002, the U.S. Department of Health and Human Services Centers for Medicare & Medicaid Services (CMS) released

This chapter is based on *Having it Your Way: Understanding State Individual Budgeting Strategies*, produced by the authors for the National Association of State Directors of Developmental Disabilities Services (NASDDDS). For further information on state individual budgeting methodologies, including in-depth profile descriptions of budgeting practices in nine states, please contact NASDDDS, 113 Oronoco Street, Alexandria, Virginia 22314. The authors gratefully acknowledge the assistance of the state officials who contributed to this study, in particular, David Maltman, Terry Cote, Margaret Zillinger, Shirley Patterson York, Lynda Kahn, Joe Gould, Wanda Seiler, Ed Campbell, Steve Wrigley, Theresa Wood, Robert Clabby, and Jon Fortune. The authors also express sincere appreciation for the editorial assistance of the volume editor, Roger Stancliffe.

a new Medicaid Home and Community-Based (HCBS) Waiver template called Independence Plus to encourage states to offer self-directed services to individuals with long-term support needs.

Although the logic of self-directed services appears to be readily accepted by service recipients and policy makers alike, the process of transitioning from program-based to individualized systems of service delivery presents state officials with significant operational, conceptual, and political challenges. Among the most difficult is the development of financing methodologies that 1) enable individuals with disabilities to control the resources allocated on their behalf; 2) provide the resources necessary to create the clinical, programmatic, and operational infrastructure required to maintain self-directed services; and 3) provide sufficient resources to ensure continuity of support for people currently receiving services. This is a difficult challenge because individual budgeting requires a degree of fiscal flexibility, accountability, and data management capacity that is unprecedented in developmental disabilities services and presents significant challenges to states making the change from traditional methods of funding and service design.

This chapter summarizes the results of a study of state individual budget development practices conducted by the National Association of State Directors of Developmental Disabilities Services in 2002–2003 (Moseley, Gettings, & Cooper, 2003). The study was designed to describe state individual budgeting activities, to identify factors that are instrumental in implementing "effective" individual budgeting methodologies, and to provide information on approaches to transitioning from traditional program funding to individual budgeting.

METHODOLOGY

Information was gathered on factors believed to be relevant to the budget-building process including the following:

- *Timing*—sequence of individual budget development activities (i.e., whether the budget was established before, during, or at the conclusion of the planning process)

- *Coverage*—identification of covered services (i.e., supports typically funded by, and those excluded from, the individual budget)

- *Rate setting*—methodologies for setting individual budgeting rates and identifying costs

- *Administrative cost coverage*—methods states use to cover administrative costs within the individual budgeting process

- *Assuring equity*—methods states use to ensure equity in their individual budgeting processes

- *Differentiating "wants" from "needs"*—mechanisms states use to separate treatment and support needs from personal preferences during the budgeting process.

In total, 43 of the 51 state developmental disabilities program agencies (84%) responded to the survey and provided data on their individual budgeting practices. The findings of this larger survey are reported in the Individual Budget Development section. In addition, nine states (Alaska, Connecticut, Kansas, Minnesota, Utah, Rhode Island, South Dakota, Vermont, and Wyoming) participated in a more in-depth analysis of individual budgeting practices. The findings from these nine states are presented later in the chapter in Implementation Strategies: Analysis of State Practice. Information on state individual budgeting practices was separated for analysis into three categories of state activity, including 1) intake, eligibility determination, and referral; 2) identification and assessment of needs, including the process for distinguishing a "need" from a "want"; and 3) establishing the amount of the individual budget. This final category includes an examination of the processes states use to equate support needs to an amount and intensity of service, to set the amount of the individual budget, and to modify an individual's budget to address new or changing needs.

Definitions

For the purposes of this study, the following definitions were used to organize and analyze the data received:

1. *Self-determination/consumer-direction/self-direction*—Belief based on the understanding that people have both the right and responsibility to exercise control over the services they receive. This belief is also based on four related principles of freedom, authority, support, and responsibility (Shumway, 1999).

    - *Freedom*—People with disabilities must be able to freely choose the events of their lives, the relationships they will have with others, the contributions they will make to their communities, and the supports or service providers they will use.

- *Authority*—People receiving support should have authority over the decisions that affect their lives, as well as over the expenditure of funds that are allocated on their behalf. People should have direct control over some, if not all, of their individual budget for services.

- *Support*—In order to responsibly exercise freedom and authority, people with disabilities, just like everyone, must have support designed to their personal strengths and needs. Within the context of self-directed services, people with disabilities must have the support they need to successfully carry out their person-centered plan.

- *Responsibility*—People directing the services they receive have responsibility for assuring that they use public funding in a useful and appropriate manner. States providing funding have a responsibility for ensuring that service systems include a safety net to respond to crisis and unanticipated need and that service dollars are used as an investment in the lives of individuals with disabilities.

2. *Individual budget*—A mechanism establishing an amount of funding available for an individual with disabilities to direct and manage the delivery of services he or she is authorized to receive. The amount of the individual budget is derived from a data-based methodology and is open to inspection and input from the individual receiving support.[1]

3. *Person-centered planning*—A process directed by the individual that is used to identify his or her strengths, capacities, preferences, and needs and the supports that will be provided to meet those needs. It is a means by which individuals are able to exercise choice and control over the process of developing and implementing a plan of care. Person-centered planning also may serve as a vehicle to enhance the ability of family members and friends to support the individual in a coherent fashion, organized around the individual's specific needs. The person-centered planning document also provides the criteria against which the adequacy and appropriateness of services and supports are measured.

---

[1]Some states use individual budgets only as a means to allocate funding to provider agencies. For the purposes of this study, *individual budget* includes the element of individual control.

Availability of Individual Budgets

The study began with a broad survey of state individual budgeting practices nationwide. An individual budgeting option was available to people receiving publicly funded specialized developmental disabilities services and supports in 75% of responding states. Within states, the availability of the individual budgeting alternative varied considerably. Individual budgets were available to *all* service recipients in only 16% of responding states. Eight states (19%) reported that an individual budgeting methodology was in use in *many* areas of the state but not statewide. Forty percent indicated that a basic individual budgeting process was in place but was being used only in *some* geographic areas of the state or only through *selected* programs. The individual budgeting process was reported to be in the *planning* stages in 23% of states, and one state (2%) had no individual budgeting activity.

Eligibility for an individual budget was influenced by the nature of the funding received and the type of program in which the person was enrolled. Of the 28 states that responded to questions on eligibility, six (21%) indicated that individual budgeting options were available to everyone receiving community developmental disabilities supports within the state. Five states (18%) reported that eligibility is limited to individuals on the state's Medicaid HCBS Waiver program for people with intellectual disabilities and/or developmental disabilities (ID/DD) or programs funded with state general revenues. Three states (11%) limited eligibility to individuals participating in the state's ID/DD HCBS Waiver program only, and six states (21%) restricted individual budgets to people participating in designated self-determined or self-directed initiatives. Individual budget availability by funding source is displayed in Table 12.1.

INDIVIDUAL BUDGET DEVELOPMENT

The sections that follow contain findings from the national survey to which 43 states responded. Of these, 32 states currently made an individual budgeting option available to service recipients, so information about individual budget methodologies came from these 32 states.

Determining an Allocation Amount

The majority of states determine the services and supports an individual is to receive and establish his or her individual budget as part of an integrated person-centered planning process. Sixty-nine percent of the states that responded to the individual budgeting survey reported that individual

Table 12.1.   Individual budget eligibility by source of funding

Individual budget eligibility limited to recipients of:	Number of states	Percent
No limitations—all eligible	6	21%
Medicaid 1915(c) waiver	3	11%
Waiver and state general fund	5	18%
State general fund	2	7%
Medicaid state plan services	0	0%
Waiver, Medicaid state plan, and general fund	2	7%
Designated projects	6	21%
Waiver, general fund, and designated projects	1	4%
General fund and designated projects	2	7%
Waiver and designated projects	1	4%
Total	28	100%

From Moseley, C., Gettings, R., & Cooper, R. (2003). *Having it your way: Understanding state individual budgeting strategies.* Alexandria, VA: NASDDDS; reprinted by permission.

budgets were determined through this *developmental* process based on discussions of the person's needs for support and assistance. These findings were supported by the study team's in-depth review of individual budgeting polices and practices in the nine target states.

Thirty-one percent of the state developmental disabilities agencies that responded to the survey separated the process of determining individual funding allocations from decisions regarding how an individual's funds will be deployed. These states typically use standardized tools, such as the Inventory for Client and Agency Planning (ICAP) (Bruininks, Hill, Weatherman, & Woodcock, 1986), the Developmental Disabilities Profile (DDP) (Brown, 1986; Brown, Hanley, Bontempo, & Manning, 1993; Brown, Nemeth, Hanley, Bontempo, & Bird, 1990), or another state-specific instrument, as part of a process of arriving at an individual funding allocation or target budget. As shown in Table 12.2, the states are almost equally divided between those that build individual budgets based on pre-established payment rates for specific categories/types of services or costs (47%) and those that do not rely on pre-established rates (53%).

Data-Based Methodology

States employ a variety of means to derive at individual budgets for the people they support. Some states determine a single target budget amount through the use of standardized assessment tools and sophisticated data analysis techniques that are designed to produce an individual rate based

Table 12.2. State individual budgeting characteristics

Budgeting characteristic	Yes	No	Total	Percent yes	Percent no
Are there individual budgets in your state?	32	11	43	74%	26%
Is the budget set by a data-based method?	11	21	32	34%	66%
Does your budget have a spending cap?	23	8	31	74%	26%
Does your budget set individual billing rates?	21	11	32	66%	34%
Is your budget set by a standard tool (e.g., Inventory for Client and Agency Planning)?	10	22	32	31%	69%
Is your budget based on a preset payment rate?	15	17	32	47%	53%
Is your budgeting process the same for all service recipients?	13	19	32	41%	59%
Is your budget determined by negotiation?	13	19	32	41%	59%

From Moseley, C., Gettings, R., & Cooper, R. (2003). *Having it your way: Understanding state individual budgeting strategies.* Alexandria, VA: NASDDDS; reprinted by permission.

on several cost and service-related variables. Other states build individual budgets through qualitative methodologies that identify services and costs through carefully structured discussions of each applicant's needs and wants within the context of the person-centered planning process. In each case, the state takes specific actions to ensure uniformity and consistency in the application of its methodology for arriving at an individual budget in order to ensure systemwide equity.

The importance of using fair, equitable, and consistent methods to develop individual budgets has been underscored at the federal level by the decision of CMS to require states applying for Independence Plus Medicaid waivers to employ individual budget development methodologies that are data based and applied in a consistent manner across the state or jurisdiction. The results of the national survey of individual budgeting practices suggest that this requirement will be a challenge faced by many states. Sixty-six percent of the responding states indicated that they do not consider the individual budgeting approach currently used in their state to be data based (see Table 12.2).

Spending Cap

The majority of state respondents (74%; see Table 12.2) reported that the process of individual budget development typically results in the establishment of a set amount of public dollars (a spending limit) to be made available to finance services for a particular eligible recipient. Alternatively referred to as the *authorized spending limit, approved funding level,* or *rate cap,* the final approved individual budget rate is expected to cover all of the person's identified needs, consistent with the provisions of his or her person-centered plan. Twenty-six percent of the responding states, in contrast, reported that spending caps are not set as a part of individual budget process.[2]

Individual Budget Variability

In most states, the use of a single individual budgeting format is still the exception to the rule. Fifty-nine percent of the responding states (19 of 32) reported that the same individual budgeting process was *not* being used with all people receiving public support in their respective jurisdictions, whereas 13 states (41%) indicated that a single or universal process was in use statewide. As illustrated in Figure 12.1, state individual budgeting procedures vary across a number of factors including funding source, provider type, and administering authority. Approximately one quarter (26%) of the states responding reported that individual budgeting practices differ according to the source/type of funding. Sixteen percent of the states reported that individual budgeting practices vary by the type of service provided. The same percentage of states noted that individual budgeting practices additionally differ according to the operational practices of the different state offices approving funding. These findings suggest that states moving to standardize their individual budget development methodologies across catchment areas should focus not only on the initial rate-setting process but also on the operational procedures that are used to pair needs with funding.

Negotiation and Approval

Over half of the states (55%) set the overall amount of the individual budget through a process of negotiation between the various parties involved in the person-centered plan. States involve people with disabili-

---

[2]The use of the term *cap* to refer to the total authorized budget amount can be misleading. Under Medicaid regulation, a beneficiary cannot be "locked-in" to a funding amount that is insufficient to cover the costs of services identified in his or her plan of care. The total amount of the individual budget is a function of the nature and intensity of the individual's needs and the costs of services to meet those needs. The person's budget may need to be increased or decreased accordingly.

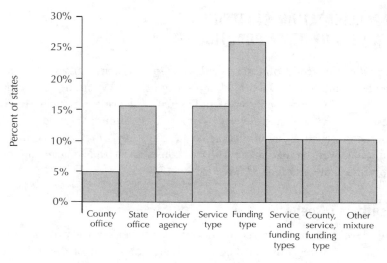

Figure 12.1. Percentage of responding states that used varying individual budget processes by service, funding, or administrative unit. (From Moseley, C., Gettings, R., & Cooper, R. [2003]. *Having it your way: Understanding state individual budgeting strategies.* Alexandria, VA: NASDDDS; reprinted by permission.)

ties in the process of developing their individual budgets in different ways. Some states, such as Connecticut, Rhode Island, and Utah, include the individual and family in virtually all funding and service-design decisions. Others separate funding decisions from the identification and selection of supports to meet identified needs.

Among responding states, final authority to approve individual budgets rests with the state (68%), with county or municipal agencies (12%), with a local committee or board (16%), and with the individual receiving support (4%). No state reported that final budget approval authority rested with the provider of service or the family.

Summary

The results of the national survey suggest that state agencies support the concept of individual budgeting and are proceeding along a number of different pathways to implement policies and procedures that both reflect the individual characteristics of each state's system of service delivery and meet emerging federal criteria for individual budgets supported via Medicaid HCBS Waiver funding. The data attest to the significant structural variability that exists between state agencies, as well as the large number of operational factors involved in the individual budgeting process.

IMPLEMENTATION STRATEGIES: ANALYSIS OF STATE PRACTICE

As part of this study, nine states (Alaska, Connecticut, Kansas, Minnesota, Rhode Island, South Dakota, Utah, Vermont, and Wyoming) participated in a more in-depth analysis of individual budgeting practices. Each of these states has policies governing access to community services that are designed to ensure that all people requesting support are treated in a fair, equitable, even-handed manner that is consistent with Medicaid and other applicable state and federal laws.

Identifying Needs

In each of the nine states receiving an in-depth review, the process of individual budget development begins with an assessment of the individual's strengths and needs for support and assistance. Although state needs-assessment methodologies differ, all of the various strategies are designed not only to identify specific needs for support, but also to achieve broader public policy objectives such as assuring: 1) equity in access to services; 2) fairness in fund distribution to provider organizations as well as to individuals receiving support; and 3) value, in terms of the cost-efficiency and effectiveness with which public funds were used.

Standardized Assessment Tools
The majority of states targeted for in-depth review (Alaska, Kansas, South Dakota, Utah, and Wyoming) assess individual needs through the use of standardized evaluations completed during the intake process (see Table 12.3). Assessment results are used to establish the amount of an individual's budget and to inform the development of the person-centered plan. Alaska, for example, uses the ICAP (Bruininks et al., 1986) to collect information on individual needs in a consistent manner across the state. Personal interviews are conducted by the state's Care Coordinators and combined with additional documentation to support the ICAP score and better identify the individual's specific support needs. Utah also uses the ICAP to assess the person's strengths and needs, but the test is administered in combination with the state's own Needs Assessment instrument to determine the applicant's position on the state's waiting list for services. Following completion of this process, Utah state officials use a state-approved protocol to discriminate wants from needs. All assessment data are integrated into a matrix that correlates functional status with the costs of supervision as part of the process of determining the amount of the individual's budget.

Table 12.3. States using standardized instruments to determine eligibility and support needs

Uses a national, standardized instrument	Uses a state instrument	Has no required instrument
Alaska	Minnesota	Connecticut
Kansas	Rhode Island	Vermont
South Dakota		
Utah		
Wyoming		

From Moseley, C., Gettings, R., & Cooper, R. (2003). *Having it your way: Understanding state individual budgeting strategies.* Alexandria, VA: NASDDDS; reprinted by permission.

South Dakota uses statistical methodologies to combine ICAP scores with predictive data on per-capita costs systemwide to arrive at service-based rates. These rates are designed to take into account the individual's functional status, systemwide average costs, and the predicted annual number of units of services the individual is likely to require. Similarly, Wyoming uses the ICAP to identify an individual's functional status and establish the level of his or her support needs. This information is translated into a resource allocation through a statistical process called DOORS that establishes the base for the individual budget (see Chapter 11). Specific needs to be addressed, as well as the required services to meet those needs, are determined by the individual's planning team.

State-Specific Assessment Instruments   Other states use state-specific instruments to evaluate need and determine individual budgets. Minnesota, for example, determines both needs and costs through the use of the state's Developmental Disabilities Screening Document. This assessment tool identifies service need based on three distinguishing factors: 1) the level of self-care support required by the individual; 2) the intensity of aggressive and/or destructive behavior, if any; and 3) the presence of a diagnosis of mental illness combined with observable destructive behavior. Similarly, Rhode Island uses a holistic process to determine the person's needs and necessary services. This approach combines data received from: 1) the state's Situational Assessment tool and the Personal Capacities Inventory; 2) information gathered through interviews with the individual requesting support, family members, and friends; and 3) professional judgment in a multifaceted process that is designed to evaluate service needs from a range of different perspectives.

No Particular Assessment Tools   Two states, Connecticut and Vermont, rely on policies and procedures to maintain conformity across the state, rather than using a standardized assessment tool to determine individual needs. In Connecticut, the Department of Mental Retardation (DMR) employs a uniform needs-assessment methodology to ensure that state DMR regional offices allocate resources to individuals using a standard distribution process based on statewide planning-list priorities, individual interests, and resource availability. New referrals are reviewed by the regional planning teams, which assign each individual a priority status based on his or her needs and the availability of resources. Funding for new services is allocated to priority levels in a triage system that targets scarce resources where they are most needed. Priority is assigned to individuals who are 1) in immediate crisis, 2) on the waiting list, 3) in need of forensic services, and 4) aging out of the secondary school system. Needs are identified through a person-centered planning process that leads the service recipient through a series of questions that attempt to separate needs from wants and to frame the request for services within the broader context of appropriateness, cost, and value. This general format also is employed by Vermont, which uses a recommended series of questions to lead eligible individuals through a process of identifying service needs. Needs and the services necessary to meet those needs are discussed in the same conversation.

Separating Needs from Wants

In this study, states described three basic approaches to establishing the amounts of funding needed by individuals to meet person-specific needs and to distinguish what is needed from what is wanted. The first method incorporated person-centered planning as the primary component of the budget development process, relying on the members of the individual's program planning team or his or her circle of support to sort out what would be needed by the individual (e.g., Connecticut, Vermont). The second approach used a standardized needs-assessment protocol to allocate statistically the amount of funding to be available to the individual based on his or her characteristics, circumstances, and other factors and to separate resource allocation from what might be viewed as more subjective discussions concerning the service needs and desires of the individual and his or her family (e.g., Alaska, Kansas, Minnesota, Wyoming). The third method combined elements of the other two approaches to inform decisions of the circle of support and individual program planning team (e.g., South Dakota, Utah).

Establishing the Individual Budget

Several states divide the individual budget development process into two separate steps, employing one methodology for determining the amount of funding the state will reimburse a county or designated provider agency for the services that are provided and another mechanism for determining the amount of the individual budget available for the person to control and manage. Three of the nine states targeted for in-depth review utilize this two-stage process: Kansas, Minnesota, and South Dakota. In Kansas, for example, nonprofit Community Developmental Disabilities Organizations are funded by the state using a tiered rate-reimbursement system individualized for each person, based on the individual's score on the DDP. The Community Developmental Disabilities Organization then works with the person and his or her circle of support to develop an individual budget based on the person's needs and preferences as identified in the person-centered plan.

The individual budgeting methodologies used in the nine states additionally differ in the sequencing of activities; that is, the order in which the various events occur in the budget-setting process. Wyoming, Kansas, South Dakota, Minnesota, and Utah establish a total amount of funding for the individual or the entity responsible for the individual's services to use to plan his or her budget at the beginning of the process, following the administration of a standardized assessment instrument, but before the development of the person-centered plan. Alaska, Connecticut, Rhode Island, and Vermont, in contrast, build the budget from the bottom up, based on the services and supports identified through the person-centered planning process. The amount of the individual budget is not set until the end of the person-centered planning process. Regardless of the sequencing of individual budgeting events, each of the nine states determined the type, scope, intensity, and duration of supports to be funded through discussions or negotiations conducted during the person-centered planning process. Person-centered planning involving the individuals receiving support, members of their families, friends, relevant professionals, and support staff, played the central role in the design of the individual's overall support plan.

The process of establishing the individual budget requires that the necessary services and supports not only be identified but also priced. In other words, state individual budgeting processes must include mechanisms for assigning costs to the various supports that are included in the service plan. Here again, state approaches differ. South Dakota, for example, reimburses providers on the basis of fixed services-based rates determined through a statistical analysis of several variables demonstrated to be related to actual service costs. Wyoming uses a similar approach. Connecticut, in contrast, builds the budget through the person-centered planning process and utilizes the department's cost standards to limit the use, frequency, and duration of some services and cap payment rates on others. In Vermont, individual budgets are derived from an estimate of the costs the Designated Agency is likely to incur to provide the particular array of services and supports identified in the individual's plan. This approach allows the budget to be adjusted upward or downward depending on the actual costs of services, taking into account staff qualifications, service availability, or the need for special expertise.

The state holds the final authority for approving individual budgets in all but one of the nine target states participating in the in-depth review. In Vermont, the funding level is set by the Designated Agency, which acts essentially as a state-designated managed care organization to manage both the cost and delivery of services to all eligible individuals in a particular geographical catchment area. Table 12.4 provides a comparison of state practices for funding individual budgets across the separate processes involved with 1) developing an individualized allocation to a local or regional agency; and 2) setting the amount of the individual budget.

Individual Budget Variability

Within-state variability in the individual budget development process was not identified as a significant issue by officials from the nine states whose individual budgeting practices were reviewed in detail. Most of the states reported using forms, processes, and decision criteria that are standard across the state. In all but one of the nine states, the authority for granting final approval of individual budgets rests with the state itself, which was in close control of the budget decision-making process. Indeed, in many cases, final budget approval rests with a small group or even a single individual within state government. That said, key informants in several of the nine states noted that differences in individual budget management and development practices do exist between state offices, counties, designated local agencies, or community provider agencies within their states and that a certain amount of variability was to be expected. Some states (e.g., Vermont, Connecticut, Wyoming) included a step in the review process that provides a second look at the budget and needs of the individual before final individual budget approval to help to ensure consistency.

In most of the nine states participating in the in-depth review (i.e., Vermont, Connecticut, Wyoming, Rhode Island, and Utah), the individual budgeting process provides latitude for the person receiving support to alter the composition of the services he or she receives, as long as the person's needs continue to be met. In such cases, the Medicaid plan of care

Table 12.4. Comparison of state practices for allocating individual funding and setting individual budgets

	Individual funding allocation			Individual budget amount				
State	Allocation set by	Allocation set through	Influenced by individual?	Set up-front?	Approved by	Influenced by individual?	Amount set through	Can person change service?
Alaska	State	Negotiate with provider	No	—	—	—	—	—
Connecticut	State	Preapproved rates	Yes	No	State	Yes	PCP negotiation	Yes
Kansas	State	DDP score	No	Yes	CDDO	Yes	PCP negotiation	Yes
Minnesota	State	State instrument	No	Yes	County	Yes	PCP negotiation	Yes
Rhode Island	State	State instrument	No	No	State	Yes	PCP negotiation	Yes
South Dakota	State	ICAP + state assessment	No	Yes	ATC	No	—	No
Utah	State	ICAP + state assessment	No	No	State	Yes	PCP negotiation	Yes
Vermont	DA	Assessment + PCP	Yes	No	DA	Yes	PCP negotiation	Yes
Wyoming	State	ICAP + state assessment	No	Yes	State	Yes	PCP negotiation	No

ATC = Adjustment Training Center (a nonprofit agency working under contract with the state to manage service delivery on a regional basis in South Dakota)

CDDO = Community Developmental Disability Organization (a nonprofit agency working under contract with the state to manage service delivery on a regional basis in Kansas)

DA = Designated Agency (a nonprofit agency working under contract with the state to manage service delivery on a regional basis in Vermont)

DDP = Developmental Disabilities Profile (an instrument to assess individual characteristics and support needs)

ICAP = Inventory for Client and Agency Planning (an instrument to assess individual characteristics and support needs)

PCP = Person-centered planning (a process involving an individual, family members, friends, and others who know the individual well to assist in identifying and securing paid and unpaid support for a safe, satisfying lifestyle that reflects individual preferences and choices)

From Moseley, C., Gettings, R., & Cooper, R. (2003). *Having it your way: Understanding state individual budgeting strategies.* Alexandria, VA: NASDDDS; reprinted by permission.

needs to be carefully worded to reflect the decision of the planning team in this regard.

OPERATIONAL ISSUES AND IMPLICATIONS

No particular budgeting approach appeared to resolve all the dilemmas involved in balancing expressed needs with inherent resource constraints. Regardless of the approach used, the result is still an approximation—an estimate—limited by time, place, and resources. Perhaps the best a state can do is to come up with a system that is 1) *logical*, in that it makes sense to those who use it; 2) *transparent*, in that decisions are based on methodologies that are easily understood; 3) *equitable*, in that the people using the system believe it gives them the same opportunity to receive assistance as anyone else, and 4) *accurate*, in that the results of the funding methodology provide resources that are sufficient to meet the person's needs.

Developmental Versus Standardized Approaches

In many states, the individual budget is built through a *developmental* process in which people receiving support and their planning teams actively participate in a series of structured decisions regarding 1) the identification of personal needs, 2) the selection of services to address those needs and, 3) the determination of the level of funding necessary to ensure that the identified needs are met. Although this budget-setting approach may appear to be a simple matter of involving people receiving support in discussions regarding the needs, services, and costs, the results of this study indicate that the processes states use are quite complicated. Indeed, as revealed by the in-depth review of state practices, those states that employ developmental methods (Connecticut, Rhode Island, Vermont) structure the budget-building process along a purposefully designed succession of decisions and support determinations that target limited resources in the most cost-effective manner possible. Table 12.5 lists the separate determinations that states may make in response to the basic questions of who will be serviced, what services will be provided, and how much the services will cost.

States employing standardized or statistical individual budgeting methodologies may address the same basic issues but do so in a different manner by assigning variable weights to factors demonstrated to be related to service costs and individual functional characteristics. The statistical analysis that is performed essentially takes the place of the step-by-step

Table 12.5. Individual budget decision process

Decision	Determinations to make: Questions to answer

Who will be served?
Outcome: Identify
   recipient
	1. Eligibility for services
	   • What are the eligibility criteria?
	   • How is eligibility determined?
	   • Is eligibility based on categorical or functional measures?
	   • Are services to be limited by eligibility category?
	
	2. Funding priorities
	   • Are services to eligible individuals restricted based on targeting criteria?

What services are
   to be provided?
Outcome: Set
   support plan
	1. Identification of needs
	   • How are needs determined?
	   • How are needs requiring support separated from those that do not?
	
	2. Identifying supports to be funded
	   • What is the process for identifying the supports to be received?
	   • Is the process consistently applied?
	   • Does the process produce valid and reliable outcomes?
	
	3. Natural supports
	   • Which identified needs are best met by existing informal supports?
	
	4. Scope of services
	   • What is the historical pattern of service funding and approval?
	   • What is the scope of services that have traditionally been provided to people at similar levels or need?
	   • What types of supports are required, restricted, or excluded?
	
	5. Preset limits and caps
	   • What types of supports or services are limited by regulation or policy?

How much will be
   paid for services?
Outcome: Set
   budget amount
	1. Assigning costs to services
	   • What is the evidence on which rates are based?
	   • Is the budget development methodology consistent throughout the state or jurisdiction?
	   • Are costs in line with historical trends?
	   • Are reimbursement rates preset or based on current costs?
	
	2. Preset limits and caps
	   • Are funds or services limited by caps or restrictions set through regulation or policy?
	
	3. Individual budget methodology
	   • Does it respond to changes in service need?
	   • Does it respond to individual choice?
	   • Does it have a process for appeals and dispute?
	   • Does it make sense to consumers and families?

From Moseley, C., Gettings, R., & Cooper, R. (2003). *Having it your way: Understanding state individual budgeting strategies.* Alexandria, VA: NASDDDS; reprinted by permission.

decision-making procedure used by states with "developmental" budgeting approaches. Wyoming offers a good example of this approach. Wyoming's individual budget development procedure begins with the administration of the ICAP (Bruininks et al., 1986) to confirm eligibility and identify the individual's functional status. ICAP data are used to derive a level of support needs through the application of the state's DOORS system, which uses multiple regression statistical techniques to set a rate formula reflecting individual needs, and the types of services required to meet those needs, based on the state's experience funding individuals with similar ICAP scores during prior years. The DOORS system does not identify particular services or service providers, but rather it sets an amount of funds that the individual can use to best meet his or her needs as determined by the planning team (see Chapter 11).

This approach essentially rearranges the sequence of activities in Table 12.5 so that each question and outcome is addressed in the following order: 1) Who will be served? 2) How much will be paid for services (individual budget amount set)? and 3) What services are to be provided? The questions of who will be served and how much will it cost are addressed through statistical or formula-driven processes.

The variability that exists in the methodologies states use to determine the support needs of eligible individuals, to equate those needs to specific services, and to set a level or amount of funding that is sufficient to pay for identified supports, reflects the individual nature of each state's developmental disabilities service system. This variability provides a great deal of information on the implications of various budget-setting methodologies to state officials interested in changing their individual budgeting methods or establishing individual budgeting capability for the first time.

State and Federal Policy Implications

The results of the individual budgeting survey raise several issues of relevance to state officials considering using the new Independence Plus templates for Section 1915(c) and Section 1115 Medicaid waiver applications. In the Independence Plus Medicaid waiver application template recently proposed by CMS for self-directed services, federal officials have set stringent criteria for individual budget development and implementation by requiring states to employ methodologies that are: 1) developed using a person-centered planning process; 2) based on actual cost and utilization data derived from reliable sources, such as those generated by the state's Medicaid Management Information system; 3) developed using a consistent process to calculate the resources available to each person; 4) open to public inspection; and 5) reviewed according to a specified method and frequency. In the draft document, CMS noted further that a state must describe how the individual receiving support and his or her family will be informed of the methodology used to calculate the individual budget, the total dollar value of services authorized, any policies that apply to the person's management of his or her budget, and, finally, the procedures that the person must follow in order to request an adjustment of the budget amount.

Evidence-Based Rates

The requirement that individual budgets be developed through a system that is based on "actual cost and utilization data" sets a standard that may be difficult for some states to meet. Although the draft materials produced by CMS in connection with the Independence Plus template do not specifically identify the type of data that would be acceptable for the development of an individual budgeting format, two thirds (66%) of the states surveyed in the course of this study reported that they did not consider their individual budgeting methodology to be data based. State officials from the nine states receiving an in-depth review offered varying responses to this question, depending on the structure of the methodology used in their respective states. Respondents whose states use standardized national or state-specific assessment tools as a part of their budget development processes opined that their state's approach was, in fact, based on cost and utilization data. Officials from states using developmental approaches, however, expressed uncertainty whether their methodologies would be considered to be data based, even though they provided a sound rationale justifying the approach and detailed descriptions of the economic basis for the decision-making processes used. This revelation suggests that states do, in fact, use cost and utilization data to design and implement their individual budgeting processes, but they may not have organized their materials into formats that could be readily assessed by external reviewers.

Concepts such as person-centered planning, self-direction, quality assurance, and even individual budgeting are, by definition, individual, variable, and subjective. As such, the structure and functioning of a self-directed program needs to be flexible in order to be tailored to the particular needs and life situations of each person receiving support. Self-directed support programs can present a challenge to traditional approaches to standardization and measurement. It is important, therefore, that states provide specific and detailed descriptions in their Independence Plus waiver applications of exactly *what* they are planning to do and *how* they are planning to do it. At the same time, CMS needs to demonstrate flexibility and a willingness to work with states to develop fair and sound methods of individual budgeting.

Consistent Process for Calculating Resources

CMS Independence Plus waiver application draft guidelines called for the development of individual budgeting processes that calculate the value of the resources available to each person in a manner that is consistent across the state or eligible population. In other materials, CMS suggested that states can meet this requirement by outlining a uniform statewide process for budget development or by establishing a process for reviewing individual budget development techniques used by subcontractors that is based on minimum criteria that must be met by all providers in the state.

Our findings suggest that this requirement might be difficult to enforce and, more importantly, may interfere with the ability of states to experiment with new and promising techniques of budget development. Almost 60% of the state respondents indicated that their state did not restrict individual budgeting formats to a single "approved" methodology. Indeed, one state official reported that current policy was to purposefully refrain from uniformity to stimulate local creativity and innovation.

The process of individual budgeting is new, complex, and evolving. It appears clear that "best" practice has not yet been identified. Permitting or even encouraging structured experimentation among state programs to identify the relative strengths of the different budgeting formats seems to make a great deal of sense.

Limiting Services and Budgets

CMS has expressed concern about attempts in some states to limit services and cap spending through the individual budgeting process. At the same time, federal officials appear to recognize that caps need to be placed on individual budgets and services to ensure that spending is contained within appropriate parameters and to provide people receiving support with a stable financial foundation. This concern is shared by states. Almost 75% of the state officials reported that their state imposed an "authorized spending limit" or cap on the amount of the budget that would be approved for an individual to cover the costs of services. Although state and federal officials alike recognize that such limits must be "soft caps" in the sense that the budget is a function of service need and may change as needs change, the final answer to the question of how much is enough is by no means clear. Continued work needs to be done by both federal and state officials in this area if self-directed services and individual budgets are to become "generic" components of Medicaid waiver services.

FINAL OBSERVATIONS

Most state ID/DD agency officials described individual budgeting as a key component of a broader system change effort aimed at implementing self-directed services by shifting control over resources to individuals receiving support. Individual budgeting has been associated with improved service outcomes and decreased costs in at least one study (Conroy & Yuskauskas, 1996; Shumway, 1999; see also Chapter 10) and is the focus of major system change activities that are underway within a number of state/local developmental disabilities service systems.

This is a critical period in the development of a national capacity to support self-directed services for people with developmental disabilities, a time when both state and federal officials must carefully sift through the lessons of long-term support policy and practice revealed by the state demonstrations of self-directed services to identify the central principles necessary for successful implementation. CMS officials are working with state representatives to craft self-directed service policies that not only reflect current state program realities but also incorporate the components of effective and appropriate practice. The problem is that national "best" practice and CMS policy regarding self-directed services are evolving at a rapid pace, making it increasingly difficult for state officials to develop programs that will meet with certainty yet-unarticulated federal expectations.

Economics and Control

Although state developmental disabilities service systems generally do not operate under managed care principles as understood in a Medicaid policy context, the fact is that service delivery operates in a tightly controlled financial environment of fixed resources regulated by both state and federal law. Competition (i.e., consumerism, in the free market sense of the term) does not exist in public ID/DD services. Where competition does occur, typically it is managed under rigid controls with the "supply" of services dependent not on "demand," as defined by the number of people who request and are able to obtain and pay for needed supports, but rather on the presence of interacting personal, social, economic, political, and legal variables. In practice, supply is a function of the amount of funding appropriated by state and federal legislatures to meet demand. Demand functions as a constant, always present, always exceeding supply. Operating within the boundaries of state policy, supply increases, rather than decreases, demand. Within this environment, states tightly manage the supply of resources, targeting services toward eligible individuals with the most urgent needs.

Traditionally, the role of state policy has been to ensure equity and fairness by managing the response to service demand through a regulated fund-allocation process and a strong relationship between the state and community service providers. Individual budgeting potentially can shift funding control to the individuals receiving support, thus enabling them to operate as consumers and choose providers who offer them the most attractive support alternatives. Under this approach, the provider now works for the individual who, as a consumer in control of portable funds, is empowered to select the provider who offers the greatest return on his or her investment. In this context, individual budgeting makes it possible for individuals to take control over the supports they receive. The presence of an individual budgeting process offers the potential for an individual to become a consumer and control the expenditure of the resources that have been allocated on his or her behalf.

But how effective a tool is individual budgeting? Do state individual budgeting strategies empower individuals with disabilities to take charge of the supports they receive (see Chapters 1, 9, and 10)? Does the move toward individual budgeting force traditional systems of service delivery to change—to increase their responsiveness to consumer needs, preferences, and desires for individual control? What role does individual budgeting play in self-direction? Finally, is individual funding the only viable approach to supporting the capacity of individuals to control their lives?

Self-Direction Challenges

Although individual budgets are but one component of a much broader plan to shift authority and responsibility to individuals receiving support, they remain at the nexus of the overall process of system change. The individual budget stands at the operational center of three long-term support policy vectors that can each function to pull state practice in different directions. These policy vectors include individual choice, entitlement, and financial accountability. Although the three concepts are treated as compatible partners in long-term support policy, each carries an operational agenda with features that can conflict with the implementation of the others. Policy initiatives in support of *individual choice and control,* for example, are designed not only to enable people receiving services to manage spending decisions through individual budgets, but also to: 1) gain authority over the expenditure of funds; 2) encourage the individual's involvement and direct participation in decisions regarding the nature, scope, and intensity of the supports received; and 3) assure choice of providers. Although initial evidence of the impact of individual budgeting on service costs suggests that state expenditures actually decrease with greater self-direction (Conroy & Yuskauskas, 1996; see Chapter 10), the issue remains contentious in some states, with service recipients and their families expressing frustration that the individual budgeting process limits choice and control through mechanisms that artificially restrict the amount of funding or the services and supports that may be purchased. In other words, for many eligible individuals and families, particularly those who have felt underserved in past years, choice means that service recipients set the limits.

The entitlement nature of the Medicaid program exerts similar pressures against cost-related limitations on access to needed services because of statutory guarantees designed to ensure that all eligible individuals receive the supports they need, regardless of the state's ability to pay. Although the administration of the broad Medicaid entitlement is relatively straightforward in the context of acute medical care, long-term support needs are, by comparison, significantly more difficult to ascertain. The need for long-term support, for example, is intermingled with the level of personal and social assistance a person receives from family, friends, and the community at large. Although state individual budgeting methodologies are designed to separate service needs that must be addressed from personal preferences that are not instrumental in achieving person-centered plan outcomes, equitable decision making is difficult to achieve with consistency.

From a narrow perspective, one can argue that when a policy emphasis on personal choice and individual control is combined with the entitlement nature of Medicaid financing, a presumption is established in favor of ever-escalating state budgets for developmental disabilities services. On the other hand, long-term supports are furnished by states within the context of a publicly financed system of human services. Every state except

Vermont is required by rule or constitutional amendment to operate under balanced annual or biennial budgets. State developmental disabilities agencies, like all state agencies, must manage expenditures within the total amount of funding approved through the legislative process. During periods of financial instability, the resources available to state programs may vary considerably from one fiscal year to the next. Although state officials usually are able to accommodate budget shortfalls by restricting or modifying the expenditure of non–program-related funds (e.g., administrative overhead expenses, travel and training costs), these steps may not balance the books during periods of extreme fiscal restraint, and, as a result, access to services may be limited.

The financing of long-term care services is a complicated matter involving many separate entities. In traditional provider-driven service designs, state funding agencies can freeze reimbursement rates; reduce funding for designated activities, such as program administration or in-service training; or take other steps to restrict outlays. Although self-directed systems of support appear to offer budget-setting methodologies that are more sensitive to individual need—and thus less apt to overfund in the beginning—once the individual budget has been set, the approach may offer fewer opportunities for states to reduce costs without directly affecting the services and supports received by the individual and/or his or her family. Individualized funding systems designed to cover the costs of supports identified as "medically necessary" by a person-centered planning process appear to be less vulnerable to resource or cost limitation—unless, of course, funding can be reduced without having an impact on the plan of care. If a state's financial status requires substantive reductions in the resources available for services, state officials committed to retaining the Medicaid waiver program would have few alternatives other than 1) amending the state's Medicaid waiver to reduce the nature or extent of services covered by the program, or 2) adjusting each individual's person-centered plan to accomplish the same service objectives through the substitution of less-expensive supports of equal quality. Such steps may or may not be acceptable to the individual who is now in charge of the supports he or she receives.

In practice, the role of the person-centered plan is critical to the funding process and functions as the fulcrum that keeps public spending and individual support needs in balance. As individual budgeting methods mature, increased attention should be directed toward the person-centered planning process to protect its integrity and utility in the support of the individual.

CONCLUSION

The results of this study offer several alternatives that can be effectively employed by states to enable people receiving support to directly control and manage the resources allocated on their behalf. The study also identifies many of the issues that must be addressed in the development and operation of an effective and appropriate individual budgeting technology. The questions (i.e., Which individual budgeting methodology is best? Which approach is appropriate for a state to use?) are not easily answered. Many variables must be considered, and the nature of each contributing factor is not consistent from one state to another.

A series of vignettes was developed and distributed to the nine states receiving in-depth reviews in an effort to assess the consistency of the various approaches used to address the same individual needs. Full analysis of these data was beyond the purview of this study. The partial assessment that was completed, when combined with the results described previously, points to several areas of future study that may significantly expand knowledge and understanding of the individual budgeting process. These areas include focused examinations of: 1) the extent that individual budgets are used to support the state's entire system of service delivery, 2) the scope of services typically included or excluded by individual budgets, 3) the evidence used by states on which to base individual funding decisions, 4) the methods used to ensure equity in access to support and funding, 5) the implementation of the individual budgeting process as perceived by the people involved, and 6) the effectiveness of individual budgets at reducing service costs.

The results of this study demonstrate the number and complexity of issues that accompany states' efforts to infuse individual budgeting practices and person-centered models of support into the mainstream of service delivery. Systematic investigations into each of the research questions identified previously would provide valuable data for states interested in making self-directed support more than a "boutique" program nested within the traditional service system. The shift to self-directed services and the implementation of individual budgeting methodologies require states to change many of the fundamental policies and practices that have sustained developmental disabilities systems over the years. The results of this study suggest that a successful transition cannot be achieved through incremental adjustments in the status quo but rather require focused attention to fundamentally alter all aspects of program delivery.

REFERENCES

Bruininks, R.H., Hill, B.K., Weatherman, R.F., & Woodcock, R.W. (1986). *Inventory for Client and Agency Planning (ICAP)*. Chicago: Riverside Publications.

Brown, C.M. (1986). *The Developmental Disabilities Profile: The design, development and testing of the core instrument*. Albany: New York State Office of Mental Retardation and Developmental Disabilities.

Brown, C.M., Hanley, A., Bontempo, A., & Manning, B.L. (1993). *The DDP and resource consumption*. Albany: New York State Office of Mental Retardation and Developmental Disabilities.

Brown, C.M., Nemeth, C., Hanley, A., Bontempo, A., & Bird, W. (1990). *Scoring the DDP*. Albany: New York State Office of Mental Retardation and Developmental Disabilities.

Conroy, J., & Yuskauskas, A. (1996). *Independent evaluation of the Monadnock Self-Determination Project*. Ardmore, PA: Center for Outcome Analysis.

Moseley, C., Gettings, R., & Cooper, R. (2003). *Having it your way: Understanding state individual budgeting strategies*. Alexandria VA: National Association of State Directors of Developmental Disabilities Services.

Shumway, D.L. (1999). Freedom, Support, Authority, and Responsibility: The Robert Wood Johnson Foundation national program on self-determination. *Focus on Autism and Other Developmental Disabilities, 14*, 28–35.

CHAPTER 13

The Economics of Deinstitutionalization

*Roger J. Stancliffe, K. Charlie Lakin, John R. Shea,
Robert W. Prouty, and Kathryn Coucouvanis*

In the United States, policy decisions about deinstitutionalization have
been made for a range of reasons related to the well-being of service recipients, litigation, funding, and political considerations. Economic factors
have not been, nor should they be, the primary basis for determining policy on developmental disability services; however, decisions about institutional downsizing and closure have economic consequences. Research-
based information about these consequences should be available to policy
makers, administrators, and advocates so that deinstitutionalization can be
planned and implemented in a rational, economically sustainable manner.
This chapter examines the research, policy, and economic context of deinstitutionalization drawing on national data on deinstitutionalization, as well
as specific examples of deinstitutionalization in California and Minnesota.

DEVELOPMENTAL AND
LIFESTYLE OUTCOMES OF DEINSTITUTIONALIZATION

When considering the relative costs of institutional and community
services for individuals with intellectual and developmental disabilities
(ID/DD), it is essential to take account of the consistently superior developmental and lifestyle outcomes experienced following movement
from institutional to community settings. Expenditures on services that
deliver unsatisfactory outcomes may reflect poor investments for society,

but more importantly, they reflect deprivation of opportunity for service recipients.

Developmental Outcomes

Solid research establishes that movement from institutions to community life has beneficial developmental outcomes. Between 1980 and 1999, 33 major studies in the United States measured changes in daily living skills or adaptive behavior associated with leaving institutions for homes in the community. A detailed review of these studies was published by Kim, Larson, and Lakin (2001). In that review, 27 studies examined changes in overall general adaptive behavior, and 6 additional studies examined major components of adaptive behavior, specifically social skills, self-care/domestic skills, and community-living skills. These 33 studies included over 3,500 total service recipients who were followed for periods ranging from 6 months to 6 years.

Figure 13.1 summarizes the findings of the deinstitutionalization studies that examined changes in overall adaptive behavior and self-care. The bar

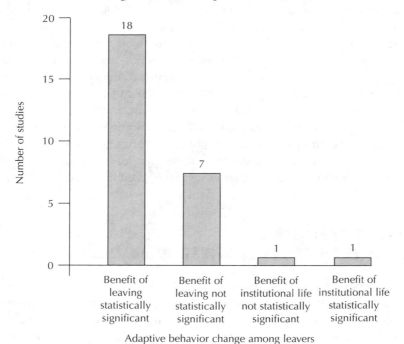

Adaptive behavior change among leavers

Figure 13.1. General adaptive behavior changes among samples leaving public institutions as compared with contrast groups or themselves.

to the far left shows that 18 of the 27 studies found statistically significant adaptive behavior growth associated with leaving institutions. Seven additional studies found improvements in adaptive behavior that did not reach statistical significance (95% confidence). One study found a statistically significant benefit, and one study found a nonsignificant benefit associated with institutional life. Together, these studies demonstrate a pattern of consistency (25 favorable and 2 unfavorable) that is extremely rare in social research and that supports the expectation that deinstitutionalization and community living are associated with positive change in general adaptive behavior.

Improvements in adaptive behavior are important in themselves, but they are also important because adaptive behavior has a strong positive relationship to many lifestyle outcomes (Stancliffe & Lakin, 1998). Studies of deinstitutionalization and the development of community-living skills, self-care and domestic skills, and social skills also showed a highly consistent pattern of benefits associated with leaving the institution for life in the community. Respectively, 100% (community living), 92% (self-care/domestic), and 100% (social) of studies showed that skills were enhanced by movement to the community (Kim et al., 2001). This consistent pattern of results from U.S. studies has also been found in reviews of research in the United Kingdom (Emerson & Hatton, 1996) and Australia (Young, Sigafoos, Suttie, Ashman, & Grevell, 1998).

Community Participation

The community participation of people living in community settings, when compared with that of people living in institutions, is impressive in its greater frequency and variety. People who live in community settings, when compared with institution residents, go to more movies, more restaurants, more stores, and more sporting events. They go on more walks off the grounds of the facility/home and have more visits to friends away from the facility. They are more likely to participate in organized sports, to have friendships with people other than those with whom they live, and to go places with their families, such as community religious services and activities (Conroy, 1998; Conroy & Bradley, 1985; Felce, de Kock, & Repp, 1986; Hill & Bruininks, 1981; Horner, Stoner, & Ferguson, 1988; O'Neil, Brown, Gordon, Schonhorn, & Green, 1981; Stancliffe & Lakin, 1998).

Relationships

People increase family involvement subsequent to leaving institutions, although most only have monthly or less frequent contact with family members (56%–70% in Eastwood, 1985; Feinstein, Lemanowicz, & Conroy, 1988; Stancliffe & Lakin, 1998). Other studies have shown considerably more frequent family contact for people in community settings who have never experienced prior institutionalization.

Other Lifestyle Outcomes

Community residents experience greater choice than individuals in institutions (Emerson & Hatton, 1996; Stancliffe & Lakin, 1998). Greater satisfaction by service recipients and by family members is associated with community services as compared with institutions (Emerson & Hatton, 1996; Larson & Lakin, 1991; Young et al., 1998).

NATIONAL TRENDS IN PUBLIC INSTITUTIONAL COSTS

Public institutions are costly enterprises. In Fiscal Year (FY) 2002, states spent, on average, $125,746 per public institution resident. In the 20 years between 1982 and 2002, the "real" (inflation adjusted) dollar cost of public institution care more than doubled from $61,117 (2002 = $1) to

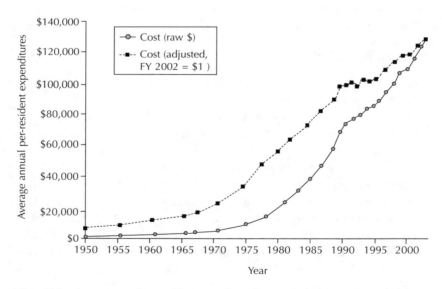

Figure 13.2. Average annual per-resident expenditures in state institutions in the United States, 1950–2002. (From Coucouvanis, K., Polister, B., Prouty, R.W., Bruininks, R.W., & Lakin, K.C. [2003]. Current populations and longitudinal trends of state residential settings [1950–2002]. In R.W. Prouty, G. Smith, & K.C. Lakin [Eds.], *Residential services for persons with developmental disabilities: Status and trends through 2002* [p. 16]. Minneapolis: University of Minnesota, Research and Training Center on Community Living, Institute on Community Integration; adapted by permission.)

$125,746 (Prouty, Smith, & Lakin, 2003). Figure 13.2 shows the average annual per-person nominal and real-dollar expenditures for public institution care between 1950 and 2002.

In the United States, rapid escalation in public institution costs began in the early 1970s. Four major factors contributed to this trend. The creation of the Intermediate Care Facility for the Mentally Retarded (ICF/MR) program in 1971 provided, for the first time, federal Medicaid cost sharing of 50%–80% of institutional costs under the condition of facilities meeting specific program, staffing, and physical plant standards. In the decade that followed, 88% of all public institution residents were living in units that met ICF/MR standards and received federal cost share. In the process, annual expenditures per resident (i.e., per diem) increased from $4,635 in 1970 to $32,759 in 1982, or in inflation-adjusted dollars from $21,458 (2002 = $1) to $61,117. This decade had the most rapid rate of increase in public institution expenditures since national data were first gathered in 1903.

ICF/MR certification costs were not the only factor in this increase. Beginning in 1968, public institution populations in the United States began to decrease steadily. In the years that followed, public institutions had to spread the fixed costs of operating the institutions (e.g., maintenance, administration, utilities) over fewer and fewer individuals. This issue is examined in more detail later in this chapter. In the 35 years following the beginning of deinstitutionalization in 1967, public institution populations decreased by 77.4% from 194,650 people to 44,066. A related phenomenon, especially in the first 20 years of institution depopulation, was the primary focus on community placement of the residents with relatively less severe impairments. As a result, the percentage of state institution residents with profound intellectual disability increased from 27.0% in 1964 (Scheerenberger, 1965) to 63.0% in 1987 (Prouty et al., 2003). The higher proportion of residents with substantial support needs demanded greater levels of direct-support staffing, as well as medical and therapeutic specialists. In addition, from the early 1970s through the mid-1990s, class action suits were filed in 38 states involving living conditions; basic freedoms; right to treatment; and other aspects of the adequacy, quality, and appropriateness of institutional services (Hayden, 1997). The required responses to these complaints often involved additional investment in institution infrastructure, increased staffing, intensified treatment programs, and/or reduced resident population—all with accompanying higher costs.

The relative impact on cost of any one of these factors is hard to determine because, for the most part, they were not only simultaneous but also interrelated. By the mid-1980s, public institutions became extremely costly in comparison with average per-person costs of 1970 (see Figure 13.2), so much so that in inflation-adjusted "real dollars" (2002 = $1), the total expenditures for state institutions in 1986 ($7.97 billion) were nearly double the real-dollar expenditures of 1970 ($4.18 billion), even though the number of average daily public institution residents had been nearly halved from 194,650 in 1970 to 100,190 in 1986. Not only were public institution expenditures in 1986 dramatically greater than they had been in 1970, but also community residential alternatives were consistently found to be only 75%–92% as costly as public institutions for comparable sets of comprehensive services (Ashbaugh & Allard, 1984; Bensberg & Smith, 1984; Jones, Conroy, Feinstein, & Lemanowicz, 1984; Minnesota Department of Public Welfare, 1979; Touche Ross, 1980).

The recognition of the greater costs and inferior outcomes of public institution services led states, from the late 1980s, not only to move public institution residents to community alternatives but also to *close* public institutions to avoid their rapidly increasing per-resident costs, often in the process relocating some residents to other institutions through consolidation plans. Between 1988 and 2002, 130 state institutions for people with ID/DD or units for people with ID/DD in other state institutions were closed (Prouty et al., 2003). In the 13 years between 1989 and 2002, state institution per-resident costs in real (2002) dollars increased by 28.9% from $97,533 to $125,746. This amount compares with a real increase of 511.8% in the 22 years between 1967 and 1989 from $15,943 to $97,533 (Prouty et al., 2003). Despite the significant efforts to better control expenditure growth within public institutions, questions continue to be asked about the benefits derived (or forfeited) by the 44,066 people still living in institutions in June 2002 and the relative costs of those benefits.

RELATIVE COSTS OF INSTITUTIONAL AND COMMUNITY SERVICES

As noted, institutional and community costs differ greatly, with average expenditure of $125,746 per public institution resident in FY 2002, as compared with $37,816 per recipient of community services financed by the Medicaid Home- and Community-Based Services (HCBS) Waiver program. But such comparisons can be misleading as institutional and community services differ in many important respects, such as the characteristics of the populations served, staff wage rates and conditions of employment, and the array of services provided. Consequently, the most meaningful comparisons of institutional and community service costs may be found in the deinstitu-tionalization costs literature in which similar groups of service recipients receive a similar array of services in institutional and community settings.

Available U.S. studies of both costs and outcomes of deinstitutionaliza-tion reveal a consistent pattern across states and over time of better out-comes and lower costs in the community (Jones et al., 1984; Knobbe, Carey, Rhodes, & Horner, 1995; Stancliffe & Lakin, 1998), which is consistent with U.S. deinstitutionalization literature on outcomes (Kim et al., 2001) and with cost-comparison research showing U.S. institutional services to be more costly than community services (e.g., Ashbaugh & Allard, 1984; Bensberg & Smith, 1984; Campbell, & Heal, 1995; Minnesota Department of Public Welfare, 1979; Schalock, & Fredericks, 1990; Touche Ross, 1980). In the three studies involving costs and outcomes (Jones et al., 1984; Knobbe et al., 1995; Stancliffe & Lakin, 1998), costs of community services ranged from 5% to 27% less than state institutional services.

Such cost differences favoring community alternatives are significant, especially in light of better outcomes, but a primary factor associated with the difference is the consistently and substantially lower wages paid to direct-support staff employed by community-service agencies. In 2000, the national average hourly wage of direct-support staff in state-operated services was $11.57 versus an estimated $8.72 (24.6% less) in nonstate community services (Polister, Lakin, & Prouty, 2003). Such wage differ-entials are consistent with previous research (e.g., Mitchell & Braddock, 1994) and are accompanied by generally better fringe benefits (e.g., health insurance, paid vacation and sick leave, educational benefits) available to state employees. Such large wage differentials have been noted as a major driver of the lower cost of nonstate community services (Campbell & Heal, 1995; Jones et al., 1984; Rhoades & Altman, 2001; Stancliffe & Lakin, 1998), especially given that staff costs are the largest component of residential and related services expenditures, generally representing about 77%–87% of total expenditures (Stancliffe & Lakin, 1998).

COSTS OF CLOSING LARGE, STATE-OPERATED FACILITIES

In economic terms, the primary challenge of deinstitutionalization is as-suring a transfer of resources from institutional to community services to accompany the ongoing movement of people. In other words, to what extent can institutional expenditures be reduced *in direct proportion* with the decrease in institutional population? The introduction and explanation of a few basic concepts may contribute to this discussion. *Variable costs* are those costs that vary with the volume of output (e.g., number of individuals served, hours of service delivered). *Fixed costs* are those that do *not* vary with output (e.g., costs of physical plant and equipment). Other costs (e.g., some food service personnel, medical records staff) are *semi-variable*, in the sense that they cannot be reduced in direct proportion with falling resident numbers but, over time, these costs also decline. Increases in *per-diem* costs (average daily expenditures per person) associated with reduced resident numbers are often called *diseconomies of reduced scale*. The greater the diseconomy of reduced scale, the more money needs to be retained to pay for the continued operation of the institution during downsizing, and the less money can be transferred from the institution budget to pay for community services.

Evidence of diseconomies of reduced scale should *not* be interpreted as showing that economies of scale operate when comparing the per-person cost of facilities of different size that are operating *at the size they were originally designed for*. The complex issue of economies of scale is examined elsewhere in this book (see Chapters 3, 6, and 7). In this section, we examine evidence for the existence of diseconomies of reduced scale associated with state institution downsizing, and we attempt to estimate the magnitude of these diseconomies.

Contrasting High-Change and Low-Change States

For 1988–2000, we contrasted trends in state institution per diems for two groups of states: 12 *high-change* states and 13 *low-change* states. The 12 high-change states (Alaska; Washington, DC; Hawaii; Maine; Michigan; Minnesota; New Hampshire; New Mexico; Oregon; Rhode Island; Vermont; West Virginia) *each* had more than a 75% overall decline in institutional population in the 12-year period. The 13 low-change states (Arkansas, Delaware, Florida, Georgia, Illinois, Kentucky, Mississippi, Missouri, Nebraska, Nevada, North Carolina, Ohio, Texas) had the most modest declines (all less than 33%) in state institution resident numbers between 1988 and 2000. Data were drawn from the University of Minnesota's *residential information system project* (RISP; e.g., see Prouty, Lakin, & Smith, 2002). The purpose of this comparison was to assess the impact of large-scale deinstitutionalization on per diems and on total expenditure on state institutions.

In Figure 13.3, the total annual state-institution population for each group of states is shown in the upper chart, expressed as a percentage of

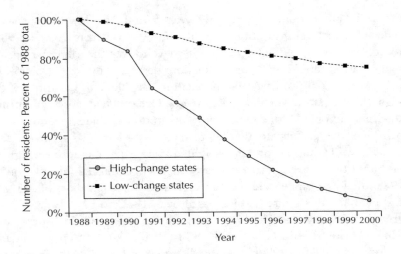

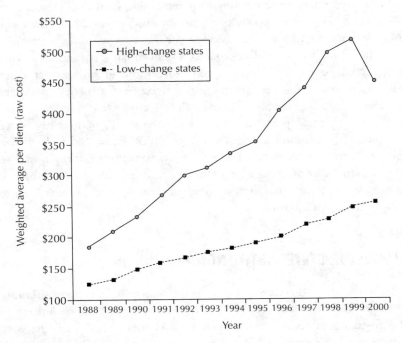

Figure 13.3. Change over time in number of state institution residents (upper chart) and average raw per diem (lower chart) by group of states.

the 1988 population. Over the 12-year period, the low-change states reduced their total institutional population by 7,613 from 28,564 (1988), to 20,951 (2000), to 73.4% of its 1988 level. Over the same period, the high-change states' institution populations decreased by 5,899 from 6,276, to 377, or to 6.0% of the 1988 population. By 2000, all but three of the high-change states (Michigan, Minnesota, Oregon) had closed all of their state institutions. With total closure, institutional resident numbers and per diems in a given state each fell to zero.

Figure 13.3 also shows the weighted average per diem for each group of states (lower chart) in current (raw) dollars not adjusted for inflation. In 1988, the low-change states had a weighted average per diem of $132.22, and by 2000, this figure had increased by $118.92 to $251.14, an 89.9% growth over 12 years. The high-change states experienced an increase of $264.09 from $184.62 (1988) to $448.71 (2000), or 143.0% over the same period, although in 1999 the weighted average was $514.46, an increase of 178.7% more than 1988's weighted average. The *decrease* in the weighted average per diem for the 12 high-change states from 1999 to 2000 was partly a consequence of Hawaii closing its last large state-operated facility in 1999, a year when the per diem for remaining Hawaiian residents (in 1999) was $733. Having no state-institution residents in 2000, Hawaii did not contribute to the weighted average per diem across states in 2000.

The 12 high-change states that experienced large reductions in their institutional populations encountered more rapid growth in per diems than the low-change states. Much of the difference in growth in per diems can be attributed to diseconomies of reduced scale.

Later in this chapter, we use the data from the 12 high-change states to estimate the magnitude of such diseconomies of reduced scale. Before doing this, we analyze detailed data from deinstitutionalization in Minnesota to examine competing explanations (i.e., other than diseconomies of reduced scale) of the rapid increase in institutional per diems during large-scale deinstitutionalization.

MINNESOTA STATE INSTITUTION PER DIEMS

Many of the states that have yet to achieve large-scale deinstitutionalization have large institutional populations and operate multiple facilities. Among the 12 high-change states shown in Figure 13.3, Minnesota had the largest state institution population, and Minnesota closed *multiple* institutions during the 1990s. We argued that diseconomies of reduced scale largely accounted for the more rapid growth in per diems in the high-change states; however, other factors could also account for growth in per diems, such as 1) inflation, 2) case mix (i.e., aggregated characteristics of the group of people served), or 3) systemwide increases in service expenditures that were not institution specific. We used deinstitutionalization in Minnesota as a case study to evaluate whether any or all of these three competing explanations could account for the rapid growth in per diems in that state.

Inflation

The trend in state institution per diems in Minnesota (Figure 13.4) mirrored the 12 high-change states' trend evident in Figure 13.3. On June 30, 1990, there were 1,337 residents in 7 state institutions in Minnesota, with an average per diem of $208, but by June 1997, only 244 residents remained, at an average daily cost of $445 ($354 expressed in 1990 dollars) (Prouty, Smith, & Lakin, 2001). Figure 13.4 shows the total Minnesota state-institution population (gray line with white circles; values shown on the left axis) together with raw and inflation-adjusted (1990 = $1) per diems (black line with black circles and dashed line with black squares; values shown on right axis) for the period of 1990–1997.

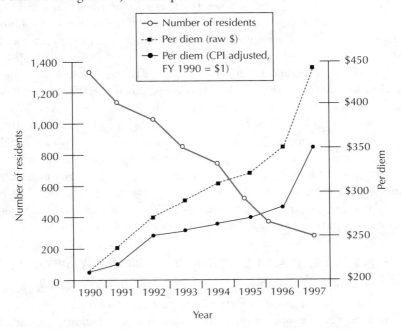

Figure 13.4.   Trends in Minnesota state institution resident numbers and per diems during downsizing.

Not surprisingly, inflation accounted for some of the increase in per diems over time. Even so, accompanying the 81.8% population decline between June 1990 and June 1997 was a 70.3% real (Consumer Price Index [CPI] adjusted) increase in average per-person daily expenditure, with a correlation between these variables of $r = -.93$, indicating a very strong association between increasing real per diems and falling institutional population.

Minnesota Longitudinal Study

Data from a longitudinal study of deinstitutionalization in Minnesota—the Minnesota Longitudinal Study—enabled us to evaluate whether case-mix factors or systemwide increases in expenditures could account for the increases in institutional per diems. This study utilized detailed annual data on services, expenditures, and outcomes for 190 residents of two Minnesota state institutions, most of whom moved to community settings during the study period of 1990 to 1997.

Case Mix: Selection Bias When Choosing Movers

If individuals with milder disabilities moved first, then as each wave of individuals with lower-support needs left the institutions, the remaining Minnesota institutional population would have had successively higher support needs, which *may* help account for higher and higher institutional per diems for individuals who stayed. To evaluate this selection-bias proposition, we compared Inventory for Client and Agency Planning (ICAP) service scores (Bruininks, Hill, Weatherman, & Woodcock, 1986) for individuals who remained institutionalized during each year ("stayers"), and for those who moved during that year ("movers"). These scores provide a valid index of the person's need for support based on a weighted combination of the ICAP adaptive behavior and challenging behavior scores. *T*-test comparisons for each year from 1991 to 1996 revealed no significant differences between movers and stayers, so increased institutional per diems over time in Minnesota could not be attributed to changes in case mix in the institutions during this period.

Changes in Per-Person Expenditure in Community Services

Rising institutional per diems may have been due to increases in expenditure related to systemwide factors, not just institution-specific cost increases; however, simple comparisons of statewide expenditure trends in institutional and community services are complicated by case-mix differences between these two service types. As noted, there were no case-mix differences for institutional and community participants in the Minnesota Longitudinal Study, and all had long histories of institutional living. We examined changes over time in CPI adjusted (real) service expenditures for study participants who moved to Minnesota community settings (both ICFs/MR and HCBS Waiver–funded services). This approach provided a fair comparison with trends in real institutional per diems because we compared individuals with similar personal characteristics and backgrounds.

Participants who remained institutionalized showed highly significant increases in real institutional per-person expenditures over time ($p < .001$), but there were no significant increases in real service costs during 3 years for those who moved to community ICF/MR or HCBS Waiver settings. These findings are consistent with the notion that, even after adjustment for inflation, rising institutional per-person expenditures are related to diseconomies of reduced scale as people moved out of the institutions and *not* to case-mix factors or systemwide increases in per diems.

MAGNITUDE OF DISECONOMIES OF REDUCED SCALE

Per diems increased about 5% per year (on average) across the country (all states) during 1988–2000 (Prouty & Lakin, 2000). In order to separate the effects on per diems of downsizing versus other factors, we subtracted 5.0 percentage points from the actual percentage change in per diems each year for the 12 high-change states. This action yields an *adjusted* change in per diems, likely attributable to *diseconomies of reduced scale* or the difficulty in reducing *fixed* and *semi-fixed* costs quickly.

On average (excluding outliers), a 6.0% annual decline in number of residents served in state institutions was associated with a 1% increase in per diem attributable to diseconomies of reduced scale. More detailed information about the computational procedures underlying this estimate may be found in Shea (2001).

Stated in this way, the effect of diseconomies of reduced scale appears small, but it should be understood that this is an *annual* estimate that *compounds* over time. For example, consider a hypothetical institution system of 1,000 residents with average annual per-person expenditure of $100,000 and movement to the community of 180 people each year. In Year 1, 180 movers represent 18% of the population, so diseconomies of reduced scale *alone* would add 3% [(18% ÷ 6%) × 1%] to the average cost of serving the remaining institutional residents. By the end of Year 3, 540 residents would have moved, and 460 would remain in institutions. In Year 4, the next 180 movers would make up 39% of the institutional population of 460, so diseconomies of reduced scale *alone* would add 6.5% [(39% ÷ 6%) × 1%] to average institutional costs in Year 4, on top of the compound effects of 3% in Year 1, 3.7% in Year 2, and 4.7% in Year 3.

As is seen in the fiscal analysis of deinstitutionalization in California presented later in this chapter, diseconomies of reduced scale can have substantial cumulative systemwide impacts over time. Understanding such impacts and taking them into account when planning and costing deinstitutionalization initiatives is important. One implication of the cumulative effects of diseconomies of reduced scale is that institutional per diems can become extremely high when only a small proportion of the original institutional population remains, as exemplified by the situation in Hawaii in 1999 mentioned previously, when per diems reached $733, or around $267,500 per person annually. Under these circumstances, a number of states have chosen to entirely close their public institutions.

The estimate of a 1% increase in per diem with a 6% annual decline in number of residents served in institutions also has other important implications. Assuming that per diems continue to increase at an average of 5% each year due to inflation and other factors, a 6% annual decrease in an institution's population would be offset by a 6% rise in per diem (5% inflation, etc. + 1% diseconomies of reduced scale). Using these assumptions, when the institutional population falls by *more than* 6% per year, total raw expenditure actually declines.

Finally, the estimate of a 1% increase in per diem with a 6% annual decline in institution resident numbers is simply an average across the 12 high-change states relative to the nation as a whole. In a given situation, the magnitude of diseconomies of reduced scale is affected by the way that the institution is downsized. As noted, the speed, scale, and completeness of deinstitutionalization all impact institutional costs. For the purposes of this chapter, we have assumed that states such as California will do much the same as the average of the 12 high-change states in reducing fixed and semi-fixed costs over time during deinstitutionalization.

TOTAL EXPENDITURES BY HIGH-CHANGE VERSUS LOW-CHANGE STATES ON INSTITUTIONS

Even though institutional per diems increased rapidly in high-change states (see Figure 13.3), this trend was more than offset in these states by the decline in state-institution population numbers. The relative (percentage) decrease in number of residents in the 12 high-change states was greater than the relative increase in per diems for all but two of the years between 1988 and 2000. Therefore, estimated *total* raw outlays on state institutions (average daily expenditures × average daily residents × 365 days) in these 12 states generally *declined* from one year to the next (see Figure 13.5). All of these states closed one or more state institutions during 1988–2000.

Raw (not adjusted for inflation) total annual expenditure on institutional services declined from $424 million (1988) to $62 million (2000) for the 12 high-change states. That is, these states had scope to reallocate a very substantial portion of the previous institutional budget to help pay for community services for former institution residents. The opposite was true for the 13 low-change states. Annual raw expenditure on state institution services in these states totaled $1,382 million in 1988, but by 2000 this amount had risen to $1,926 million, despite a 26.6% fall in institu-

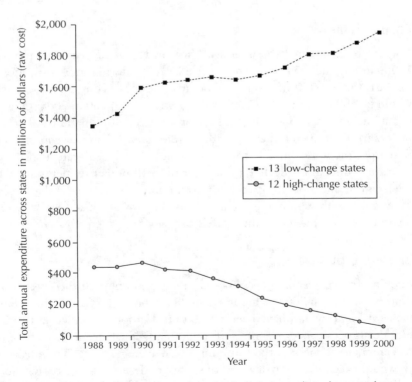

Figure 13.5. Change over time in total annual raw state institution expenditures by group of states.

tional population during this time. Five of these 13 states (Arkansas, Delaware, Mississippi, Nebraska, Nevada) had no closures of state institutions at all. These opposing trends in total annual raw expenditure for the two groups of states are shown in Figure 13.5.

ECONOMICS OF DEINSTITUTIONALIZATION IN CALIFORNIA

As noted previously, major downsizing and closure of state institutions has mostly taken place in smaller states with relatively small state-institution systems. Shea (2001) undertook a detailed fiscal analysis of California Assembly Bill 896 (AB896) (2001) that called for the closing of at least three of the state's five large developmental centers over a 7-year period. That bill was unsuccessful, but other legislators have subsequently introduced similar bills. The fiscal analysis of AB896 remains of considerable interest, however, because it examines the fiscal consequences of large-scale deinstitutionalization within a very large state-institution system.

Assumptions

For the purposes of fiscal analysis, Shea made a series of assumptions. From among the 3,700 residents of five large California state institutions in 2001, the net shift of residents from institutions to community settings would be 500 per year from 2002 to 2007 with a final 200 in 2008. Ongoing annual increases in raw expenditure associated with inflation and other factors were assumed to be 5%, with an additional 1% increase in institutional per diem attributable to diseconomies of reduced scale associated with each annual 6% decline in number of institutional residents served. The nature and operating costs of community services were based on experience with community placements for former California state-institution residents under the Coffelt Settlement Agreement.

Operating Outlays

Looking first at *operating* (as opposed to *capital*) outlays, if these assumptions held, then in 2002, some $81.2 million (about half federal; half state General Fund) would have been freed up in California to meet expenditure needs occasioned by a net shift of 500 individuals from developmental centers to services in the community. On average, these 500 individuals would have received half a year of service at developmental centers and half a year in the community. Before any adjustment for *diseconomies of reduced scale*, one half of the $81.2 million would have been used at developmental centers (i.e., $40.6 million), and one half in the community (i.e., $40.6 million). Of the latter $40.6 million, $6.3 million is needed to cover average cost increases occasioned by *diseconomies of reduced scale* in the institutions. This figure is calculated by multiplying $1,827 per person ($164,043–$162,216), by the reduced average number of residents (3,450) (see Table 13.1). The annual cost of diseconomies of reduced scale will rise from $6.3 million annually in 2002 to about $40 million per year by 2007 (see Table 13.2). Clearly, this issue represents one important factor in the overall planning for and costing of deinstitutionalization.

A fundamental issue for the economic viability of large-scale institutional downsizing, as envisaged by AB896, is the extent to which funding used to pay for institutional services can be transferred to finance community services as residents move to community settings. This issue is examined in Table 13.2. The top row of this table shows that, with 5% annual budget growth due to inflation and other factors, the institutional budget would rise from $600.2 million in 2002 to $804.3 million in 2008 if the institutional population remained unchanged at 3,700. Under the assumptions described previously, as institution residents moved to community services, a variety of costs would need to be met. These include the continued operation of the downsized institutions for the residents who remain, additional costs associated with diseconomies of reduced scale, and funding of extra transition assistance from institutional staff. The cost of community services for the former institution residents also needs to be met: one-time start-up costs, operating costs of community services, and additional case-management and transition assistance by community case managers. Even after all of these factors were taken into account, Shea's analysis showed that some funds would not be expended and could be used to fund enhanced community services, such as meeting the urgent, unmet service needs of others. Funds available for enhanced community services are shown in the bottom row of Table 13.2 and rise from $5.9 million in 2002 to $294.6 million in 2008.

The analysis summarized in Table 13.2 indicates that, overall, the institutional downsizing proposed by AB896 would be cost neutral, with the possible exception of some generic service funding in the short run. In terms of the operating costs of the institutional and community disability services involved, all of the changes could be funded out of the funds currently used to provide services in the institutions. That is, the proposed AB896 was found to be economically sustainable and cost neutral (or better). On the basis of this analysis, the current failure to proceed with large-

Table 13.1. Projected operating costs (raw cost, not adjusted for inflation) at California State Institutions in comparison with *Status Quo* assumptions, from 2002 to 2008

Item	2002	2003	2004	2005	2006	2007	2008
Status quo							
1. Institution operating expenditures to serve 3,700 people (in millions of dollars)	$600.2	$630.2	$661.7	$694.8	$729.5	$766.0	$804.3
Proposed change							
2. Average number of residents	3,450	2,950	2,450	1,950	1,450	950	750
3. Annual percent of change in average number of residents	−6.8%	−14.5%	−16.9%	−20.4%	−25.6%	−34.5%	−21.1%
4. Assumed percent of change in cost per resident-year:							
4a. Attributable to diseconomies of reduced scale only	1.1%	2.4%	2.8%	3.4%	4.3%	5.7%	3.5%
4b. Attributable to other factors only	*	5.0%	5.0%	5.0%	5.0%	5.0%	5.0%
Overall, combined (or total)	1.1%	7.4%	7.8%	8.4%	9.3%	10.7%	8.5%
5. Projected cost per resident-year:							
5a. Attributable to diseconomies of reduced scale only (in dollars)	$164,043	$168,005	$172,751	$178,627	$186,261	$196,965	$203,876
5b. Attributable to other factors only (in dollars)	$162,216*	$170,327	$178,843	$187,786	$197,175	$207,034	$217,385
Overall, combined (or total) (in dollars)	$164,043	$176,208	$189,996	$205,958	$225,058	$249,245	$270,453
6. Total institutional expenditures, ignoring diseconomies of reduced scale only (in millions of dollars)	$559.6	$502.5	$438.2	$366.2	$285.9	$196.7	$163.0
7. Amount available in the budget (if ½ state and ½ federal) to serve deflections and movers to the community (net shift)** (in millions of dollars)	$40.6	$127.7	$223.5	$328.6	$443.6	$569.3	$641.3

From Shea, R. (2001). *Fiscal analysis of Assembly Bill 896. California's developmental services system unification, finance and economic issues.* Napa, CA: Allen, Shea, & Associates; adapted by permission.

Note: *Status quo* institution operating expenditures assume a constant number of residents (3,700) and a projected increase in unit costs (per-diem or per-annum cost for each person) of 5% per year, starting with a per-annum cost of $162,216 per person in 2002. The values in Row 4a are calculated by dividing the numbers in Row 3 by 6.0, without regard to sign. The values in Row 4b reflect an assumption that unit costs attributable to "factors other than diseconomies of reduced scale" will rise by 5% per year beyond the budgeted year of 2002.

*Budgeted costs reflect various factors affecting costs in 2002, except for diseconomies of reduced scale.

**500 for half-year in 2002; 500 for half-year in 2003, plus 500 for full-year in 2003; and so forth.

Table 13.2. Projected use of budget (in millions of raw dollars) for institutional and community services by year, assuming 50% federal financial participation

Item	2002	2003	2004	2005	2006	2007	2008
Institutions' status quo operating expenditures to serve 3,700 residents	$600.2	$630.2	$661.7	$694.8	$729.5	$766.0	$804.3
Institutional services—subtract							
a. Money for institution services (ignoring diseconomies of reduced scale)	$559.6	$502.5	$438.2	$366.2	$285.9	$196.7	$163.0
b. Money for diseconomies of reduced scale	$6.3	$17.3	$27.3	$35.4	$40.4	$40.1	$39.8
c. Money for extra transition assistance from institution staff	$2.5	$2.6	$2.8	$2.9	$3.0	$3.2	$1.3
Budget remaining to fund community services	**$31.8**	**$107.8**	**$193.5**	**$290.3**	**$400.2**	**$526.1**	**$600.1**
Community services—subtract							
a. Money for one-time, added start-up costs	$5.2	$5.4	$5.7	$6.0	$6.3	$6.6	$1.8
b. Money for operating costs in the community for former institution residents	$17.9	$56.2	$98.4	$144.7	$195.3	$250.7	$296.8
c. Money for additional community case manager, case management, and transition assistance	$2.8	$3.7	4.6	$5.6	$6.7	$7.9	$6.9
Budget remaining to fund enhanced community services[a]	**$5.9**	**$42.5**	**$84.8**	**$134.0**	**$191.9**	**$260.9**	**$294.6**

From Shea, R. (2001). *Fiscal analysis of Assembly Bill 896. California's developmental services system unification, finance, and economic issues.* Napa, CA: Allen, Shea, & Associates; adapted by permission.

Notes: Status quo DC operating expenditures assume constant number of residents (3,700) and a projected increase in unit costs (per-diem or per-annum cost for each person) of 5% per year, starting with a per annum cost of $162,216 per person in 2002.

[a]Detail may not add exactly due to rounding.

scale deinstitutionalization in California was not due to fiscal impediments (see Shea, 2001, for details).

Capital Expenditures

In some states, including California, physical plant needs of aging institutions are a factor in deinstitutionalization. In 1997, a firm (i.e., Vanir Construction Management) was retained by the State of California to study physical facility needs at California's five large, state-operated facilities. In 1998, the *Vanir Report* (Vanir Construction Management, 1998) estimated the cost of capital improvements at the five developmental centers to meet accessibility (as dictated by the Americans with Disabilities

Act [ADA] of 1990, PL 101-336), seismic safety, and building code standards—and to make modest program improvements—at $0.9–$1.4 billion.
More money would be needed today to accomplish this work. Based on
data provided by California's Department of Developmental Services and
a set of working assumptions (e.g., time sequence of outlays, which developmental centers would be closed and when, the impact of consolidation
within developmental centers staying open), Shea estimated that approximately half ($750 million–$1.0 billion) of the $1.5–$2.0 billion in construction outlays could be avoided by passage of AB896.

IDENTIFYING AND REPLACING INSTITUTIONAL FUNCTIONS

Public institutions have served many social functions. Wolfensberger
(1975) wrote compellingly about these functions and depicted U.S. public
institutions as passing through three periods of social function/justifica-
tion prior to 1925: 1) making the "deviant" person "undeviant"; 2) shel-
tering the "deviant" person from society; and 3) protecting society from
the "deviant" person. By 1925, Wolfensberger argued that the public institution had entered a period characterized by a "loss of rationales," when
institutional placements grew largely on the basis of momentum.

The era of deinstitutionalization brought reconsideration of the purposes that institutions fulfilled. In that era, institutions were viewed

- As places for people who could not adjust to community life

- As locales for people who needed the concentrated attention of specialists in health care, behavioral therapy, and other disciplines

- As settings to train people in the skills needed for successful community living

- As placements of last resort for people who no one else will serve

- As locations for people who were considered "a danger to themselves
  and others"

- As areas for people who were thought to be too expensive to serve in
  the community

As populations of public institutions have continued to fall, increasingly
specialized roles have been ascribed to institutions. With ultimate closure of
public institutions, states must identify the roles and services that the public
institutions are providing so that alternative sources can be established. This
process often requires systematic analysis of each institutional admission and
readmission. Frequently, the roles/services sustaining the institution have

relatively little to do with the characteristics and "treatment" needs of individuals and more to do with their life circumstances. For example, many
public institutions serve as the one place where there is always an open "bed"
in times of crisis (e.g., death or illness of the primary care provider, unex-
pected and immediate demission from community settings). Identifying
such roles/services provided by institutions that will still be needed after
their closure is an important aspect of the closure process. Likewise, designing those features into the system of community supports as programs or
enhanced capacities is an important aspect of institutional closure and represents an additional cost. Probably the most commonly identified func-
tion/service needed in support of public institution closure is community-
based behavioral support and crisis response (see Hanson, Wieseler, &
Lakin, 2002), but the nature of the community service needed depends on
analysis of the roles and functions of the specific institution to be closed.

CONCLUSION

In any analysis of public expenditures, including expenditures for services
for people with ID/DD, ultimately the resources expended are determined
much more by resource-allocation traditions than by inherent costs.
Attempting modest control for diseconomies of reduced scale, the five
states (Georgia, Illinois, Iowa, Missouri, Nebraska) with state-institution
population reductions from 1980 to 2002 in the range of 42.0% to 48.0%
had average daily state-institution per-diem costs in FY 2002 that ranged
from $235 (Missouri) to $334 (Illinois). Nine states (California, Delaware,
Montana, New Jersey, Ohio, Tennessee, Texas, Virginia, Wisconsin) with
state-institution population reductions from 1980 to 2002 that ranged
from 50.0% to 62.0% had average per-diem costs that ranged from $253
(Texas) to $589 (Tennessee). Similarly, combining Medicaid ICF/MR and
HCBS Waiver expenditures for states showed that, in FY 2003, states had
average combined annual per-person expenditures that ranged from less
than $35,000 in nine states to more than $70,000 in six states. That is,
there is enormous variability between states in the cost of ID/DD services.

    Because there is no "right amount" that services should cost, the
amounts services do cost are affected by various factors. One set of factors that
may well substantially affect expenditures in the next few years is the cost of
direct-support workers. We noted previously the wage differential between
direct-support workers in public institutions and community-service settings.
Perhaps more relevant to the long-term costs of community alternatives is the
differential between community support workers and workers in general.

In 2000, the average wages of nonstate direct support workers were just 55.4% of the average for all workers (Polister et al., 2003). Direct-support staff vacancies are a growing reality in community services. At some point, worker shortages may begin to exert a substantial pressure on wages. Because ultimately the prices paid for services are constrained by government allocations for them, and with states currently experiencing great difficulty in even maintaining the status quo, the ultimate outcomes of wage pressures are hard to predict. If pressures are sufficient to cause substantial worsening of workforce stability, governments may intervene with improved compensation for workers (voluntarily, through regulatory agencies requiring improved workforce performance, or through court challenges). Should such pressures lead to essentially the same wages being available for community direct support as for institutional direct support, the price advantages for community services would be substantially reduced, if not reversed. What would remain of course are the well-established benefits in quality of life, social relationships, and community participation that are experienced by people living in community settings.

REFERENCES

Americans with Disabilities Act (ADA) of 1990, PL 101-336, 42 U.S.C. §§ 12101 *et seq.*

Ashbaugh, J., & Allard, M.A. (1984). *Comparative analyses of the cost of residential, day and other programs within institutional and community settings.* Cambridge, MA: Human Services Research Institute.

Bensberg, G., & Smith, J.J. (1984). *Comparative costs of public residential and community residential facilities for the mentally retarded.* Lubbock: Texas Tech University, Research and Training Center in Mental Retardation.

Bruininks, R.H., Hill, B.K., Weatherman, R.F., & Woodcock, R.W. (1986). *Inventory for Client and Agency Planning (ICAP).* Chicago: Riverside Publications.

California Assembly Bill 896 (2001).

Campbell, E.M., & Heal, L.W. (1995). Prediction of cost, rate, and staffing by provider and client characteristics. *American Journal on Mental Retardation, 100,* 17–35.

Conroy, J.W. (1998). *Are people better off? Outcomes of the closure of Winfield State Hospital.* Report submitted to the Kansas Council on Developmental Disabilities. (Available from the Center for Outcome Analysis, Ardmore, PA)

Conroy, J.W., & Bradley, V.J. (1985). *The Pennhurst longitudinal study: A report of five years of research and analysis.* Philadelphia: Temple University Developmental Disabilities Center.

Coucouvanis, K., Polister, B., Prouty, R.W., Bruininks, R.W., & Lakin, K.C. (2003). Current populations and longitudinal trends of state residential settings (1950–2002). In R.W. Prouty, G. Smith, & K.C. Lakin (Eds.), *Residential services for persons with developmental disabilities: Status and trends through 2002* (pp. 3–16). Minneapolis: University of Minnesota, Research and Training Center on Community Living, Institute on Community Integration. Also available on-line at http://rtc.umn.edu

Eastwood, E.A. (1985). *Community living study: Three reports of client development, family impact, and the cost of services among community-based and institutionalized persons with mental retardation.* Belchertown, MA: Belchertown State School.

Emerson, E., & Hatton, C. (1996). Deinstitutionalization in the UK and Ireland: Outcomes for service users. *Journal of Intellectual & Developmental Disability, 21,* 17–37.

Feinstein, C., Lemanowicz, J., & Conroy, J. (1988). *A survey of family satisfaction with regional treatment centers and community services to persons with mental retardation in Minnesota.* Philadelphia: Temple University, Developmental Disabilities Center.

Felce, D., de Kock, U., & Repp, A.C. (1986). An eco-behavioral analysis of small community-based houses and traditional large hospitals for severely and profoundly mentally handicapped adults. *Applied Research in Mental Retardation, 7,* 393–408.

Hanson, R., Wieseler, N., & Lakin, K.C. (Eds.). (2002). *Crisis prevention and response in the community.* Washington, DC: American Association on Mental Retardation.

Hayden, M.F. (1997). Class-action, civil rights litigation for institutionalized persons with mental retardation and other developmental disabilities: A review. *Mental and Physical Disabilities Law Reporter, 21*(3), 411–423.

Hill, B.K., & Bruininks, R.H. (1981). *Family, leisure, and social activities of mentally retarded people in residential facilities.* Minneapolis: University of Minnesota, Department of Educational Psychology.

Horner, R.H., Stoner, S.K., & Ferguson, D.L. (1988). *An activity-based analysis of deinstitutionalization: The effects of community re-entry on the lives of residents leaving Oregon's Fairview Training Center.* Eugene: University of Oregon, Specialized Training Program, Center on Human Development.

Jones, P.A., Conroy, J.W., Feinstein, C.S., & Lemanowicz, J.A. (1984). A matched comparison study of cost-effectiveness: Institutionalized and deinstitutionalized people. *Journal of The Association for the Severely Handicapped, 9,* 304–313.

Kim, S., Larson, S.A., & Lakin, K.C. (2001). Behavioural outcomes of deinstitutionalisation of people with intellectual disability: A review of U.S. studies conducted between 1980 and 1999. *Journal of Intellectual & Developmental Disability, 26,* 35–50.

Knobbe, C.A., Carey, S.P., Rhodes, L., & Horner, R.H. (1995). Benefit–cost analysis of community residential versus institutional services for adults with severe mental retardation and challenging behaviors. *American Journal on Mental Retardation, 99,* 533–541.

Larson, S.A., & Lakin, K.C. (1991). Parent attitudes about residential placement before and after deinstitutionalization: A research synthesis. *Journal of The Association for Persons with Severe Handicaps, 16,* 25–38.

Minnesota Department of Public Welfare. (1979). *Residential care study.* St. Paul, MN: Author.

Mitchell, D., & Braddock, D. (1994). Compensation and turnover of direct care staff. In M.F. Hayden & B.H. Abery (Eds.), *Challenges for a service system in transition: Ensuring quality community experiences for persons with developmental disabilities* (pp. 289–312). Baltimore: Paul H. Brookes Publishing Co.

O'Neil, J., Brown, M., Gordon, W., Schonhorn, R., & Green, E. (1981). Activity patterns of mentally retarded adults in institutions and communities—a longitudinal study. *Applied Research in Mental Retardation, 2,* 267–379.

Polister, B., Lakin, K.C., & Prouty, R. (2003). Wages of direct support professionals serving persons with intellectual and developmental disabilities: A survey of state agencies and private residential provider trade associations. *Policy Research Brief, 14*(2). (Available from the University of Minnesota, Institute on Community Integration, Minneapolis, or on-line at http://rtc.umn.edu)

Prouty, R.W., & Lakin, K.C. (Eds.). (2000). *Residential services for persons with developmental disabilities: Status and trends through 1999.* Minneapolis: University of Minnesota, Research and Training Center on Community Living, Institute on Community Integration. (Available on-line at http://rtc.umn.edu)

Prouty, R.W., Lakin, K.C., & Smith, G. (Eds.). (2002). *Residential services for persons with developmental disabilities: Status and trends through 2001.* Minneapolis: University of Minnesota, Research and Training Center on Community Living, Institute on Community Integration. (Available on-line at http://rtc.umn.edu)

Prouty, R.W., Smith, G., & Lakin, K.C. (Eds.). (2001). *Residential services for persons with developmental disabilities: Status and trends through 2000.* Minneapolis: University of Minnesota, Research and Training Center on Community Living, Institute on Community Integration. (Available on-line at http://rtc.umn.edu)

Prouty, R.W., Smith, G., & Lakin, K.C. (Eds.). (2003). *Residential services for persons with developmental disabilities: Status and trends through 2002.* Minneapolis: University of Minnesota, Research and Training Center on Community Living, Institute on Community Integration. (Available on-line at http://rtc.umn.edu)

Rhoades, J.A., & Altman, B.M. (2001). Personal characteristics and contextual factors associated with residential expenditures for individuals with mental retardation. *Mental Retardation, 39,* 114–129.

Schalock, M., & Fredericks, H.D.B. (1990). Comparative costs for institutional services and services for selected populations in the community. *Behavioral Residential Treatment, 5,* 271–286.

Scheerenberger, R. (1965). A current census of state institutions for the mentally retarded. *Mental Retardation, 3*(1), 4–6.

Shea, R. (2001). *Fiscal analysis of Assembly Bill 896. California's developmental services system unification, finance and economic issues.* Napa, CA: Allen, Shea, & Associates.

Stancliffe, R.J., & Lakin, K.C. (1998). Analysis of expenditures and outcomes of residential alternatives for persons with developmental disabilities. *American Journal on Mental Retardation, 102,* 552–568.

Touche Ross. (1980). *Cost study of the community-based mental retardation regions and the Beatrice State Developmental Center.* Lincoln, NE: Department of Public Institutions.

Vanir Construction Management. (1998). *Condition assessment and master planning: DDS developmental centers, final report summary: Vol. 1. Report prepared for the California Department of Developmental Services (DDS) and the California Department of General Services (DGS), Residential Services Division (RESD), Project Management Branch (PMB).* Sacramento, CA: Author.

Wolfensberger, W. (1975). *The origins and nature of our institutional models.* Syracuse, NY: Syracuse University, Human Policy Press.

Young, L., Sigafoos, J., Suttie, J., Ashman, A., & Grevell, P. (1998). Deinstitutionalisation of persons with intellectual disabilities: A review of Australian studies. *Journal of Intellectual & Developmental Disability, 23,* 155–170.

CHAPTER 14

Expenditures and Outcomes

Directions in Financing, Policy, and Research

K. Charlie Lakin and Roger J. Stancliffe

In January 2003, a National Goals Conference on Intellectual and Developmental Disability was held in Washington, D.C. The conference was sponsored by 9 federal agencies and 16 other professional, advocacy, and research organizations. Its purpose was to identify and examine national goals for individuals with intellectual and/or developmental disabilities (ID/DD) and the knowledge and policy development needed to achieve them. By examining national laws, regulations, judicial decisions, executive orders, consensus conference findings, and other sources, conference participants identified six broad commitments made to people with ID/DD in the United States. These included to (National Goals Conference, 2003):

- Increase self-determination and personal control in decisions affecting oneself and one's family

- Provide opportunities to live, participate, and receive needed services in one's own community

- Improve the quality of life for individuals and families as they define it for themselves

- Support families as the most permanent unit of development, protection, and assistance

- Invest in each individual's developmental potential and capacity to contribute in age-related roles as productive and respected community members

- Ensure access to sufficient, high-quality health and social supports to protect the health, safety, rights, and essential well-being of each individual

Although many sources of these national goals and commitments were identified, one law stood out together with a subsequent clarification by the U.S. Supreme Court and Executive Order by the President for its full implementation. This combination included the Americans with Disabilities Act (ADA) of 1990 (PL 101-336), the Supreme Court's interpretation in *Olmstead v. L.C.* (1999), and the President's New Freedom Initiative.

In *Olmstead*, the U.S. Supreme Court ruled that Title II of the ADA required states to provide the services, programs, and activities developed for people with disabilities in the "most integrated setting appropriate." The Supreme Court also concluded that states were obligated to place qualified individuals with disabilities in community settings, rather than in institutions, 1) when treatment professionals determined that a community placement was appropriate; 2) when the individuals themselves did not oppose an appropriate community placement; and 3) when the state in which the person lived could reasonably accommodate the community placement, taking into account the resources available and the needs of others with disabilities.

In June 2001, President George W. Bush signed an Executive Order committing the Executive Branch of the U.S. government to the principal findings of *Olmstead* that "unjustified isolation or segregation of qualified individuals with disabilities through institutionalization is a form of disability-based discrimination prohibited by Title II of the Americans with Disabilities Act of 1990 (ADA)." The Executive Order stipulated that, "the United States is committed to community-based alternatives for individuals with disabilities and recognizes that such services advance the best interests of Americans."

With the national legislative, judicial, and administrative branches fully committed to community lives for people with ID/DD, needed supports for fully integrated, satisfying lives for individuals with ID/DD seem nearly guaranteed. In reality, no guarantee of adequate community support is presently being enforced, and the challenges associated with fulfilling that promise continue to grow. The promise of community as opposed to institution living is still more associated with individual state actions than expressed national commitments. In 10 states in June 2002, more than 30% of all residential-support recipients with ID/DD were housed in developmental disability institutions of 16 or more residents (increasing to

14 states when nursing home residents with ID/DD are included). In contrast, in 11 states fewer than 5% of all residential-support recipients were housed in institutions of 16 or more residents. Because many states vary substantially in the sufficiency of their allocation of resources to support people eligible for and seeking services, the number of people waiting for services ranges from virtually none in a few states to thousands in others (Prouty, Smith, & Lakin, 2003).

INCREASING PREVALENCE OF DISABILITY

As states struggle to simply maintain current levels of spending for individual services, substantial new challenges are emerging on state capacities to do so. A primary factor in the likelihood of future expectations of greater cost effectiveness and cost containment is the rapidly increasing overall prevalence of disability in the United States and other industrial nations. Although these increases will be most noticed within programs of support for people with ID/DD, their effects on the overall demand and expense of long-term supports in general will clearly affect people with ID/DD.

The 1997 National Health Interview Survey (NHIS) used the presence of limitations in Activities of Daily Living (for which personal assistance is needed as the definition of disability) to determine that 55% of the 9.3 million people within the United States with "significant" disabilities were 65 years and older (see Figure 14.1). Within the noninstitutionalized population, people 65 years and older make up 13% of the total population and 55% of the people with limitations that require assistance. People older than 80 years make up 3% of the population and 27% of the people with functional limitations requiring personal assistance. Clearly, the size of the population older than 65 years, and especially older than 80 or 85, is a major factor in long-term support demands in the United States. As shown in Figure 14.2, the U.S. population of people 65 years and older is projected to increase from 36.4 million in July 2004 to 39.7 million in 2010, to 46.0 million in 2015, to 53.7 million in 2020, and to 62.6 million in 2025—that is, 72% in a single generation!

According to the National Nursing Home Survey of 1997 and the National Home Health and Hospice Care Survey of 1998, about one in four people 85 years or older in the United States receives nursing, assisted living, or home health services. Between 2000 and 2025, the number of people 85 years and older is estimated to increase from 4.2 million to 7.4 million,

General population = 263 million

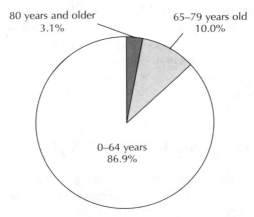

People with significant disabilities = 9.35 million

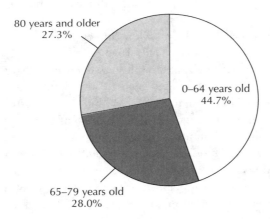

Figure 14.1. Breakdown of general population and population with Activities of Daily Living and Instrumental Activities of Daily Living limitations and requiring assistance in the United States by age group in 1997. *Source:* University of Minnesota, 1997.

more than 75%. In just 15 years, between 2025 and 2040, the number of people 85 and older will nearly double again to 14.3 million (see Figure 14.3). Dramatic increases in the number of older people in the United States are going to have very substantial effects on demand for long-term care services and on the overall costs of supporting people with disabilities.

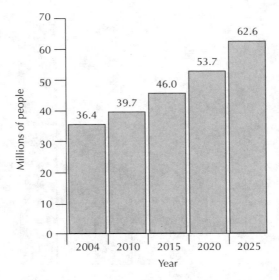

Figure 14.2. Projections of growth in members of the U.S. population who are 65 years and older. *Source:* U.S. Census Bureau, 2001.

Between 2000 and 2020, the number of individuals age 65 or older with significant limitations in major life activities can be projected to increase by about 5.6 million people. Using present ratios of people with significant limitations to actual long-term services and support recipients, these demographic shifts can be expected to increase long-term service and support demand by about 1.6 million people by 2020. This demand is about three times the current number of U.S. residents with ID/DD using Medicaid Intermediate Care Facility for the Mentally Retarded (ICF/ MR), Medicaid Home and Community-Based Services (HCBS) Waiver programs, and nursing-home services altogether.

Of course, many other factors are likely to affect the prevalence of disability in the future. Increased survival rates from trauma and prematurity contribute to increased demand for disability-related supports; so, too, does the increasing longevity of people with ID/DD. Braddock and colleagues (Chapter 2) reported that the mean age at death of people with ID/DD increased from 59 years in the 1970s to 66 years in 1993 and that increased life expectancy alone accounts for an estimated 10%–20% of the growth in demand for residential services since 1970. These changes in longevity are most dramatic in statistics from the Centers for Disease Control and Prevention that indicate that in the past generation the median age of death of people with Down syndrome increased from 1 year

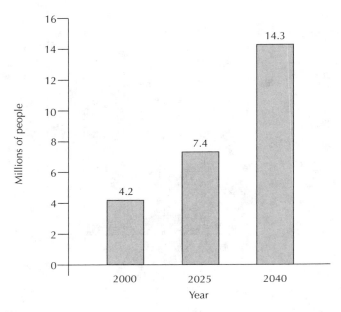

Figure 14.3. Projected growth among 85-year-old and older Americans between 2000 and 2040. *Source:* U.S. Census Bureau, 2001.

to 49 years and the average life span increased from 25 years to 50 years (Friedman, 2001; Yang, Rasmussen, & Friedman, 2002).

Rapidly growing demand for long-term services and supports (LTSS) is unavoidable. Although most of that demand can be expected to come from people who are aging, the overall capacity of the nation to continue to fund services for people with ID/DD at previous levels of increase seems substantially in jeopardy.

CURRENT FINANCING CHALLENGES

Long-range demographic pressures are not the only financial challenges in supporting LTSS for people with ID/DD. With almost all states reacting to substantial budget shortfalls in the economic slowdown evident in Fiscal Year (FY) 2002 and after, budget-containment proposals and initiatives have been a priority. Budget restrictions are evident in almost every state and affect expenditures for people with ID/DD. Figure 14.4 shows a notable reduction in FY 2003 in the rate of growth of expenditures for Medicaid-funded ICF/MR and HCBS Waiver programs.

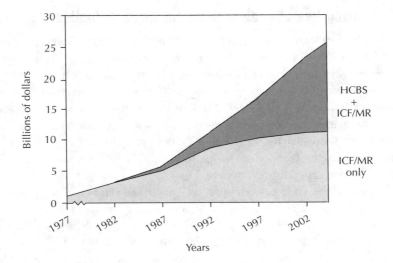

	1977	1982	1987	1992	1997	2002	2003
HCBS	0.000	0.003	0.294	1.655	5.965	13.365	14.039
ICF/MR	1.611	3.610	5.501	8.830	9.996	10.747	11.485

Figure 14.4. Total Intermediate Care Facility for the Mentally Retarded (ICF/MR), and Home and Community-Based Services (HCBS) Waiver expenditures from 1977 to 2003. *Source:* University of Minnesota, 2004.

Although the rate of growth in Medicaid expenditures between 1992 and 2002 was truly remarkable, it slowed dramatically in 2003. From average annual increases of more than 25% per year between 1992 and 2002, HCBS Waiver expenditures increased about 6% in 2003. Because of the lag between budget development and appropriation and actual spending, changes in expenditure patterns are estimated to be most notable in FY 2004 and beyond. Whatever the specific long-term effect on state spending, the large increases of the past are unlikely to be replicated soon. Substantial focus on cost effectiveness and cost containment will be evident for the foreseeable future. Cost effectiveness and cost containment in service financing require three key primary commitments: 1) maximizing the use of federal cost-sharing opportunities consistent with overall reduction in state and local expenditures and desired support outcomes; 2) closing institutions in a manner that reduces overall inefficiencies; and 3) supporting rather than supplanting families as primary support providers.

Maximizing Use of Federal Government Participation

Since the 1990s, most states have exhibited a remarkable capacity to expand federal Medicaid cost share for community services, frequently for services previously financed exclusively with state funds. Often, the "savings" obtained by states from shifting half or more of the cost of existing state-funded services to federal Medicaid programs were then reinvested in new services that were again cost-shared with the federal government. As a result, between FY 1991 and FY 2000, real-dollar federal contributions for community services for people with ID/DD increased by 227% whereas state expenditures increased by 46%.

During the same period, inflation-controlled state and federal service expenditures for all institutional and community services for people with ID/DD increased by 45% from $20.34 billion to about $29.5 billion, with state expenditures (in real 2000 dollars) increasing from $12.7 billion to $14.72 billion (15.9%) and federal expenditures increasing from $7.64 billion to $14.78 billion (93.5%) (Braddock, Hemp, Rizzolo, Parish, & Pomeranz, 2002; Lakin & Prouty, 2003). Although the success of previous efforts to maximize federal financial participation has left most states with relatively little in state expenditures that are "unmatched" by federal expenditures, 14 states were identified in FY 2002 as still having 20% or more of their total state spending for developmental disabilities services unmatched by federal cost-sharing programs. Nationally, an estimated $5 billion in state expenditures were unmatched (Rizzolo, Hemp, Braddock, & Pomeranz-Essley, 2004). Continued efforts to claim all appropriate federal cost–share is a primary responsibility of state officials. Of course, their notable past success in doing so leaves most state agencies in the more difficult position of requiring new state monies to be generated in order to increase expenditure for LTSS for people with ID/DD. This situation poses a substantial challenge in today's budgetary environment. It causes states to focus greater attention on the efficiency with which currently appropriated funds are used as a key aspect of meeting LTSS demand.

Closing Institutions Efficiently

In the United States (and possibly other countries as well), the cost of public institutions and the cost of community services are noticeably different. Differences in per-person costs are very large, with the average cost of 1) state institutions in FY 2002 about $126,000 per year, 2) community HCBS about $38,000, and 3) private community ICFs/MR about $67,000 per year (Prouty et al., 2003; Rizzolo et al., 2004; see also Chapter 13). Although such differences are dramatic, important factors contribute to these differences, including the case mix (characteristics) of service recipients and the comprehensiveness of services included. Even so, Stancliffe et al. (Chapter 13) concluded that the cost of comprehensive community services ranged from 73% to 95% of public institution costs.

Studies comparing institution and community-service costs in the United Kingdom reported that community services typically cost more than institutions (see Chapter 3). In the United Kingdom, recently established residential campuses, which have replaced some older traditional institutions, also have lower costs than community housing (see Chapter 7). The reasons for this difference between costs in the United States and the United Kingdom have not been studied directly. Two notable factors may be involved. First, U.S. public institutions in almost all instances operate today with resident populations that are far lower than the number of people for whom the institutions were designed and once housed.

Stancliffe et al. (Chapter 13) examined the phenomenon of diseconomies of reduced scale as public institutions were downsized. They concluded that per-person expenditures rise during downsizing because fixed and semi-fixed costs cannot be reduced in proportion to the declining number of residents. For example, Minnesota's Fergus Falls Regional Treatment Center once accommodated as many as 2,800 people, but in 2003, it housed about 100. Heat and utilities for the campus cost $940,000 in 2003 (Franklin, 2003). This fixed cost was distributed across the current 100 residents, yielding per capita expenditures for utilities alone that were $9,400. Other diseconomies of reduced scale no doubt were present in cost centers such as buildings and grounds maintenance, administration, and professional support services. Reduced scale is the important element in this circumstance; such diseconomies should not be assumed to apply to facilities that are operating at the size they were designed for.

Another factor contributing to the cost difference between institutional and community supports in the United States is the substantial differential in compensation paid to state institution staff and nonstate community staff in the United States that is not found in the United Kingdom. In the United States, community direct-support personnel have average wages that are about 74% of those of state employees, with state employees also more often enjoying substantially better benefit programs (Lakin et al., 2003). The disparity between the U.S. and the U.K. findings highlights the need for care when interpreting cost data from different countries.

There are, however, no disparities between countries regarding the outcomes of institutional and community living. Reviews of research in the United Kingdom (Emerson & Hatton, 1996), the United States (Kim, Larson, & Lakin, 2001), and Australia (Young, Sigafoos, Suttie, Ashman, & Grevell, 1998) all reveal better outcomes in community settings.

Emerson et al. reported a distinct pattern of better quality of care and quality of life in community housing than in residential campuses (institutions) and concluded that "the additional costs associated with dispersed housing schemes (15% greater than residential campuses) may be justified in the light of the substantial benefits" (2000, p. 98). That is, even in circumstances where community-living services cost more than institutions, the benefits are worth the additional expenditure.

The lower cost of community services in a U.S. context, together with the internationally confirmed benefits of such services, make a compelling case for much poorer cost effectiveness of U.S. institutions and the consequent imperative to continue to close them. Stancliffe et al.'s (Chapter 13) demonstration of how per-person costs rise as institutions are downsized, means that steadily paced total institutional closure is the best approach for service recipients and taxpayers alike. The common practice of downsizing (i.e., size reduction but not closure) at a leisurely pace not only deprives "residual" service recipients access to more effective opportunities and better quality of life but also subjects taxpayers to prolonged periods of paying inordinately high prices for inferior outcomes.

Support Families as Primary Support Providers

Less than 20% of all people identified as having ID/DD at any one time, and less than one third of adults 18 years and older, receive residential services outside their family home (Jaskulski, Lakin, & Zierman, 1995; Larson et al., 2002). Without question, the entire service system for people with ID/DD is dependent on sustaining high levels of family support. Lewis and Johnson (Chapter 4) showed that an important factor in the lower cost of family-based care is subsidization by the family itself combined with lesser access to services. Lakin, Hewitt, Larson, and Stancliffe (Chapter 5) demonstrated that supports for people with ID/DD who are living with family members have costs to public programs that average about 41% of the costs of adults supported in nonfamily settings. Too often, however, there is a naïve expectation on the part of service systems that these benefits can be obtained easily. Increased support and financial incentives to families who provide for family members with disabilities in their family home are essential aspects of policy that respond to the cost-containment needs of services systems.

The family home is almost always the most favorable living arrangement for children with ID/DD, and it is very often also the most favorable for adults. But often, public policy favors less advantageous circumstances that cost much more. As Lewis and Johnson (Chapter 4) noted, "the proportion of individuals in residential placement outside the family home depends largely on the availability of financial support and outside services to the family" (p. 82). Family support for people with ID/DD must be viewed as an investment in and a partnership with families that need assistance to succeed in a role on which society is dependent. Policy makers since the 1990s have acknowledged the importance of providing specific supports to families with members with ID/DD living at home. In 2002, states spent an estimated $1.38 billion dollars to assist families of people with ID/DD, an increase from $1.05 billion just 2 years earlier (see Chapter 2).

SETTING SIZE AND SERVICE COST

Intellectual disability services are staff intensive. As a result, human services do not behave like manufacturing industries with regard to economies of scale. As we noted in Chapter 1, previous research on economies of scale showed a weak or nonexistent relationship between residential setting size and per-person expenditures. Interpreting this research can be complex, particularly when including public institutions. The largest service settings—state institutions—are typically the most costly, but size per se does not necessarily cause costs to be higher. A 26% average wage salary differential between state-institution and community-service employees (Lakin et al., 2003), the fact that operation of most state institutions is far below design capacity, and the extensive regulation of state institutions based on ICF/MR standards and requirements enforced by courts (see Chapter 2) have all contributed to the difference. Among community services, factors such as the model of residential support, standards associated with funding programs, and differences in direct-support staff wages between state and nonstate community-services staff appear to be much more important determinants of expenditure than setting size (Stancliffe & Lakin, 1998). Nerney, Conley, and Nisbet (1990) did report some evidence of diseconomies of very small scale in the smallest group homes, but their findings supported the observation that economies of scale appear to be model dependent and largely evident among very small congregate facilities with 24-hour paid staffing.

Felce and Emerson (Chapter 3) reviewed evidence of economies of scale in residential services in the United Kingdom and likewise concluded that, except for small settings with continuous staff presence, no economies of scale were evident. Felce and Emerson observed that increased per-resident costs for staffing arise only when the staff ratio can no longer be held constant as resident numbers fall. The crucial point occurs beyond the stage when resident numbers are such that only one staff member at a time is required on duty. Further reduction of staff (below one) is not possible when continuous staffing is needed, so if resident numbers drop still further, staffing cannot be reduced proportionally and staffing ratios and per-resident staff costs usually rise (Felce, Jones, Lowe, & Perry, 2003; see also Chapters 3 and 6). Such diseconomies of very small scale apply only in residential services where the service model or the residents' support needs require continuous paid staff presence. For settings that do not involve full-time staff, staffing ratios (and costs) can be held constant as resident numbers fall (see Chapters 6 and 7). Similarly in support arrangements that do not involve 24-hour payment even if 24-hour support is provided, as in adult foster/host family support, companion models, and supported living with some unpaid natural support, economies of small scale may not affect costs.

The available evidence suggests that economies of scale play little or no role in the cost of many community residential services and only have a significant influence in very small settings with continuous paid staffing. That is, all things being equal, a consequence of operating very small residences with full-time paid staffing is likely to be somewhat higher per-person costs than larger settings supporting people with the same needs. But all things are rarely equal, and other factors, such as the effects of service model and regulatory requirements, strongly influence costs in these settings. However, the ability to reduce staffing to less than full time through development of independence, use of natural supports, non-hourly payments for support, and technology for monitoring can moderate per-person costs for individuals living alone or with one or two companions.

These findings, taken together with the trend toward more individualized services and provision of individual budgets, indicate that substantially more individualized supports can be provided without necessarily increasing average per-person costs, but that this is unlikely to be accomplished exclusively through smaller and smaller residences with full-time staffing.

SERVICE MODELS AND FUNDING PROGRAMS

Comparisons of outcomes and costs of community-support models appear to follow a pattern similar to those of institutional and community services: Outcomes appear consistently better as the relative restrictiveness of settings decreases and as average costs tend to consistently decrease along with the intensity of staff support provided.

Intermediate Care Facilities for the Mentally Retarded and Home and Community-Based Services Waivers

Lakin and colleagues (Chapter 5) and Hewitt, Larson, and Lakin (2000) noted that, in Minnesota, combined packages of health, social, and vocational supports for ICF/MR and HCBS Waiver recipients were about 28% more expensive for ICF/MR residents. In this comparison, the individuals living in ICFs/MR were more likely to have severe or profound intellectual disabilities (54.9% to 36.3%), but people receiving HCBS Waivers were slightly more likely to have reported challenging behavior (e.g., 12.4% of ICF/MR residents were reported to exhibit "severe physical aggression" as compared with 14.0% of HCBS Waiver recipients). Other factors were significant but uncontrolled in the comparison, including that 14.5% of HCBS Waiver recipients lived with family members and 10.6% of HCBS Waiver recipients versus 0.2% of ICF/MR residents were children whose schooling was paid for by local school districts. Of course, the much wider array of service options that allows individuals to receive needed support in the family home and to participate in generic services of the community is a design feature of HCBS Waiver programs.

Comparisons of outcomes between community ICFs/MR and HCBS Waiver–funded residences have shown better self-determination, better integration, increased quality of life, less challenging behavior, and better adaptive behavior outcomes in HCBS settings (Conroy, 1998; Stancliffe, Abery, & Smith, 2000; Stancliffe, Hayden, Larson, & Lakin, 2002; Stancliffe & Lakin, 1998). Comparisons of community ICFs/MR and other community residences have also shown better outcomes in non-ICF/MR settings (Conroy, 1996). Overall, the available cost information and outcome studies are consistent with the notion that ICFs/MR are less cost effective than residential settings financed with more flexible HCBS Waiver options. By no coincidence, numbers of residents in community ICFs/MR were static (a 1% national decline) between 2001 and 2002, whereas people living in nonfamily residential arrangements with HCBS Waiver financing grew rapidly (a 15% national increase) between 2001 and 2002 (Prouty et al., 2003).

Supported Living and Semi-Independent Living

Emerson and colleagues (Chapter 7) found no significant cost differences between supported living and traditional small-group homes (also see Emerson et al., 2001) in the United Kingdom; however, for the same cost, supported-living program participants exercised more choice, including greater choice over where and with whom they lived, and experienced more community participation than did residents of small-group homes with three or fewer residents. These results were congruent with U.S. supported-living findings (Howe, Horner, & Newton, 1998) that have reported similar costs to traditional community-living services but better results on resident choice and community participation.

Similar findings were also reported for comparisons between semi-independent living and group homes in Australia (Stancliffe & Keane, 2000; see also Chapter 6). Individuals living semi-independently enjoyed more choice, greater independence, and more participation in domestic activities. U.S. comparisons between group homes and semi-independent living have also shown more favorable outcomes in semi-independent settings (Burchard, Hasazi, Gordon, & Yoe, 1991; Stancliffe et al., 2000). Of course, because semi-independent living by definition involves at least some time in the day or night when service recipients are not supervised, the markedly lower-paid staffing levels in semi-independent living are associated with lower service costs (see Chapter 6).

Emerson and colleagues (Chapter 7) noted that using options that are more oriented to independence (e.g., supported living) can put residents at greater risk in some areas than their group home counterparts. In the United States, concerns have been raised about the effectiveness of efforts made to assure adequate protections of people in the less strictly regulated programs financed by HCBS Waivers (General Accounting Office, 2003; Hewitt et al., 2000). Traditional quality assurance systems have not been expanded and/or been sufficiently well redesigned to meet the rapid growth and dispersal of community residential settings. Such findings also remind us that with the increased freedom comes community-life risk, and that risk must be attended to with as much planning as opportunities for social relationships, community participation, and integrated employment.

Individual Needs-Based Funding

Lakin and colleagues (Chapter 5) described how, in 1996, Minnesota implemented a four-level Waiver Allocation Structure (WAS) to allocate funding for new entrants in the HCBS Waiver program based on diagnostic, functional, behavior, and health status. The level of resource allocation determined through each individual's assessment is added to the local government's pool of authorized spending with discretion left to the local government to develop, price, and authorize each individual's service plan.

Analysis revealed a relatively weak relationship between the four established WAS funding levels and the actual expenditures for individual HCBS (see Chapter 5). The WAS accounted for only 3.1% of variability in all individual HCBS Waiver expenditures, or 8.4% of variability for those individuals assessed under the WAS system. This difference indicates that needs-based funding initiatives are more effective in making the funding system more needs based if they are applied to all service recipients rather than being restricted to new entrants in the system. Lakin and colleagues (Chapter 5) found that, when employed in addition to the WAS categories, recipients' personal characteristics accounted for an additional 15.3% of variability in individual HCBS Waiver expenditures. Adaptive behavior and challenging behavior were the strongest predictors. In other words, the same characteristics that were used to place people in one of the four WAS categories, when reemployed as continuous scales (rather than a few discrete levels), were much more predictive of expenditures than the four WAS categories derived from them.

Campbell and colleagues (Chapter 8) found when they examined expenditures in four Western states (Montana, Nebraska, South Dakota, and Wyoming) that personal characteristics accounted for 33% of variability in individual expenditures. This finding was similar in magnitude to the 34% of variance associated with living and day activity arrangements and other services received. Although these findings indicated that the four states studied had systems with somewhat greater association between costs and service recipients' individual characteristics than Minnesota did, the association was still of moderate strength.

Fortune and colleagues (Chapter 11) described the problems experienced in the 1990s in Wyoming with a system involving five payment levels similar to Minnesota's WAS levels. Wyoming subsequently moved to an individualized funding model, the DOORS model, which is based on each person's objectively assessed individual characteristics and his or her service utilization. The DOORS model directly provides a unique individual budget amount (IBA) to pay for each person's services. Following the implementation of the DOORS model, Wyoming successfully realized its goal of substantially increasing the association between individual service recipients' assessed support needs and the amounts of funding provided to meet those needs. With the introduction of DOORS, the proportion of variability in individual funding associated with individual characteristics rose from 37% to 47%, and the proportion of variability explained by the total DOORS model increased from 52% to 75%.

Several factors appear to be involved in the different outcomes in Wyoming and Minnesota, and we may tentatively conclude that funding is most effectively needs-based when: 1) needs-based funding systems are applied to all service recipients, not just those entering the system for the first time; 2) continuous individualized funding amounts are provided (rather than a small number of discrete funding levels); 3) a specified amount allocated to pay for services is received by the individual rather than infusing it into an overall pool to be managed by an intermediate agency for multiple service recipients; and 4) desired variations in allocated amounts to reflect different circumstances (e.g., people living with family members versus in residential settings; children who are enrolled in public schools) are integrated into the individual rate-setting formula and not treated as matters of local discretion. Funding arrangements that are based on individual assessment of support needs offer a basis of rational and equitable allocation for public money that may be increasingly important as public funding encounters greater scrutiny and restriction.

Moseley, Gettings, and Cooper (Chapter 12) reported that in 2002 some form of individual budget was in place in nearly three fourths of the 43 states they surveyed; however, the development and use of individual budgeting varied considerably from state to state. In some states, individual budgets were established for all service recipients, whereas in other states they were used on a much more limited basis, usually for individual service recipient–directed support options. In some states, allocations made on behalf of individuals are passed through to local governments or service providers to be managed. In other states, the control of the individual amounts allocated is retained by individuals and/or their families. Although there is great variation in application, individual budgets are rapidly becoming a mainstream funding mechanism in the United States. In some states they are already the dominant approach. Other states are making substantial commitments to design, develop, and implement rational, reliable, and acceptable methodologies to establish individualized needs-based budgets.

A growing number of states are employing individual budget–generating mechanisms that are valid and reliable. The federal government is also setting expectations for such mechanisms. The new Independence Plus waiver template allows states a relatively streamlined means of obtaining authorized self-directed services within the Medicaid HCBS Waiver program, but states participating in the Independence Plus option are required to use consistent, data-based methods to determine individual budgets. The further development, evaluation, and refinement of procedures to establish rational, reliable, and appropriate levels of funding for individuals needing support will be an important task for researchers, funders, and policy makers for the foreseeable future. Its importance will grow with the growth of service recipient–controlled budgets for self-directed/family-directed supports.

Individual/Family Controlled Budgets

One of the primary and most rapidly growing applications of individual budget-setting methodologies is to establish the budget for consumer-directed supports (CDS). In CDS programs individuals and/or families not only have individual allocations of amounts of money to spend for services, but they also have the primary control over the specific uses of those resources. Within the amount of funding available in their individual budgets, individuals and/or families determine the services they will purchase, who will provide those services, the price they will pay, and so forth, usually with considerable latitude to operate outside the standards and limitations of traditional services for people with ID/DD. Head and Conroy (Chapter 10) suggest that better outcomes can be achieved at slightly lower cost through controlling the amounts of funding allocated to individual budgets and allowing substantial control by "consumers" of those funds. One of the salient features of CDS (often identified as "self-determination") is the opportunity to "de-professionalize" and "de-program" supports using neighbors as support staff and community education service providers, and neighborhood resources as worksites and recreation.

Consumer-directed services were promoted in the self-determination demonstration projects financed by the Robert Wood Johnson Foundation but have also been carried out in a wide range of related initiatives in other states. Head and Conroy's (Chapter 10) results support the goals of the self-determination program and extend the findings of an evaluation of the initial "Self-Determination" demonstration in New Hampshire (Conroy & Yuskauskas, 1996).

The human service system in America is steadily embracing CDS as an important option for individuals and families. As CDS expand, identifying those choices and opportunities available through the freedom and flexibility of CDS that are directly related to desired outcomes and/or efficient use of available resources will become important. Stancliffe and Lakin (Chapter 9) demonstrated the value of distinguishing the control of one's budget from the choices made on the basis of that control by showing that owning or renting one's own home was more highly associated with control over daily decisions than was simply having control of one's own budget. Such a finding does not diminish the importance of budgetary control, but reminds us that it is not opportunity that creates outcomes, it is what one does with opportunity.

FINANCING THE ESSENTIAL INFRASTRUCTURE OF COMMUNITY SUPPORTS

The studies reported in this volume have demonstrated with considerable consistency that the most cost-effective community services tend to be those that maximize individual control and choice, sustain the engagement of a family role in providing support, and minimize the use of small congregate settings with full-time staffing. These important aspects of a cost-effective system of supports are ones that depend substantially on the ability of individuals, families, and formal and informal support providers to operate outside the framework of traditional agencies providing congregate services. Nurturing the opportunity for these factors to affect outcomes and expenditures in the ways desired requires an infrastructure of support for individualized services. It requires investment by administrative and advocacy agencies to assure that the essential conditions for cost-effective, individualized supports exist. Five areas of high importance for this investment are: access to information; support for person-centered planning; fair, transparent, individualized resource allocation; development of a qualified direct-support workforce; and quality monitoring and improvement.

Access to Information

The freedom to choose is of relatively little benefit without understanding the choices available. Traditional service providers are easily able to explain to service recipients what they provide. For more independent community-support users, the nature of the choices is substantially affected by knowledge and perceived viability of the options. Individuals and families need assistance in learning of options from the service providers who wish to sell those options to them, from other individuals and families who have created their own options, and from other sources of information that provide catalogs and how-to descriptions of creative responses to individual needs that can be adopted or adapted.

Support for Person-Centered Planning

As individuals and families are given greater opportunities to create supports in an individualized manner, they should be encouraged to reflect carefully and honestly on the needs and desires of the individual to be supported and the breadth and capacities within the individual's support network to provide what is needed. Facilitated person-centered planning is an extremely helpful means of assuring that people attend to the individual in the planning process. It also provides the planning process with a facilitator who is experienced with techniques to identify capacities, needs, and preferences; who is familiar with the experiences of others in trying different approaches to meet individual needs; and who knows the resources of the community that may assist in accommodating the needs and/or fulfilling the desires of the individual.

Fair, Transparent, Individualized Resource Allocation

Frequently throughout this volume, the benefits of equitable, understandable, and transparent means of establishing individual expenditure authorizations have been noted. The financing of supports for people with ID/DD has a well-established, well-entrenched history of relative financial incentives to the most costly, inefficient, and disempowering services. To change this requires a substantial commitment within states to assuring that resources are allocated in ways that reflect the support needs of individuals and not the costs of the places in which they are being placed.

Development of a Qualified Direct-Support Workforce

Community support of people with ID/DD faces unprecedented challenges in recruiting, training, and retaining direct-support professionals (DSPs). High turnover within the DSP workforce has been consistently linked to low pay, which in the United States averages about 55% of average pay for all workers and provides an annual income at the poverty level for a family of four (Lakin et al., 2003). Larson, Hewitt, and Lakin (in press) found that family and case manager ratings of service quality were lower in settings in which staff earned relatively lower wages. Turnover rates of DSPs are consistently reported to average between 40% and 75% of the workforce each year. Finding replacements is difficult due to low wages, high job demands, and poor understanding and preparation for the work role (Larson, Lakin, & Hewitt, 2002).

The problems of workforce recruitment, training, and retention have largely been left to the individual agencies employing DSPs. Individuals with ID/DD increasingly live in settings in which DSPs work with little supervision and greatly enhanced responsibility. Growing numbers of families are accepting responsibility for recruiting, retaining, and training the individuals supporting their family members with no background in recruitment, training, or supporting worker retention. As these trends are encouraged, infrastructures need to be created within states and localities to recruit adequate pools of potential DSPs, to match support providers with those needing support, to train DSPs when other training is not available or convenient to the DSPs' work schedules, to assist DSPs in advancing within the field, and so forth. Without a sufficiently large and well-prepared workforce, the commitments of community living and increased self-determination made to individuals and families cannot be kept. Keeping those promises is sufficiently important to demand investments in and commitments to workforce development programs.

Quality Monitoring and Improvement

As noted previously, the number of settings in which people with ID/DD live and work has been growing at a phenomenal rate, more than doubling from about 49,500 to 125,400 between 1992 and 2002. Systems of traditional quality assurance based on teams of government employees visiting service sites to assure compliance with existing standards have not grown commensurately. Even when they do, too often they create conditions that are contrary to the factors identified in this volume as predictive of greater choice, higher quality of life, and lower cost. The failures of the traditional system of quality assurance to protect people with ID/DD in community settings have been recognized for some time (General Accounting Office, 2002; Wyden, 1993). The challenges for the future are to integrate and support broader consortia of stakeholders to work with designated government employees in quality assurance and improvement programs; to assure that quality assurance resources are efficiently targeted most intensely on individuals most in need of protection; to assure participation and coordination of people in various roles around quality assurance functions, including family members, service coordinators, and health and therapy specialists; to build individual quality assurance plans as part of lifestyle and service planning practices; and to make certain that quality assurance findings are linked to useful ways of improving the quality of services, not just in areas of inadequacy, but in all areas of importance to individual and family quality of life and self-determination.

FUTURE DIRECTIONS FOR COSTS AND OUTCOMES RESEARCH

We have identified a number of challenges for financing and policy in developmental disability service systems as they move toward the commitments identified by the National Goals Conference. Researchers also face challenges. They can continue to play a valuable role in family support through ongoing monitoring of the growth in national and state family-support expenditures, evaluation of the equity with which these expenditures are distributed, and assessment of their effectiveness in yielding desired outcomes for families, for people with ID/DD, and for service systems.

High-quality research information on outcomes and costs will be essential as stakeholders continue to struggle with the issue of how best to allocate available funding. In addition, state funding arrangements will need to be scrutinized carefully to assess whether they meet basic tests of fairness and consistency. Identifying, refining, and evaluating valid methods for determining individual funding levels will continue to challenge researchers and policy makers alike.

As noted by Lakin and colleagues (Chapter 5), evaluation of HCBS Waiver funding in Minnesota showed that introduction of funding policies that were intended to be needs based did not necessarily result in a funding system that actually was substantially needs based. Fundamental research is called for into what is meant by needs-based funding and supports: Which needs? Identified how? and By whom? At present, operational identification of "needs" frequently tends to be synonymous with personal characteristics such as adaptive and challenging behavior, existing service use, and/or availability of unpaid support (usually through living with family). In the absence of agreed criteria for "needs" and "needs-based expenditures," current indicators of need are often validated by demonstrating that they are related to existing expenditures on individual services and supports, even though such expenditures are seen as being less needs based than desired.

Self-determination and personal control have received much attention through systems-change initiatives, such as the Robert Wood Johnson Foundation–funded demonstration projects, and related activities in other states. Initial research findings on service recipient outcomes and costs from such projects are encouraging (see Chapter 10), but there is limited research information available about the specific nature and effects of the changes in service and support arrangements associated with individual budgets and service recipient–directed services. It is important to identify the specific arrays of support practices and the service-provision infrastructure that best enable service recipients and their families to take advantage of the opportunities afforded by an individual budget and service recipient–directed services. For example, what difficulties are encountered by individuals and families when recruiting and retaining support staff? Lakin and colleagues (Chapter 5) reported substantial unexpended funds for family support services in Minnesota, in part due to the nonavailability of staff. Likewise, some individuals and families will choose not to become involved in managing budgets or directing services. How will these individuals fare during the continued evolution toward more individualized service and support arrangements?

Relatively little research has addressed outcomes and costs in service models such as semi-independent and supported living. Current information suggests that better outcomes are being achieved at similar or lower costs than in traditional services such as group homes, but how these better outcomes are achieved is not clear. Findings of better outcomes associated with the more individualized support models, as well as the findings of better outcomes for people controlling their own budgets (see Chapter 10), raise questions about which factors are associated the most with the differences in outcomes. For research to contribute to outcomes in more flexible, service recipient–controlled environments, it must examine the specific support options people select and/or the effectiveness of support practices within these options. For example, research on organizational methods and staff activities associated with the active support model in the British literature (Felce, Jones, & Lowe, 2002) could contribute to establishing better outcomes in residential service settings at no increased cost. Of course, consistent with the commitments identified by the National Goals Conference, research on outcomes needs to give better attention to health and safety outcomes.

Growing demands for services and supports, particularly in economic environments that are seeking to constrain the growth of public expenditures, create increased pressure for accountability for costs and outcomes in community supports. Increasingly, support systems will be explicitly challenged to increase cost effectiveness (i.e., obtain better outcomes at lower or equal cost, or equal outcomes at lower cost). Although there is much left to learn in increasing cost-effectiveness, there is a promising foundation of research and experience to guide these efforts. The challenge will be to adopt these promising practices in systems that are slow to change.

REFERENCES

Americans with Disabilities Act (ADA) of 1990, PL 101-336, 42 U.S.C. 12101 *et seq.*

Braddock, D., Hemp, R., Rizzolo, M., Parish, S., & Pomeranz, A. (2002). *The state of the states in developmental disabilities: 2002 study summary.* Boulder: University of Colorado, Coleman Institute for Cognitive Disabilities.

Burchard, S.N., Hasazi, J.E., Gordon, L.R., & Yoe, J. (1991). An examination of lifestyle and adjustment in three community residential alternatives. *Research in Developmental Disabilities, 12,* 127–142.

Conroy, J.W. (1996). The small ICF/MR program: Dimensions of quality and cost. *Mental Retardation, 34,* 13–26.

Conroy, J.W. (1998). Quality in small ICFs/MR versus waiver homes. *TASH Newsletter, 24*(3), 23–24, 28.

Conroy, J.W., & Yuskauskas, A. (1996). *Independent evaluation of the Monadnock Self-Determination Project.* Ardmore, PA: Center for Outcome Analysis.

Emerson, E., & Hatton, C. (1996). Deinstitutionalization in the UK and Ireland: Outcomes for service users. *Journal of Intellectual & Developmental Disability, 21,* 17–37.

Emerson, E., Robertson, J., Gregory, N., Hatton, C., Kessissoglou, S., Hallam, A., Järbrink, K., Knapp, M., Netten, A., & Walsh, P. (2001). The quality and costs of supported living residences and group homes in the United Kingdom. *American Journal of Mental Retardation, 106,* 401–415.

Emerson, E., Robertson, J., Gregory, N., Hatton, C., Kessissoglou, S., Hallam, A., Knapp, M., Järbrink, K., Walsh, P.N., & Netten, A. (2000). Quality and costs of community-based residential supports, village communities, and residential campuses in the United Kingdom. *American Journal on Mental Retardation, 105,* 81–102.

Felce, D., Jones, E., & Lowe, K. (2002). Active support: Planning daily activities and support for people with severe mental retardation. In S. Holburn, & P.M. Vietze (Eds.), *Person-centered planning: Research, practice, and future directions* (pp. 247–269). Baltimore: Paul H. Brookes Publishing Co.

Felce, D., Jones, E., Lowe, K., & Perry, J. (2003). Rational resourcing and productivity: Relationships among staff input, resident characteristics, and group home quality. *American Journal on Mental Retardation, 108,* 161–172.

Franklin, R. (2003, February 16). What to do with a city of ghosts? *Minneapolis Star Tribune,* pp. B1, B9.

Friedman, J.M. (2001). Racial disparities in median age of death of persons with Down syndrome—United States, 1968–1997. *Morbidity and Mortality Weekly Report, 50*(22), 463–465.

General Accounting Office. (2003). *Federal oversight of growing Medicaid Home and Community-Based Waivers should be strengthened* (GAO-03-576). Washington, DC: U.S. General Accounting Office.

Hewitt, A., Larson, S.A., & Lakin, K.C. (2000). *An independent evaluation of the quality of services and system performance of Minnesota's Medicaid Home and Community-Based Services for persons with mental retardation and related conditions.* Minneapolis: University of Minnesota, Research and Training Center on Community Living/Institute on Community Integration.

Howe, J., Horner, R.H., & Newton, J.S. (1998). Comparison of supported living and traditional residential services in the State of Oregon. *Mental Retardation, 36,* 1–11.

Jaskulski, T., Lakin, K.C., & Zierman, S.A. (1995). *The journey to inclusion.* Washington, DC: President's Committee on Mental Retardation.

Kim, S., Larson, S., & Lakin, K.C. (2001). Behavioural outcomes of deinstitutionalisation of people with intellectual disability: A review of U.S. studies conducted between 1980 and 1999. *Journal of Intellectual & Developmental Disability, 26,* 35–50.

Lakin, K.C., Polister, B., & Prouty, R.W. (2003). Wages of non-state direct support professionals lag behind those of public direct support professionals and the general public. *Mental Retardation, 41*(2), 178–182.

Lakin, K.C., & Prouty, R.W. (2003). *Medicaid Home and Community Based Service: The first 20 years. Embarking on a new century.* Washington, DC: American Association on Mental Retardation.

Larson, S.A., Hewitt, A.S., & Lakin, K.C. (in press). Multi-perspective analysis of work force challenges and their effects on consumer and family quality of life. *American Journal on Mental Retardation.*

Larson, S.A., Lakin, K.C., & Hewitt, A. (2002). Direct support professionals: 1975 to 2000. In R. Schalock, P. Baker, & M.D. Croser (Eds.), *Embarking on a new century* (pp. 203–220). Washington, DC: American Association on Mental Retardation.

National Goals Conference. (2003). *Keeping the promises: Findings and recommendations.* Silver Spring, MD: The Arc of the United States.

Nerney, T., Conley, R., & Nisbet, J. (1990). *Cost analysis of residential systems serving persons with severe disabilities: New directions in economic and policy research.* Cambridge, MA: Human Services Research Institute.

Olmstead v. L.C. (1999), 119 S. Ct. 2176

Prouty, R.W., Smith, G., & Lakin, K.C. (Eds.). (2003). *Residential services for persons with developmental disabilities: Status and trends through 2002.* Minneapolis: University of Minnesota, Research and Training Center on Community Living, Institute on Community Integration. Also available on-line at http://rtc.umn.edu

Rizzolo, M.K., Hemp, R., Braddock, D., & Pomeranz-Essley, A. (2004). *The state of the states in developmental disabilities.* Boulder: University of Colorado, Coleman Institute for Cognitive Disability.

Stancliffe, R.J., Abery, B.H., & Smith, J. (2000). Personal control and the ecology of community living settings: Beyond living-unit size and type. *American Journal on Mental Retardation, 105,* 431–454.

Stancliffe, R.J., Hayden, M.F., Larson, S., & Lakin, K.C. (2002). Longitudinal study on the adaptive and challenging behaviors of deinstitutionalized adults with intellectual disability. *American Journal on Mental Retardation, 107,* 302–320.

Stancliffe, R.J., & Keane, S. (2000). Outcomes and costs of community living: A matched comparison of group homes and semi-independent living. *Journal of Intellectual & Developmental Disability, 25,* 281–305.

Stancliffe, R.J., & Lakin, K.C. (1998). Analysis of expenditures and outcomes of residential alternatives for persons with developmental disabilities. *American Journal on Mental Retardation, 102,* 552–568.

University of Minnesota. (1997). *National Health Interview Survey.* Unpublished analysis. Minneapolis: Author.

University of Minnesota. (2004). *National Residential Information System Project.* Unpublished data.

U.S. Census Bureau. (2001). *Statistical abstract of the United States: 2001.* Washington, DC: U.S. Department of Commerce, Economics and Statistics Administration.

Wyden, R. (Chair). (1993). *Growth of small residential living programs for the mentally retarded and developmentally disabled. Hearing before the Subcommittee on Regulation, Business Opportunities and Technology of the Committee on Small Business, U.S. House of Representatives* (Serial No. 103-8). Washington, DC: U.S. Government Printing Office.

Yang, Q., Rasmussen, S.A., & Friedman, J.M. (2002). Mortality associated with Down's syndrome in the USA from 1983–1997: A population based study. *Lancet, 23,* 1019–1025.

Young, L., Sigafoos, J., Suttie, J., Ashman, A., & Grevell, P. (1998). Deinstitutionalisation of persons with intellectual disabilities: A review of Australian studies. *Journal of Intellectual & Developmental Disability, 23,* 155–170.

Index

Page numbers followed by *f* indicate figures; those followed by *t* indicate tables.